# Diagnosing Non-small Cell Carcinoma in Small Biopsy and Cytology

Andre Luis Moreira • Anjali Saqi
Editors

# Diagnosing Non-small Cell Carcinoma in Small Biopsy and Cytology

Springer

*Editors*
Andre Luis Moreira, MD, PhD
Department of Pathology
Memorial Sloan Kettering Cancer Center
New York, NY, USA

Anjali Saqi, MD, MBA
Department of Pathology and Cell Biology
Columbia University Medical Center
New York-Presbyterian Hospital
New York, NY, USA

ISBN 978-1-4939-1606-1 ISBN 978-1-4939-1607-8 (eBook)
DOI 10.1007/978-1-4939-1607-8
Springer New York Heidelberg Dordrecht London

Library of Congress Control Number: 2014950416



Printed on acid-free paper

Springer is part of Springer Science+Business Media (www.springer.com)

# Preface

Lung cancer is the leading cause of cancer-related deaths worldwide, but its recognition at an early stage and diagnosis with minimally invasive procedures can decrease morbidity and mortality. In fact, within the past decade, enormous strides to detect, sample, and treat lung cancer have been made. After many years of no clear progress in therapy for lung cancer, the last decade has witnessed a large paradigm shift on the treatment and management of patients with non-small cell lung cancer (NSCLC). Most of the changes have occurred in adenocarcinoma with the identification of driver mutations that can be targeted with a specific therapy and introduction of new chemotherapeutic drugs.

Though promising, this progress is not without challenges. As the number of minimally invasive procedures and treatment options is increasing, the sizes of the tissue samples upon which diagnoses are rendered and molecular tests are conducted are decreasing. This shift has resulted in unprecedented significance centered upon small samples, such as fine-needle aspirates (FNAs) and core biopsies, often the only tissue from patients.

These challenges have affected many professionals in the field of pulmonary oncology especially pathologists, who are now required to diagnose and subclassify NSCLC into adenocarcinoma or squamous cell carcinoma and triage specimens for molecular pathology and other ancillary tests on small biopsy material. The subclassification of NSCLC has a direct impact on patient's clinical management. In response to these challenges, many professionals of multidisciplinary groups including pathologists, pulmonologists, oncologists, surgeons, and radiologists have worked together to propose new recommendations and the classification of NSCLC.

This book provides an up-to-date practical yet comprehensive guide to manage the shift in the diagnosis of lung cancer from large resections to small samples, including cytology and core biopsy specimens. Specifically, it outlines various available minimally invasive modalities and presents algorithms to optimize and maximize sample collection and processing beginning at the time of tissue acquisition during the procedure. More importantly, the book provides an overview and practical applications of the multidisciplinary new recommendations for the classification of small biopsies and cytology proposed by the International Association for the Study of Lung Cancer, American Thoracic Society, and European Respiratory Society (IASLC/ATS/ERS) and molecular triage for pulmonary adenocarcinoma proposed by the College of American Pathologists, International Association for the Study of Lung Cancer, and Association for Molecular Pathology (CAP/IASLC/AMP).

We would like to thank all the authors that have contributed and shared their experience and expertise in pulmonary pathology, interventional pulmonology/radiology, and oncologic pathology. Without them, this work would not be possible. We would also like to thank the editorial staff for their tremendous patience and excellent guidance throughout the preparations of this book.

New York, NY, USA Andre Luis Moreira
New York, NY, USA Anjali Saqi

# Contents

# Contributors

**William Bulman, MD** Department of Medicine, Columbia University Medical Center, New York, NY, USA

**John P. Crapanzano, MD** Department of Pathology and Cell Biology, Columbia University Medical Center, New York-Presbyterian Hospital, New York, NY, USA

**Gilda da Cunha Santos, MD, PhD, FRCPC, FIAC** Department of Laboratory Medicine and Pathobiology, University of Toronto, University Health Network, Toronto, ON, Canada

**Sanja Dacic, MD, PhD** Department of Pathology, University of Pittsburgh Medical Center, Pittsburgh, PA, USA

**Alexander Drilon, MD** Department of Medicine, Thoracic Oncology Service and Developmental Therapeutics, Memorial Sloan Kettering Cancer Center, New York, NY, USA

**Juliana Eng, MD** Department of Medicine, Thoracic Oncology Service, Memorial Sloan Kettering Cancer Center, New York, NY, USA

**Elena Lucas, MD** Department of Pathology, University of Texas Southwestern Medical Center, Dallas, TX, USA

**Sara E. Monaco, MD** Department of Pathology, University of Pittsburgh Medical Center, Pittsburgh, PA, USA

**Andre Luis Moreira, MD, PhD** Department of Pathology, Memorial Sloan Kettering Cancer Center, New York, NY, USA

**Daisuke Nonaka, MD** Department of Histopathology, The Christie Hospital, Manchester, United Kingdom

**Paul K. Paik, MD** Department of Medicine, Thoracic Oncology Service, Memorial Sloan Kettering Cancer Center, New York, NY, USA

**Sunati Sahoo, MD** Department of Pathology, University of Texas Southwestern Medical Center, Dallas, TX, USA

**Anjali Saqi, MD, MBA** Department of Pathology and Cell Biology, Columbia University Medical Center, New York-Presbyterian Hospital, New York, NY, USA

**William D. Travis, MD** Department of Pathology, Memorial Sloan Kettering Cancer Center, New York, NY, USA

**David F. Yankelevitz, MD** Department of Radiology, Mount Sinai Medical Center, Mount Sinai Hospital, New York, NY, USA

# Chapter 1
# Histologic Classification and Its Need for Treatment of Lung Cancer

**Andre Luis Moreira and William D. Travis**

## Introduction

Lung cancer is the most commonly diagnosed cancer worldwide representing 13 % of all cancer diagnosis and is still the one with the highest cancer-related death, representing 1 in 5 deaths to cancer, approximately 20 % of all cancer-related death globally [1, 2]. Due to the high mortality rate, the incidence to fatality ratio is 0.87. In the United States, it is estimated that lung cancer would account for over 228,190 new cases and 159,480 cancer deaths in 2013 [3].

The diagnosis of lung cancer is made by evaluation of tissue either by excision of the tumor or sampling by small biopsy or cytology specimens from the primary tumor or metastatic sites [4–6].

Therapy for lung cancer is highly influenced by disease stage and other tumor characteristics. Surgery with curative intent is offered to patients with stage I disease. Adjuvant therapy following resection is recommended for patients in stages II and III. The majority of patients, however, present with advanced stage disease at diagnosis (stage IV); therefore, only small biopsy specimens and/or cytology are available for diagnosis and determination of prognostic and predictive markers. Surgery is not a valid therapeutic option for these patients.

A.L. Moreira, M.D., Ph.D. (✉) • W.D. Travis, M.D.
Department of Pathology, Memorial Sloan Kettering Cancer Center,
1275 York Ave., New York, NY 10065, USA
e-mail: moreiraa@mskcc.org



A.L. Moreira, A. Saqi (eds.), *Diagnosing Non-small Cell Carcinoma in Small Biopsy and Cytology*, DOI 10.1007/978-1-4939-1607-8_1

Contrary to the vital importance of biopsy/cytology for the diagnosis and treatment of lung cancer, the World Health Organization (WHO) classifications of lung tumors through the 1999 edition [7–9] were based on resection specimens only and did not address lung cancer diagnosis based on small biopsies and cytology. Cytologic features for the diagnosis of lung cancer were addressed for the first time in the 2004 WHO classification [10].

Traditionally there have been four major histologic types of lung cancer based on resection specimen. These include small cell lung carcinoma (SCLC), adenocarcinoma, squamous cell carcinoma, and large cell carcinoma. For the diagnosis in small biopsy material, including cytology, the latter three categories were often grouped as non-small cell lung carcinoma (NSCLC), since there was no difference in clinical management of patients with the diagnosis of NSCLC. In addition, squamous cell carcinoma and adenocarcinoma are basically the only histologic subtypes of NSCLC that could be diagnosed in small biopsy and cytologic specimens. The diagnosis of large cell carcinoma cannot be established with certainty in small biopsy material, since the entity is defined as a poorly differentiated carcinoma without histologic evidence of adenocarcinoma (gland formation) or squamous cell carcinoma (keratinization), and therefore this diagnosis required examination of a resected tumor to exclude these differentiation features [10].

Historically, the most important diagnostic distinction was between SCLC and NSCLC [10] due to significant differences in clinical presentation, spread of tumor, and response to therapy. Contrary to NSCLC, the diagnosis SCLC precluded a surgical approach. The tumor was generally diagnosed at advanced stages and was treated differently than NSCLC. Previously, there was no evidence for histologic type to influence a specific chemotherapeutic approach to NSCLC.

However, over the past decade, new studies have shown that the response to some chemotherapeutic agents, as well as targeted therapies directed at specific molecular alterations present in the tumor, is dependent upon histologic subtype.

This paradigm shift brought many new challenges to our understanding of pulmonary carcinoma, especially to pathologists that are now required to subclassify NSCLC in small biopsy material [11–14]. In response to this challenge, a multidisciplinary group of lung cancer specialists including pathologists, radiologists, oncologists, and surgeons joined forces under the leadership of three professional societies, namely, the International Association for the Study of Lung Cancer (IASLC), the American Thoracic Society (ATS), and the European Respiratory Society (ERS), to reevaluate the histologic classification of lung cancer and integrate the classification with clinical and radiographic information [15]. These professionals have recommended major changes in the structure of the previous 2004 World Health Organization classification either in excised tumors, but more importantly, in small biopsies and cytologic material.

This chapter discusses the changes that lead to the modification of the lung cancer classification, as well as the application of the new classification to small biopsies and cytology specimens.

## Histology-Based Therapy for Lung Cancer

In older studies the role of chemotherapy in advanced NSCLC showed only a weak association between histology and therapeutic outcomes, but none showed an interaction between different regimens of therapy and histologic subtypes of NSCLC. Therefore, there was no clear evidence that histology had a prognostic (independent of treatment) or a predictive role (associated with the effectiveness of a specific treatment) for patients with NSCLC. All NSCLC cases were treated in the same manner, thereby limiting the relevance of histologic NSCLC subtyping in routine clinical practice. However, as new chemotherapeutic agents became available, studies showed for the first time a difference in response or toxicity in patients with specific histologic subtypes of NSCLC.

Bevacizumab is a humanized anti-vascular endothelial growth factor (VEGF) monoclonal antibody that has been used in several solid tumors. The combination of bevacizumab with chemotherapy has showed a significant benefit in progression-free survival and overall survival in patients with non-squamous NSCLC [16]. It is important to notice that the terminology "non-squamous NSCLC" is not recommended to be used for pathology diagnosis. It is reported as such in clinical studies to indicate that only tumors with the histologic diagnosis of squamous cell carcinoma were excluded. Bevacizumab is contraindicated in squamous cell carcinoma because of an increased risk of severe pulmonary hemorrhage [17, 18]. Therefore, in patients with advanced disease, a biopsy diagnosis of squamous cell carcinoma will preclude the inclusion of this efficient drug in the treatment plan.

Another drug that has been shown to have different efficacy according to histologic type of lung cancer is pemetrexed, which is a very active cytotoxic agent and is a powerful inhibitor of folate-dependent enzymes including thymidylate synthase. This drug is indicated only for the treatment of non-squamous NSCLC because it has showed no antitumor activity in patients with the histologic diagnosis of SQCC [19–21].

Therefore, an accurate tumor classification in biopsy/cytology specimen is directly implicated with patient's clinical management and the choice of chemotherapeutic drugs used for systemic therapy.

## Tumor Classification for Molecular Targeted Therapy

The discovery that activating mutations in the *epidermal growth factor receptor* (*EGFR*) are associated with response to treatment with the small molecule tyrosine kinase inhibitors (TKI) has revolutionized the field of thoracic oncology [22–24]. Gefitinib, erlotinib, and more recently afatinib, TKI drugs approved for the treatment of patients with lung adenocarcinoma, have been shown to significantly extend progression-free and overall survival in patients that harbor activating *EGFR* mutations [25–27].

The presence of mutation is closely associated with the histologic diagnosis of adenocarcinoma and tumors with an adenocarcinoma component such as adenosquamous carcinoma and combined high-grade neuroendocrine carcinoma (small cell carcinoma or large cell neuroendocrine carcinoma) with an adenocarcinoma component, but not other pure histologic subtypes.

Another important molecular alteration discovered in pulmonary adenocarcinoma is *ALK* rearrangement. Soda et al. described that a subset of pulmonary adenocarcinomas showed an inversion within chromosome 2 that resulted in a transforming fusion kinase between *echinoderm microtubule-associated protein-like 4* (*EML4*) in 2p21 and *anaplastic lymphoma kinase* (*ALK*) in 2p23.2 [28]. This fusion results in constitutive activation of ALK kinase. *ALK* rearrangement is the second driver oncogene in pulmonary carcinoma that can be targeted by specific therapy. *ALK* rearrangement appears to be restricted to patients with the histologic diagnosis of adenocarcinoma. Patients with ALK rearranged tumors are eligible to be treated with crizotinib, another TKI that has been shown to be an efficient drug in the treatment of ALK-positive tumors. Therefore, mutations in the *EGFR* gene and rearrangements of ALK are two molecular alterations that can be targeted by specific therapies and are recommended based on histologic and molecular profile of the tumor [22–35].

Several other molecular alterations have been identified in adenocarcinomas, and few are undergoing clinical trials with molecular targeted agents (see chapter on new discoveries for a detailed description of these alterations).

Based on these advances, correct histologic diagnosis and molecular characterization of adenocarcinoma are prerequisite for optimal therapy and triage of pathologic specimens for molecular diagnostic tests.

## Subtyping of NSCLC in Small Biopsy Material and Cytology

The 2011 classification of adenocarcinoma [15] recommends that subtyping of NSCLC should be performed in a small biopsy material and cytology. Moreover, the subclassification of NSCLC should still be based on histologic criteria. Therefore, if a tumor has histologic features of adenocarcinoma, such as gland (acinar) and papillary formation, this should be classified as an adenocarcinoma (Fig. 1.1). Other patterns of adenocarcinoma such as micropapillary and lepidic can be seen in small biopsy specimens but may be difficult to be recognized in cytologic material [36–39]. In the latter, a cell block preparation may be very helpful in identifying histologic patterns of adenocarcinoma that cannot be recognized on smears [37]. Similarly if a tumor shows keratinization and the presence of intercellular bridges, which are hallmarks of squamous cell carcinoma, the tumor should be classified as a squamous cell carcinoma (Fig. 1.2, Table 1.1). When clear differentiation features are present, there is no need to further characterize these lung tumors by immunohistochemical stains.

On cytology specimens, a precise histologic subtype of NSCLC is feasible using well-described criteria; the issue has been addressed in several studies [40–46].

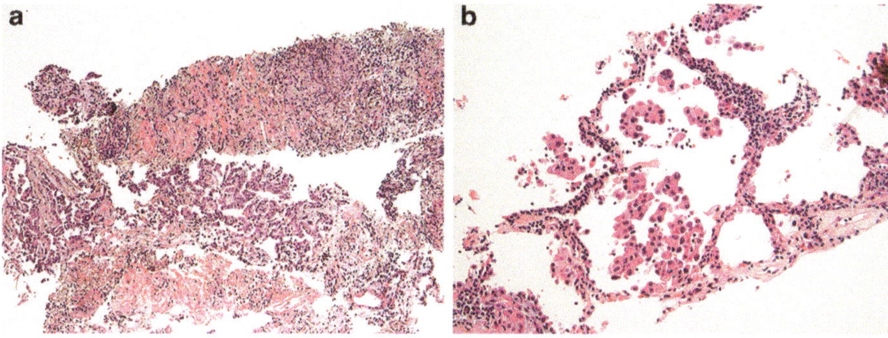


**Fig. 1.1** Photographs of H&E-stained slides diagnosed as adenocarcinoma in core biopsy specimens. (**a**) Adenocarcinoma with papillary pattern (original magnification×100). (**b**) Adenocarcinoma with micropapillary pattern (original magnification×200). As per current nomenclature, there is no need to perform immunohistochemical stains for further classification unless a metastatic adenocarcinoma is suspected

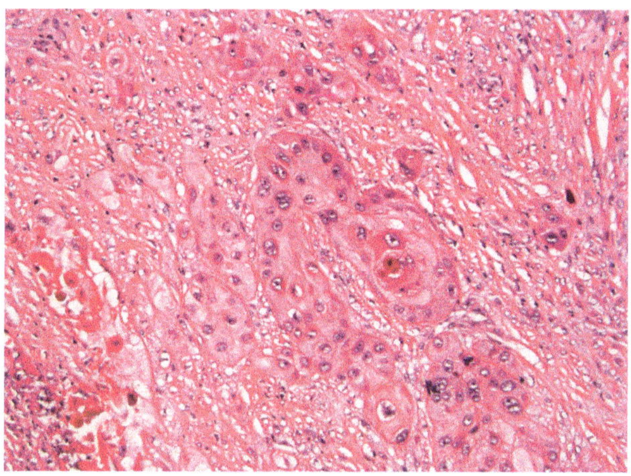

**Fig. 1.2** Photograph of an H&E-stained slide diagnosed as squamous cell carcinoma. Note the presence of keratinization and intracellular bridges, hallmarks of keratinizing squamous cell carcinoma. As per current nomenclature, there is no need to perform immunohistochemical stains for further classification of this tumor (original magnification×200)

As demonstrated by Rekhtman et al. [40], a subclassification of NSCLC into adenocarcinoma and squamous cell carcinoma in cytology specimens can be achieved in approximately 93 % of the cases using cytomorphologic criteria only. However, the subclassification of NSCLC can be a problem in paucicellular specimens and in poorly differentiated carcinomas where no clear histologic differentiation is present. In these situations, the distinction between adenocarcinoma and squamous cell carcinoma cannot be made by morphologic features alone. For example, solid-type adenocarcinomas can show squamoid features such as nested appearance and glassy eosinophilic cytoplasm (Fig. 1.3), although there is no clear

**Table 1.1** Proposed nomenclature for the diagnosis of NSCLC in small biopsy/cytology material

| | Histologic criteria | 2 markers IHC profile |
|---|---|---|
| Adenocarcinoma | Presence of acinar, papillary, lepidic, or micropapillary patterns | Not recommended[a] |
| Squamous cell carcinoma | Presence of keratinization and intracellular bridges | Not recommended |
| NSCC favor adenocarcinoma | Solid pattern, no other evidence of differentiation | Any TTF-1 positivity, negative for p63/p40 |
| NSCC favor squamous cell carcinoma | Solid pattern, no other evidence of differentiation | Diffuse and strong positivity for p63 or p40. Negative for TTF-1 |
| NSCLC not otherwise specified (NOS) | Solid pattern, no other evidence of differentiation | Double positivity for TTF-1 and p63 or p40 either focal or diffuse Double-negative stain for TTF-1[a] and p40 |

[a]TTF-1 may be useful to confirm lung origin. If TTF-1 negative, markers for metastases from other sites such as the breast, gastrointestinal, or genitourinary tract may be useful if clinically indicated

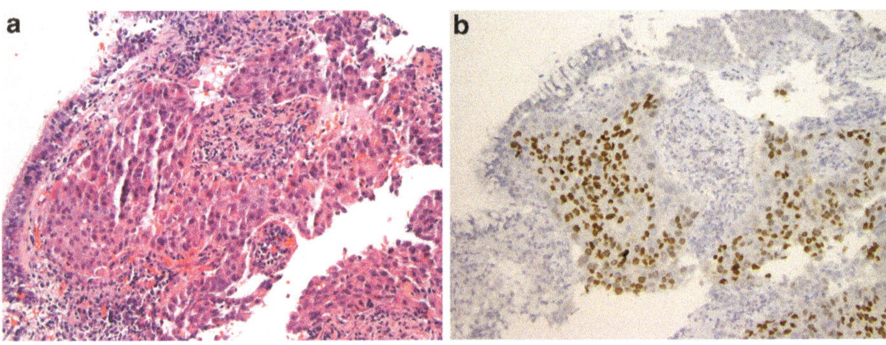


**Fig. 1.3** Photograph of a poorly differentiated carcinoma diagnosed as NSCLC favor adenocarcinoma. (**a**) H&E-stained section showing a solid growth pattern without evidence of glandular or squamous differentiation. Note the squamoid appearance (original magnification × 200). (**b**) Immunohistochemical stains show the tumor cells are diffusely positive for TTF-1, whereas negative for p40 (not showed). This pattern of immunoreactivity supports the diagnosis

keratinization or presence of intracellular bridges. This can be seen either on cytology or small biopsy material and can be confused with squamous cell carcinoma. Knowledge of this pitfall can greatly reduce misclassification of NSCLC.

It is recommended that in cases of a poorly differentiated carcinoma without any clear morphologic evidence of glandular or squamous differentiation, immunohistochemical markers should be used to help in the tumor classification.

There are many studies in the medical literature that attempted to identify the best panel of immunohistochemical stains to be used for the separation of adenocarcinoma and squamous cell carcinoma in small biopsy material [42–45]. Considering the need to save tissue for molecular studies that are indicated in adenocarcinomas, a consensus for the use of a minimal panel has been recommended by the IASLC/

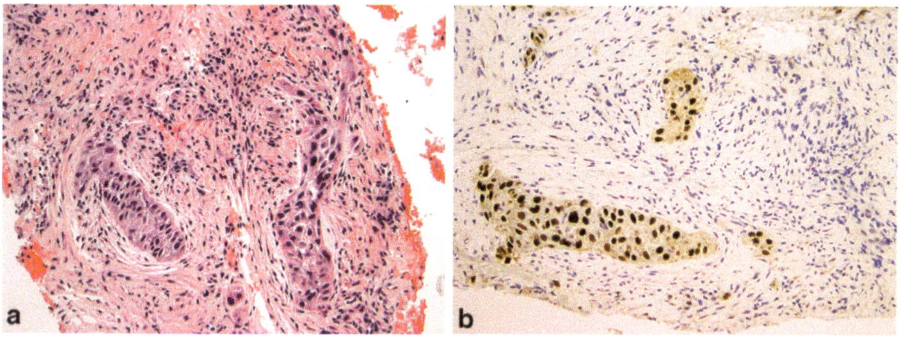


**Fig. 1.4** Photograph of a poorly differentiated carcinoma diagnosed as NSCLC favor squamous cell carcinoma. (**a**) H&E-stained section showing a solid growth pattern without evidence of glandular or squamous differentiation. Note the squamoid appearance. (**b**) Immunohistochemical stains show the tumor cells are diffusely positive for p40, whereas negative for TTF-1 (not showed). This pattern of immunoreactivity supports the diagnosis (original magnification × 100)

ATS/ERS classification [15] and adopted by the World Health Organization. This minimal panel of antibodies includes 2 markers, TTF-1 (thyroid transcription factor-1) and p63 or p40 (an isoform of p63 that seems to be more specific than p63 for the detection of squamous lesions) [47, 48]. Up to 20–30 % of lung adenocarcinomas, including those positive for TTF-1, can be positive for p63, but in virtually all of these cases p40 will be negative [47, 48].

Several studies have shown that TTF-1, although not specific, is a good marker for adenocarcinomas of the lung. Therefore, any staining pattern of TTF-1, either focal or diffuse, is a good indication of adenocarcinoma differentiation. As per the IASLC/ATS/ERS recommendation, tumors that are poorly differentiated but show immunohistochemical features of adenocarcinoma should be classified as NSCLC favor adenocarcinoma (Fig. 1.3). In contrast, poorly differentiated tumors that show immunophenotype consistent with a squamous cell carcinoma, which is defined by a strong and diffuse positivity for P63 or P40 and negative reactivity for TTF1, should be classified as NSCLC favor squamous cell carcinoma (Fig. 1.4).

Although this proposition seems straightforward, there are still some difficulties in classifying tumors that defies this binary approach. For instances, what to do with tumors that show reactivity for both markers or are negative for both markers? The 2011 classification recommended that these tumors should be classified as NSCLC-NOS meaning that the specific subtype cannot be determined in the biopsy specimen with certainty [15]. In the case of a double-negative tumor or a carcinoma with ambiguous immunophenotype based on the two markers, it is imperative to correlate the findings with clinical history. In case of a history or the possibility of a metastatic tumor, additional immunohistochemical stains should be added to the panel to rule out metastatic disease and/or a non-epithelial tumor such as melanoma, sarcoma, and lymphoma. Awareness of the limitations of the two antibody panel, clinical pitfalls, and source, specificity, and sensitivity of the clone of antibodies used are essential to avoid misclassification of lung tumors.

In studies that evaluated the immunophenotype of adenocarcinomas and squamous cell carcinomas in resections, specimens using the binary model of immunoreactivity (TTF-1/p63) have demonstrated that adenocarcinomas have great variability in their staining pattern [42], whereas squamous cell carcinomas are more homogenous with universal strong and diffuse expression of p63 and/or p40 with negative stain for TTF-1. Therefore, it can be concluded that a negative stain for p63/p40 tends to exclude the diagnosis of squamous cell carcinoma [42, 47, 48]. In addition, tumors that are double positive (TTF-1+/p63+ or p40+) or double negative (TTF-1−/p63− or p40−) have the same pattern of mutation as other adenocarcinomas that follow the more common immunoreactivity pattern (TTF-1+/p63− or p40−). In some of the cases where both TTF-1 and p40 are positive, if different populations of tumor cells are expressing these markers, a comment can be made that this could represent an adenosquamous carcinoma; however, that diagnosis requires a resection specimen. For practical purposes, the diagnosis of a NSCLC favor adenocarcinoma or NSCLC-NOS in a small biopsy material should be regarded as equivalent to the diagnosis of adenocarcinoma for therapeutic decision and or triage for molecular studies.

In patients with a resectable tumor, the diagnosis of NSCLC-NOS may correlate with the diagnosis in a resected specimen of an adenocarcinoma with a predominant solid pattern or a large cell carcinoma, if no definite differentiation is identified after examination of the entire tumor. In reality, the proposed classification for small biopsy material gives the pathologists some leeway on how to address evolving concepts, such as large cell carcinoma as a histologic independent entity and uncertainties on diagnosis due to sampling issues.

Critics of this biopsy classification have pointed out that the use of the term "favor" adenocarcinoma or a squamous cell carcinoma can generate concern and confusion among treating physicians since the term "favor" may be interpreted as doubt about the diagnosis. One possible scenario is that clinicians faced with the diagnosis of NSCLC favor adenocarcinoma may be reluctant to treat the patient appropriately with drugs that can be used in adenocarcinomas because there is the concern that there might be an underlining squamous cell carcinoma in the biopsy. Therefore, in order to apply this terminology, there must be clear communication with the treating physician on what the diagnosis implies.

Another concern for the term of "NSCLC favor" is triaging of cases for molecular diagnostic tests. This important issue has been addressed by the recent molecular testing guidelines for pulmonary adenocarcinoma recommended by the College of American Pathologists (CAP), the International Association for the Study of Lung Cancer (IASLC), and the Association for Molecular Pathology (AMP) [49]. In order to reduce the chances of missing a targetable mutation, all tumors with diagnosis of NSCLC-NOS or NSCLC favor adenocarcinoma in a small biopsy material should be submitted for molecular tests. Only tumors with the histologic diagnosis of squamous cell carcinoma and NSCLC favor squamous cell carcinoma (diffuse and strong nuclear stain for p63 or p40) should not be sent routinely for molecular diagnostic tests [49].

Alternatively, the diagnosis of adenocarcinoma can be rendered in the cases of NSCLC favor adenocarcinoma (no histologic evidence of gland formation and immunohistochemical profile of TTF-1+/P63-/p40-) and NSCLC-NOS (no histologic evidence of gland formation and double-negative immunoreactivity profile TTF-1-/p63-or p40) based on the variability of reactivity patterns seen in adenocarcinoma [42], the molecular profile similarities to that of adenocarcinoma [50], and the levels of confidence of the pathologists rendering the diagnosis.

## Conciliation of the Histologic Classification of Adenocarcinoma in Resected Material and in Biopsy Specimens

The 2011 IASLC/ATS/ERS classification of pulmonary adenocarcinoma recognizes that adenocarcinomas are histologic heterogeneous and that different histologic patterns are associated in prognostic significance [15]. Therefore, the recommendation indicates that an invasive adenocarcinoma should be classified based on the predominant histologic pattern. All other histologic patterns present in the tumor should be indicated in the report (Table 1.2).

In patients with stage 1 disease, invasive adenocarcinomas with a predominant lepidic pattern have a good prognosis with approximately 92 % 5-year recurrence-free survival. Tumors with predominant papillary and acinar pattern have an intermediate recurrence-free survival of approximately 84 % in 5 years, and those with predominant

**Table 1.2** New proposed classification of pulmonary adenocarcinoma and its implication to small biopsy specimens

| Resection | Small biopsy | Cytology |
|---|---|---|
| Adenocarcinoma in situ (AIS) | Lepidic pattern[a] | Flat sheets[a] (strips on cell blocks [37]) |
| Minimally invasive adenocarcinoma (MIA) | Lepidic pattern[a] | Flat sheets[a] (strips on cell blocks [37]) |
| Lepidic predominant (LPA) | Lepidic pattern may be present | Flat sheets (strips on cell blocks [37]) |
| Papillary predominant | Papillary pattern may be present | Papillary clusters may be present |
| Acinar predominant | Acini may be present | Acini may be present |
| Solid predominant | Solid pattern may be present | – |
| Micropapillary predominant | Micropapillae may be present | Small clusters may be present[b] |

[a]AIS and MIA cannot be diagnosed in a small biopsy material or cytology. A comment about the differential diagnosis (AIS, MIA, LPA) can be mentioned

[b]Small tight clusters have been reported as cytologic correlates for micropapillary pattern; however, this feature has low sensitivity and specificity for the diagnosis of micropapillary pattern in resection specimen

solid or micropapillary patterns have approximately 73 % recurrence-free survival at 5 years. The latter shows approximately 30 % change of recurrence or death of disease in 5 years [51–53]. Some studies have also suggested that the prognostic stratification by histologic pattern is also effective in patients with advanced stage [53–55] and in patients receiving adjuvant therapy. These results are still preliminary and there is no current recommendation for a differential treatment of lung adenocarcinoma with systemic therapy based on predominant histologic pattern or tumor grade.

The new classification also recognizes two new categories, adenocarcinoma in situ and minimally invasive adenocarcinoma. Both tumors in these categories have excellent prognosis with 100 % recurrence-free survival in 5 years if the tumor is completely resected [51]. Both tumors are characterized by a predominant lepidic growth pattern without significant invasion. However, these tumors cannot be diagnosed in biopsy material, since it is required by definition that the entire tumor must be examined in order to render the diagnosis.

The next challenge to the pathologists is how to address the issue of determining the predominant type or subtypes of adenocarcinoma in invasive tumors on small biopsies and cytology. There are no studies on a direct correlation of predominant histologic types between small biopsy material and resection specimen. The difficulty in these studies may rest on sampling issues, since a biopsy may not contain all growth patterns present in the tumor and may not be representative of the predominant type either. Although no formal recommendation exists, it is possible that, similarly to the resection specimen, the pathologist should list the growth patterns seen in the biopsy. This is particularly important for histologic patterns such as micropapillary, where even a small proportion may be an indication of a high risk for recurrence [56].

In cytology, the issue has been taken up recently. The conclusion is that the determination of predominant type or subtyping of adenocarcinoma in cytology material is not feasible [36–38]. Rudomina et al. [36] showed that the presence of acinar structures in cytology preparations had a predictive value of 94 % when correlated with the presence of acinar pattern in resection specimens. Acinar is the most common pattern in adenocarcinomas [51, 52]. However, the presence of papillary clusters with fibrovascular cores had a predictive value of 75 %, and the presence of micropapillary tufts had a predictive value of 64 % for micropapillary pattern on excised specimens. The authors found no cytologic features that correlated with solid pattern. Rodriguez et al. [37] demonstrated that in approximately 40 % of cases, an acinar or papillary type can be attributed in cytology material, but there are no reliable cytomorphologic features that correlate with a solid or micropapillary-type adenocarcinoma. The latter two are very important histologic patterns that are associated with poor prognosis. Therefore, as of the writing of this chapter, subtyping of adenocarcinomas in cytology materials is not recommended.

In summary, the IASLC/ATS/ERS classification of pulmonary adenocarcinoma has changed the way pathologists diagnose and classify lung cancer and requires a great integration with other professionals in the field of pulmonary oncology for diagnosis and management with patients with lung cancer. For pathologists, the main challenge is the subclassification of NSCLC into adenocarcinomas and squamous cell carcinomas as well as the need to perform molecular profiling of adenocarcinomas in small biopsy material and cytology. Luckily a series of recommendations on how to triage tumors for molecular characterization, a panel of immunohistochemical markers that can help in the classification, in association with proposed terminology that offer flexibility in reporting complex cases have helped pathologists navigate this evolving field. It is imperative that pathologists become familiar with these important recommendations in order to continue to provide the necessary care of patients suffering from this devastating disease.

## References

1. Ferlay J, Soerjomataram I, Ervik M, Dikshit R, Eser S, Mathers C, Rebelo M, Parkin DM, Forman D, Bray F. GLOBOCAN 2012 v1.0, Cancer incidence and mortality worldwide: IARC CancerBase No. 11 [Internet]. Lyon, France: International Agency for Research on Cancer; 2013. Available from: http://globocan.iarc.fr.
2. Bray F, Ren JS, Masuyer E, Ferlay J. Estimates of global cancer prevalence for 27 sites in the adult population in 2008. Int J Cancer. 2013;132(5):1133–45. doi:10.1002/ijc.27711. Epub 2012 Jul 26.
3. Siegel R, Naishadham D, Jemal A. Cancer statistics, 2013. CA Cancer J Clin. 2013;63(1): 11–30.
4. Nizzoli R, Tiseo M, Gelsomino F, et al. Accuracy of fine needle aspiration cytology in the pathological typing of non-small cell lung cancer. J Thorac Oncol. 2011;6(3):489–93.
5. Travis WD, Brambilla E, Noguchi M, et al. Lung cancer diagnosis in small biopsies and cytology: implications of the 2011 IASLC/ATS/ERS lung adenocarcinoma classification. Arch Pathol Lab Med. 2013;137(5):668–84.
6. Travis WD, Brambilla E, Noguchi M, et al. Diagnosis of lung adenocarcinoma in resected specimens: implications of the 2011 International Association for the Study of Lung Cancer/American Thoracic Society/European Respiratory Society Lung Classification. Arch Pathol Lab Med. 2013;137(5):685–705.
7. WHO. Histological typing of lung tumours. Geneva: World Health Organization (WHO); 1967.
8. WHO. Histological typing of lung tumors. Geneva: World Health Organization (WHO); 1981.
9. Travis WD, Colby TV, Corrin B, Shimosato Y, Brambilla E. Histological typing of lung and pleural tumors. Berlin: Springer; 1999.
10. Travis WD, Brambilla E, Muller-Hermelink HK, Harris CC. Pathology and genetics. Tumours of the lung, pleura, thymus and heart. Lyon, France: IARC Press; 2004.
11. Hirsch FR, Spreafico A, Novello S, Wood MD, Simms L, Papotti M. The prognostic and predictive role of histology in advanced non-small cell lung cancer: a literature review. J Thorac Oncol. 2008;3:1468–81.
12. Travis WD, Rekhtman N, Riley GJ, et al. Pathologic diagnosis of advanced lung cancer based on small biopsies and cytology: a paradigm shift. J Thorac Oncol. 2010;5:411–4.
13. Travis WD, Rekhtman N. Pathological diagnosis and classification of lung cancer in small biopsies and cytology: strategic management of tissue for molecular testing. Semin Respir Crit Care Med. 2011;32:22–31.
14. Moreira AL, Thornton RH. Personalized medicine for non-small cell lung cancer: implications of recent advances in tissue acquisition for molecular and histologic testing. Clin Lung Cancer. 2012;13:334–9.
15. Travis WD, Brambilla E, Noguchi M, et al. The New IASLC/ATS/ERS international multidisciplinary lung adenocarcinoma classification. J Thorac Oncol. 2011;6(2):244–85.
16. Sandler A, Gray R, Perry MC, Brahmer J, Schiller JH, Dowlati A, Lilenbaum R, Johnson DH. Paclitaxel-carboplatin alone or with bevacizumab for non-small cell lung cancer. N Engl J Med. 2006;355:2542–50.

17. Johnson DH, Fehrenbacher L, Novotny WF, et al. Randomized phase II trial comparing bevacizumab plus carboplatin and paclitaxel with carboplatin and paclitaxel alone in previously untreated locally advanced or metastatic non-small- cell lung cancer. J Clin Oncol. 2004;22:2184–91.
18. AVASTIN® (bevacizumab) Solution for intravenous infusion [package insert]. South San Francisco, CA: Genentech, Inc.; 2011
19. Scagliotti G, Brodowicz T, Shepherd FA, et al. Treatment-by-histology interaction analyses in three phase III trials show superiority of pemetrexed in nonsquamous non-small cell lung cancer. J Thorac Oncol. 2011;6:64–70.
20. Scagliotti G, Hanna N, Fossella F, et al. The differential efficacy of pemetrexed according to NSCLC histology: a review of two Phase III studies. Oncologist. 2009;14:253–63.
21. Alimta® (pemetrexed disodium) [package insert]. Indianapolis, IN: Eli Lilly and Company; 2009.
22. Lynch TJ, Bell DW, Sordella R, Gurubhagavatula S, Okimoto RA, Brannigan BW, Harris PL, Haserlat SM, Supko JG, Haluska FG, et al. Activating mutations in the epidermal growth factor receptor underlying responsiveness of non-small-cell lung cancer to gefitinib. N Engl J Med. 2004;350:2129–39.
23. Paez JG, Janne PA, Lee JC, Tracy S, Greulich H, Gabriel S, Herman P, Kaye FJ, Lindeman N, Boggon TJ, et al. EGFR mutations in lung cancer: correlation with clinical response to gefitinib therapy. Science. 2004;304:1497–500.
24. Pao W, Miller V, Zakowski M, Doherty J, Politi K, Sarkaria I, Singh B, Heelan R, Rusch V, Fulton L, et al. EGF receptor gene mutations are common in lung cancers from "never smokers" and are associated with sensitivity of tumors to gefitinib and erlotinib. Proc Natl Acad Sci USA. 2004;101:13306–11.
25. Fukuoka M, Yano S, Giaccone G, Tamura T, Nakagawa K, Douillard JY, Nishiwaki Y, Vansteenkiste J, Kudoh S, Rischin D, et al. Multi-institutional randomized phase II trial of gefitinib for previously treated patients with advanced non-small-cell lung cancer (The IDEAL 1 Trial) [corrected]. J Clin Oncol. 2003;21:2237–46.
26. Maemondo M, Inoue A, Kobayashi K, Sugawara S, Oizumi S, Isobe H, Gemma A, Harada M, Yoshizawa H, Kinoshita I, et al. Gefitinib or chemotherapy for non-small-cell lung cancer with mutated EGFR. N Engl J Med. 2010;362:2380–8.
27. Mok TS, Wu YL, Thongprasert S, Yang CH, Chu DT, Saijo N, Sunpaweravong P, Han B, Margono B, Ichinose Y, et al. Gefitinib or carboplatin-paclitaxel in pulmonary adenocarcinoma. N Engl J Med. 2009;361:947–57.
28. Soda M, Choi YL, Enomoto M, et al. Identification of the transforming EML4-ALK fusion gene in non-small-cell lung cancer. Nature. 2007;448:561–6.
29. Pao W, Girard N. New driver mutations in non-small-cell lung cancer. Lancet Oncol. 2011;12:175–80.
30. Rikova K, Guo A, Zeng Q, Possemato A, et al. Global survey of phosphotyrosine signaling identifies oncogenic kinases in lung cancer. Cell. 2007;131:1190–203.
31. Pao W, Chmielecki J. Rational, biologically based treatment of EGFR-mutant non-small-cell lung cancer. Nat Rev Cancer. 2010;10:760–74.
32. Felip E, Gridelli C, Baas P, et al. Metastatic non-small-cell lung cancer: consensus on pathology and molecular tests, first-line, second-line, and third-line therapy: 1st ESMO Consensus Conference in Lung Cancer; Lugano 2010. Ann Oncol. 2011;22:1507–19.
33. Ellis PM, Blais N, Soulieres D, et al. A systematic review and canadian consensus recommendations on the use of biomarkers in the treatment of non-small cell lung cancer. J Thorac Oncol. 2011;6:1379–91.
34. Kwak EL, Bang YJ, Camidge DR, et al. Anaplastic lymphoma kinase inhibition in non-small-cell lung cancer. N Engl J Med. 2010;363:1693–703.
35. Shaw AT, Yeap BY, Solomon BJ, et al. Effect of crizotinib on overall survival in patients with advanced non-small cell lung cancer harbouring ALK gene rearrangement: a retrospective analysis. Lancet Oncol. 2011;12:1004–12.

36. Rudomina DE, Lin O, Moreira AL. Cytologic diagnosis of pulmonary adenocarcinoma with micropapillary pattern: does it correlate with the histologic findings? Diagn Cytopathol. 2009;37:333–9.
37. Loukeris K, Vazquez MF, Sica G, et al. Cytological cell blocks: predictors of squamous cell carcinoma and adenocarcinoma subtypes. Diagn Cytopathol. 2012;40:380–7.
38. Rodriguez EF, Monaco SE, Dacic S. Cytologic subtyping of lung adenocarcinoma by using the proposed IASLC/ATS/ERS adenocarcinoma classification. Cancer Cytopathol. 2013;121:629–37.
39. Moreira AL. Subtyping of pulmonary adenocarcinoma in cytologic specimens: the next challenge. Cancer Cytopathol. 2013;121:601–4.
40. Rekhtman N, Brandt SM, Sigel CS, et al. Suitability of thoracic cytology for new therapeutic paradigms in non-small cell lung carcinoma: high accuracy of tumor subtyping and feasibility of *EGFR* and *KRAS* molecular testing. J Thorac Oncol. 2011;6:451–8.
41. Sigel CS, Moreira AL, Travis WD, et al. Subtyping of non-small cell lung carcinoma. A comparison of small biopsy and cytology specimens. J Thorac Oncol. 2011;6:1849–56.
42. Rekhtman N, Ang DC, Sima CS, et al. Immunohistochemical algorithm for differentiation of lung adenocarcinoma and squamous cell carcinoma based on large series of whole-tissue sections with validation in small specimens. Mod Pathol. 2011;24:1348–59.
43. Loo PS, Thomas SC, Nicolson MC, et al. Subtyping of undifferentiated non-small cell carcinomas in bronchial biopsy specimens. J Thorac Oncol. 2010;5:442–7.
44. Righi L, Graziano P, Formari A, et al. Immunohistochemical subtyping of non-small cell lung cancer not otherwise specified in fine-needle aspiration cytology: a retrospective study of 103 cases with surgical correlation. Cancer. 2011;117:3416–23.
45. Mukhopadhyay S, Katzenstein AL. Subclassification of non-small cell lung carcinoma lacking morphologic differentiation on biopsy specimens; utility of an immunohistochemical panel containing TTF-1, napsin-A, p63, and CK5/6. Am J Sur Pathol. 2011;35:15–25.
46. Da Cunha Santos G, Lai SW, Saieg MA, et al. Cyto-histologic agreement in pathologic subtyping of non-small cell lung carcinoma: review of 602 fine needle aspirates with follow-up surgical specimens over a nine year period and analysis of factors underlying failure to subtype. Lung Cancer. 2012;77:501–6.
47. Bishop JA, Teruya-Feldstein J, Westra WH, Pelosi G, Travis WD, Rekhtman N. p40 is superior to p63 for the diagnosis of pulmonary squamous cell carcinoma. Mod Pathol. 2012;25:405–15.
48. Pelosi G, Fabbri A, Bianchi F, Maisonneuve P, Rossi G, Barbareschi M, Graziano P, Cavazza A, Rehktman N, Pastorino U, Scanagatta P, Papotti M. DeltaNp63 (p40)and thyroid transcription factor-1 immunoreactivity on small biopsies or cell blocks for subtyping non-small cell lung cancer: a novel two-hit, sparing-material approach. J Thorac Oncol. 2012;7:281–90.
49. Lindeman NI, Cagle PT, Beasley MB, et al. Molecular testing guideline for selection of lung cancer patients for EGFR and ALK tyrosine kinase inhibitors: guideline from the College of American Pathologists, International Association for the Study of Lung Cancer, and Association for Molecular Pathology. J Thorac Oncol. 2013;8:823–59.
50. Rehktman N, Tafe LJ, Chaft JE, Wang L, Arcila ME, Colanta A, Moreira AL, Zakowski MF, Travis WD, Sima CS, Kris MG, Ladanyi M. Distinct profile of driver mutations and clinical features in immunomarker-defined subsets of pulmonary large cell carcinoma. Mod Pathol. 2013;26:511–22.
51. Yoshizawa A, Motoi N, Riely GJ, Sima CS, Gerald WL, Kris MG, Park BJ, Rusch VW, Travis WD. Impact of proposed IASLC/ATS/ERS classification of lung adenocarcinoma: prognostic subgroups and implications for further revision of staging based on analysis of 514 stage I cases. Mod Pathol. 2011;25:653–64.
52. Sica G, Yoshizawa A, Sima CS, et al. A grading system of lung adenocarcinomas based on histologic pattern is predictive of disease recurrence in stage i tumors. Am J Surg Pathol. 2010;34:1155–62.
53. Warth A, Muley T, Meister M, et al. The novel histological IASLC/ATS/ERS classification system of lung adenocarcinoma is a stage independent predictor of survival. J Clin Oncol. 2012;30:1438–46.

54. Russel PA, Wainer Z, Wright GM, Daniels M, Conron M, Williams RA. Does lung adenocarcinoma subtype predict patient survival? A clinicopathologic study based on the new International Association for the Study of Lung Cancer/American Thoracic Association/European Respiratory Society international multidisciplinary lung adenocarcinoma classification. J Thorac Oncol. 2011;6:1496–504.
55. Campos-Parra AD, Aviles A, Contreras-Reyes S, Rojas-Marin CE, Sanchez-Reyes R, Borbolla-Escoboza RJ, Arrieta O. Relevance of the novel IASLC/ATS/ERS classification of lung adenocarcinoma in advanced disease. Eur Respir J. 2014;43:1439–47.
56. Nitadori J, Bograd AJ, Kadota K, Sima CS, Rizk NP, Morales EA, Rusch VW, Travis WD, Adusumilli PS. Impact of micropapillary histologic subtype in selecting limited resection vs lobectomy for lung adenocarcinoma of 2 cm or smaller. J Natl Cancer Inst. 2013;105: 1212–20.

# Chapter 2
# Advances in Nonsurgical Sampling Techniques for the Diagnosis and Staging of Lung Cancer

**David F. Yankelevitz and William Bulman**

## Introduction

Intrathoracic malignancy can present with symptoms, as an incidental finding on imaging performed for an unrelated reason or as a finding during lung cancer screening. Radiographic findings are judged in the context of clinical and historical features, allowing the clinician to characterize the overall picture as low, intermediate, or high suspicion for malignancy. Further radiology or laboratory testing provides clues as to the type and possible stage of malignancy. Ultimately the clinician must decide whether intervention or radiographic monitoring is indicated. In many patients, some form of pathologic sampling is required to determine the diagnosis and, if it is a malignancy, the stage of the malignancy. Depending on the tumor cell type, it may also be critically important to obtain the molecular profile, which has implications for prognosis or treatment.

There are multiple ways to sample lesions in the thorax. Suspected primary or metastatic parenchymal lesions may be amenable to percutaneous CT-guided needle biopsy. Primary and metastatic lesions can be accessed bronchoscopically with saline lavage or washing, cytologic brushing, forceps biopsy, or needle aspiration. Multiple surgical options are available, including mediastinoscopy, video-assisted thoracoscopic biopsy, and open thoracotomy. Selecting from among these options can be challenging, but the overriding goal should be to obtain all of the information

D.F. Yankelevitz, M.D.
Department of Radiology, Mount Sinai Medical Center, Mount Sinai Hospital, New York, NY, USA

W. Bulman, M.D. (✉)
Department of Medicine, Columbia University Medical Center, 161 Fort Washington Ave., New York, NY 10032, USA
e-mail: wab10@cumc.columbia.edu



A.L. Moreira, A. Saqi (eds.), *Diagnosing Non-small Cell Carcinoma in Small Biopsy and Cytology*, DOI 10.1007/978-1-4939-1607-8_2

**Table 2.1** Nonsurgical sampling techniques employed for suspected intrathoracic malignancies

| Sampling technique | Site(s) accessible | Staging procedure | Real-time imaging and sampling | Complication risk | Specimen(s) attainable |
|---|---|---|---|---|---|
| Wang | Central | Yes | No | + | FNA and biopsy |
| Radial EBUS | Central and peripheral | Yes[a] | No | + | FNA |
| Convex EBUS | Central | Yes | Yes | + | FNA |
| CT | Central and peripheral | No | +/– | ++ | FNA and biopsy |
| Navigational | Central and peripheral | No | +/– | + | FNA and biopsy |

[a]Radial EBUS is now most commonly used for guidance of sampling peripheral nodules; its use in sampling mediastinal lymph nodes for diagnostic and staging purposes has largely been supplanted by Convex EBUS

needed for diagnosis and staging with the least risk to the patient. For a patient with suspected thoracic nodal metastasis, the ideal procedure is one in which diagnosis and staging are performed in a single step.

This chapter will address some of the more commonly used nonsurgical sampling techniques employed for suspected intrathoracic malignancies (Table 2.1). Selecting the sampling modality must take into account the current and future needs of the patient. The optimal paradigm for care of the patient with lung cancer involves multidisciplinary coordination, and the cytologist or pathologist should fully understand the rationale for and the limitations of each of these techniques in order to fully participate in this care. Although they may not be directly involved in the choice of a sampling modality or the performance of the actual procedure, pathologists play a critical role beyond simply providing a cytologic, histologic, or molecular diagnosis. It is essential that the pathologist provides regular feedback as to the quality and quantity of the specimen to the bronchoscopist, radiologist, or surgeon who is collecting tissue samples.

The sampling targets in the chest can be roughly divided into central lesions and peripheral lesions. Over 70 % of patients with non-small cell lung cancer (NSCLC) will have nodal involvement at the time of their initial presentation [1]; therefore, many patients will have both peripheral and central targets to choose from. The various nonsurgical techniques for sampling available can be broadly divided into bronchoscopic and radiologic techniques, although some modalities combine both bronchoscopic and radiologic approaches to obtain pathologic specimens. This chapter addresses three bronchoscopic techniques, including endobronchial ultrasound-guided transbronchial needle aspiration (EBUS-TBNA) using convex probe technology (CP-EBUS), endobronchial ultrasound-guided sampling of peripheral nodules using radial probe technology (RP-EBUS), and electromagnetic navigational bronchoscopy (ENB). It also discusses CT-guided techniques for the sampling of parenchymal lung nodules, including CT-guided needle aspiration (CTNA) and CT-guided biopsy (CTNB).

In this chapter, "sampling" refers to the group of procedures available to clinicians for tissue diagnosis in suspected thoracic malignancy. Physicians and patients alike use the word "biopsy" when referring to these procedures. While the latter term may be useful in discussing various options with patients, it is incorrectly applied to brushings and fine-needle aspirates which result in a cytologic sample and not a histologic one. The distinction is an important one for the clinician; it is important to understand the kind of information obtainable from the samples derived from the different procedures. An excellent example would be the case of pulmonary lymphoma. Cytologic sampling with EBUS-TBNA combined with flow cytometry may establish a diagnosis of lymphoma, but the added information obtained from histologic sample, which has greater preservation of nodal architecture than a cytologic sample, may be useful for guiding treatment decisions. Knowledge of these differences may guide procedural choices in certain clinical circumstances.

## General Principles of Lung Cancer Management Pertaining to Pathologic Sampling

Multiple guidelines exist to aid in clinical decision-making for the care of a patient with suspected lung cancer. For instance, the American College of Radiology recently proposed the Lung Imaging Reporting and Data System to standardize management of lung nodules identified on screening based on the size of the nodule, presence of a solid component, and growth characteristics [2]. Once the decision to sample a target has been made, the optimal modality for sampling has to be determined. Characteristics of the lesion and clinical features of the case must be factored into an analysis of the risks and benefits of each potential approach. Some techniques are more suitable for lesions with particular characteristics, and many factors, including the location, size, and differential diagnosis, must be taken into account when choosing a sampling modality. It is important for the clinician to understand the sensitivity and the limitations of the available sampling techniques, particularly when choosing between them.

Multiple approaches may yield the correct pathologic diagnosis, but clinicians must look at the broad context of each individual's current and future care needs with respect to diagnosis, staging, and future treatment. The American College of Chest Physicians (ACCP) recently updated its guidelines for clinicians who deal with lung cancer (Diagnosis and Management of Lung Cancer, 3rd ed: American College of Chest Physicians Evidence-Based Clinical Practice Guidelines). In the article entitled "Establishing the Diagnosis of Lung Cancer," Rivera and colleagues [3] outline the basic principles that should guide clinicians in their decision-making with respect to the selection of various diagnostic interventions. The clinician should strive to establish a pathologic diagnosis in the safest and least invasive way possible. Suspected solitary metastases should be confirmed pathologically. In patients with radiographic evidence for multiple metastatic foci in which pathologic sampling of extrathoracic disease would be problematic or difficult, sampling of the primary focus of intrathoracic disease is appropriate. Suspected malignant effusions should be confirmed pathologically. For patients with suspected mediastinal involvement and no evidence on imaging for extrathoracic disease, the guideline emphasizes that the diagnosis should be established by the "least invasive and safest method," and bronchoscopy with TBNA, EBUS-TBNA, esophageal ultrasound-guided TBNA (EUS-TBNA), and transthoracic needle aspiration (TTNA) are listed as options.

An important consideration in undiagnosed patients is minimizing the number of procedures they undergo during the course of their management, seeking wherever possible to perform staging and diagnosis in a single step. It may be tempting to perform a CT-guided biopsy of a large peripheral mass, but if this patient is later found to have suspicious N3 nodes on a subsequent PET and requires a subsequent EBUS-TBNA to pathologically establish nodal involvement, the patient may have undergone an unnecessary intervention. This principle requires that full radiographic staging be undertaken before deciding which intervention is optimal. Patients are often very anxious and want a definitive diagnosis as soon as possible, but in the majority of cases, it is far better to have the right information than to do something right away.

An important distinction between the diagnosis and staging of NSCLC and small cell lung cancer (SCLC) should be mentioned. In NSCLC, radiographic staging should guide pathologic sampling, so that the patient's true stage is established definitively to inform prognosis and guide therapy. In SCLC, which can often be suspected radiographically in a finding of bulky, central mediastinal tumor on imaging, the diagnosis can be established by sampling whichever site using whatever intervention is easiest and safest; staging of the disease is then determined radiographically [3]. In simplest terms, in NSCLC, radiology dictates pathologic sampling to establish a stage, whereas in SCLC, staging is usually radiographic.

## Sampling Central Lesions

In patients with central targets, either masses or adenopathy in the mediastinum or parenchymal masses adjacent to the central airways from the trachea to the hila, bronchoscopic sampling is a consideration. "Blind" techniques for transbronchial needle aspiration (TBNA) of mediastinal lymph nodes were developed by Wang and colleagues [4, 5] at John Hopkins over 30 years ago. Yield and safety of this technique are limited by the blind nature of the procedure, but in expert hands, it is a safe and effective tool. Wang reported an overall diagnostic yield for malignancy of 85 %. Sensitivities for the procedure have been reported ranging from 39 to 89 % [6]. Prior to the development of EBUS-TBNA, the technique was usually employed only for large subcarinal (station 7) and precarinal (station 4R) lymph nodes and was, for the most part, performed routinely only by small percentage of pulmonologists [7]. Although newer technologies have largely supplanted blind TBNA,

Wang and others [4, 5] strongly advocate that this procedure still has a role to play in the diagnosis and staging of lung cancer, citing its benefits as minimal discomfort, decreased cost, reduced risk, and widespread availability.

## Radial and Convex Probe EBUS

Radial ultrasound was first developed for the field of gastroenterology in the 1980s and was adapted to bronchoscopy as more miniaturized components were developed in the 1990s. Modern radial probe endobronchial ultrasound (RP-EBUS) (Olympus) utilizes an ultrasound processor and a reusable 20 MHz ultrasound probe that is inserted through the working channel of a standard bronchoscope with a minimum working channel diameter of 2.0 mm. The radial probe uses mechanical radial scanning from a rotating transducer which, when placed in contact with the airway wall, generates a 360° B-Mode Doppler image of the layers of the bronchial wall and deeper structures adjacent to the airway. The image produced is one perpendicular to the long axis of the probe. The 20 MHz frequency allows for high resolution of the separate layers of the airway wall while providing visualization to a depth of approximately 5 cm [8]. For larger, more central airways, the probe can be covered in a sheath which has water-filled balloon at the distal tip. This can be used to facilitate circumferential contact with the airway wall for 360° imaging, allowing for imaging of the central airways and airway wall as well as central peribronchial structures such as mediastinal lymph nodes and central parenchymal lesions. The probe's small diameter (1.4 mm at the distal tip) allows for probe access to areas of the lung periphery beyond the wedge position of the bronchoscope. It is this feature which allows it to be of use in localizing peripheral lung nodules for pathologic sampling, as will be discussed later.

Early reports of performance characteristics of this tool as a means of guiding conventional TBNA of mediastinal lymph nodes suggested that in expert hands, RP-EBUS guidance improved the overall yield of TBNA over the conventional techniques. Diagnostic yield for TBNA with RP-EBUS guidance has been shown to be superior to blind TBNA, although this comparison is colored by the fact that many studies of blind TBNA did not employ rapid on-site evaluation (ROSE) [6]. In a prospective randomized trial in 200 patients, Herth and colleagues [9] reported an overall yield of 80 % for RP-EBUS-guided TBNA versus 71 % with standard TBNA ($p<0.05$). The superiority of RP-EBUS was derived from improved yield in nodal stations other than the subcarinal station 7; at station 7, no significant difference was seen [9]. The main disadvantage of the radial probe EBUS is that real-time pathologic sampling is not possible. The probe must be withdrawn from the working channel of the bronchoscope in order to allow for the insertion of a brush, needle, or forceps. This technique has the same final limitation of blind TBNA: after identification of a target lesion, the probe is removed, and the subsequent needle stick remains a blind procedure. The probe can be deployed inside a 2.0 mm diameter guide sheath, which can be left in place after ultrasound localization of a target, facilitating placement of a sampling tool and allowing for multiple passes at an identified target. Other disadvantages of the radial probe EBUS are its lack of color Doppler visualization of blood flow for the identification of vessels, as is possible with convex probe technology, and mechanical frailty of the probes. Although reusable, the delicate radial EBUS probes have a limited lifetime of up to 75 uses when handled with care [10].

## Convex Probe EBUS

Despite its demonstrated superiority over conventional, blind TBNA for sampling central targets, RP-EBUS did not gain widespread use because of the development and introduction of curvilinear or convex probe ultrasound (CP-EBUS) technology. CP-EBUS represents an advance over radial probe technology in that it permits real-time pathologic sampling during ultrasound imaging. The convex probe technology uses a series of ultrasound transducers arranged in a curvilinear pattern at the distal end of a dedicated CP-EBUS bronchoscope. Multiple manufacturers of bronchoscopic systems currently offer a CP-EBUS platform. On the Olympus EBUS bronchoscope, the most widely used system, the curvilinear array provides a 60° field of view which is parallel to the long axis of the bronchoscope. The convex EBUS probe uses multiple quad-frequencies of 5, 7.5, 10, and 12 MHz, allowing for a depth of penetration of the ultrasound image to 5 cm, although the resolution is insufficient to differentiate the layers of the airway wall. The EBUS convex probe scope has a working channel with a diameter of 2.2 mm which terminates just proximal to the ultrasound probe head and which is angulated distally 35°, allowing the TBNA needle to pass over the probe in the plane of the ultrasound image. This permits real-time TBNA, with visualization of the needle in the target structure, representing a significant advantage over RP-EBUS. Other advantages include the optional color Doppler visualization of blood flow for the identification of vessels.

There are several disadvantages of the EBUS convex probe bronchoscope. The ultrasound transducer in the tip of the bronchoscope is distal to the light source and viewing port, and the direction of view is angulated 35° forward, parallel to the vector of the needle as it exits the scope, in contrast to the head-on field of view of standard bronchoscopy. This obliquely angulated view, which does not include the ultrasound transducer in the field, can make learning to use the EBUS convex probe scope difficult and perhaps raises the risks of traumatic injury to airway structures during bronchoscopy. Passage of the scope through the vocal cords can be particularly difficult and should be done with extreme care, as vocal cord injuries have been reported [11].

The EBUS convex probe bronchoscope is also larger than standard bronchoscopes, with an outer diameter of 6.9 mm. For this reason, EBUS convex probe bronchoscopy is done via the oral route, and airways smaller than 6.9 mm cannot be accessed. The size of the scope typically permits EBUS-TBNA of hilar nodal stations 11 and 12, however, as noted below [8]. The scope has a maximum flexion range (angulation up) of 120° and a maximum extension range (angulation down) of 90°. With the needle in the working channel, some degree of flexion is lost, and directing the scope into apically directed segments can be challenging. Airway wall contact can be facilitated by using a water-fillable disposable balloon which fits over the transducer head. This can be particularly useful in the trachea and the mainstem bronchi, where contact with the wall can be made difficult by limits in scope flexion, particularly with the needle and sheath in place, and by the irregular contours of the tracheal rings.

Another disadvantage of the EBUS convex probe bronchoscope is its lack of a video processor. The apparatus of the ultrasound transducer occupies space in the distal end of the bronchoscope which normally houses the video processor in a modern video bronchoscope. An EBUS scope utilizes older fiberoptic technology which has lesser image quality. The size of the scope, which limits access to more distal airways, along with the fact that the field of view is both obliquely angled and of lesser quality than a standard scope, mandates the need for a full inspection with a standard scope, before or after the EBUS bronchoscopy, in those patients with suspected NSCLC who are yet unstaged, to look for endobronchial disease or other foci of neoplasm. With the convex probe EBUS bronchoscope, sampling can be done of airway-adjacent parenchymal lesions and upper paratracheal (2 L and 2R), lower paratracheal (4 L and 4R), subcarinal (7), hilar (10 L and 10R), interlobar (11 L and 11R), and lobar (12 L and 12R) nodal stations. The prevascular/retrotracheal (3), subaortic (5), para-aortic (6), paraesophageal (8), and pulmonary ligament (9) nodal stations are not accessible via the tracheobronchial tree with the CP-EBUS [8]. Studies have shown that EBUS-TBNA using convex probe technology can be used in combination with endoscopic esophageal ultrasonography (EUS) to access the additional stations at 8 and 9, and some authors have used the CP-EBUS itself in the esophagus for this purpose [12].

The convex probe EBUS bronchoscope uses disposable needles available from multiple manufacturers. The needles are designed to be anchored to the bronchoscope and have an inner stylet, a movable sheath, and a stopping mechanism that limits needle travel to a fixed distance. The inner stylet serves to minimize the chances that a plug of bronchial wall will occlude the distal lumen of the needle. The needles have a movable sheath which can be deployed into the visual field of view prior to needle deployment to ensure that the needle leaves the working channel at the 35° angulation which will allow it to clear the ultrasound transducer and minimize the chance of a costly deployment into the transducer itself. The needles have a dimpled tip that serves to make them more echogenic, enhancing visualization in the ultrasound image. 21- and 22-gauge needles are now available. The larger inner diameter of the 21-gauge needle can provide larger samples at the expense of increased stiffness; this may allow for easier needle penetration but can limit scope mobility. Studies comparing the yield and complication rates of the 21- and 22-gauge needles have shown similar yields with slightly bloodier specimens obtained with the larger gauge [13, 14]. Use of the 21-gauge needle has been shown to result in fewer needle passes per aspirated node, and some have suggested that it may be superior with regard to better preservation of histologic architecture as well as quantity of tissue obtained [14]. The latter may have important ramifications when it comes to having adequate tissue for molecular testing in NSCLC, although data on this point is lacking.

A thorough ultrasonographic survey of the mediastinum at the time of CP-EBUS-TBNA is essential. Multiple studies of the performance characteristics of CP-EBUS-TBNA have identified PET-negative lymph nodes which were found to have malignant invasion on TBNA. Herth and colleagues showed that CP-EBUS can identify micro-metastasis in patients with lung cancer and a radiographically normal mediastinum [15]. Although the percentage of cases in which CP-EBUS-TBNA upstages patients from their radiographic staging is small, they do occur, and these cases highlight the need for a full ultrasound assessment of accessible nodes and a full sampling from N3 to N2 to N1 nodes, irrespective of PET status, whenever possible in unstaged patients. In certain circumstances, however, targeted sampling is sufficient. In patients with radiographic stage 4 disease and difficult to access metastases, for example, a targeted EBUS-TBNA to establish a diagnosis may be wholly appropriate [3].

Target identification should begin before the procedure, with a careful analysis of the imaging. During the actual procedure, target identification with ultrasound should be done before the needle is inserted into the bronchoscope. The needle/sheath apparatus is then inserted and locked into place, and the sheath is deployed into the field of view and locked into place, ensuring that the needle will leave the bronchoscope at the proper angle, missing the transducer. After re-identifying the target lesion, the distance to the target (i.e., the distance of desired needle deployment) must be estimated or calculated using x and y axis centimeter markings on the view screen and the Pythagorean theorem. The stop mechanism on the needle handle is then set to this distance. Color Doppler visualization can be used to determine if blood vessels lie in the needle path. A variety of needle deployment techniques and sample collection techniques have been described. Firm deployment of the needle with the inner stylet in place can facilitate smooth needle penetration through the bronchial wall. Pitfalls at this stage often involve obstructing tracheal or bronchial rings, which can necessitate scope repositioning. After needle deployment, agitation of the stylet, ensuring that it is pushed as far distally as possible, can help to discharge a bronchial plug if one has been collected. Some operators use a suction technique, with suction ranging up to negative 20 cc, while others use no suction. A locking suction syringe is included with the Olympus EBUS needle package. The needle is then pushed in and pulled out across the span of the target, with care taken not to pull the tip of the needle out of the tissue, which could result in aspiration of the specimen into the suction syringe. Some operators use as many as 10–15 passes across a target lesion. Suction, if used, is then turned off, the needle is pulled fully into the sheath, the sheath is retracted, and the needle is removed from the bronchoscope.

It is important for the bronchoscopist to spend a moment to focus on the patient immediately after the TBNA. The puncture site should be visually observed for hemostasis. The puncture site should also be inspected for its location with respect to the desired target determined by careful examination of the imaging; was the intended target truly sampled? Precision in this regard is critical to prevent inadvertent upstaging or downstaging, as could be the case if a 10R hilar node was sampled instead of an intended nearby mediastinal 4R lymph node.

Although institutional protocol or physician preference may drive decisions regarding the type of sedation used for EBUS-TBNA, the procedure can be performed with either general anesthesia (GA), anesthesia-monitored deep sedation, or with topical anesthetic agents and moderate sedation. Results from the American College of Chest Physicians Quality Improvement Registry, Education, and Evaluation (AQuIRE) Registry, a 6-center, prospective study involving over 1,200 patients published in 2013, showed that using GA or deep sedation for EBUS-TBNA has the potential to improve patient comfort and results in the sampling of a greater number of nodal stations, possibly allowing for (or reflective of) a more systematic or thorough sampling of thoracic nodes [16, 17]. Some studies have shown that use of moderate sedation resulted in lower overall procedural yield [16]. In the AQuIRE Registry data set, the use of GA did not affect complication rates for the procedure, but it increased procedure time and the likelihood of a need for escalation of care post procedure [18]. EBUS-TBNA done with moderate sedation has the advantages of not requiring an operating room or anesthesiologist, which could lower overall procedural cost.

## Performance Characteristics of EBUS-TBNA

Until CP-EBUS-TBNA became widely available, surgical mediastinoscopy was the procedure of choice for the sampling of mediastinal lymph nodes to establish a diagnosis and/or to stage the disease in patients with suspected stage II or stage III NSCLC. Multiple studies throughout the early years of EBUS-TBNA have reported similar or superior sensitivity and specificity to surgical mediastinoscopy. Adams and colleagues performed a meta-analysis of the CP-EBUS-TBNA studies published through 2008, finding a pooled specificity of 1.00 (95 % CI 0.92 to 1.00) and a pooled sensitivity of 0.88 (95 % CI 0.79 to 0.94) [19]. Gu and colleagues performed a meta-analysis which included a total of 11 studies with 1,299 patients, finding that EBUS-TBNA had a pooled sensitivity of 0.93 (95 % CI, 0.91–0.94) and a pooled specificity of 1.00 (95 % CI, 0.99–1.00) [20]. Yasufuku and colleagues published results of a prospective trial in which 159 patients underwent CP-EBUS-TBNA followed by mediastinoscopy under GA. They showed CP-EBUS-TBNA to have a sensitivity, negative predictive value, and accuracy of 81 %, 91 %, and 93 % respectively, compared to 79 %, 90 %, and 93 % for surgical mediastinoscopy [21]. The potential advantages of CP-EBUS over mediastinoscopy go beyond issues of sensitivity and negative predictive value. Whereas mediastinoscopy requires general anesthesia, EBUS can be performed with either general anesthesia, anesthesia-monitored deep sedation, or with topical anesthetic agents and moderate sedation. Lung cancer staging and diagnosis using EBUS-TBNA results in lower overall procedural risk compared to mediastinoscopy [22] and can result in lower overall healthcare costs [23, 24]. As noted above, EBUS-TBNA has a greater range of nodal stations that can be sampled compared to mediastinoscopy.

Expert interventional pulmonologists and thoracic surgeons performed the majority of published studies on the sensitivity of EBUS-TBNA for lung cancer, and the majority of the studies were conducted exclusively in patients under GA. Even in expert hands, procedural yield can vary greatly from center to center. In the AQuIRE registry, which included 6 hospitals, diagnostic yield (with yield defined as TBNA providing a specific diagnosis) ranged from 37 % to 54 % [17]. The performance characteristics of EBUS as a tool in widespread clinical use are not well known, and some operators may struggle to replicate the results seen in clinical trials.

Complications can occur with CP-EBUS-TBNA as with any bronchoscopy. As noted, there are multiple features of the CP-EBUS bronchoscope and the CP-EBUS-TBNA technique which make it more challenging to master than standard bronchoscopy. A significant majority of the published studies examining the performance characteristics of CP-EBUS-TBNA report no complications with the procedure. However, vocal cord injury [25], pneumothorax [26], pneumomediastinum [6], mediastinitis [27, 28], empyema [29], nonfatal hemorrhage [30], and fatal hemorrhage [31] have been published or presented. Despite these, the overall complication rate for CP-EBUS-TBNA is indeed low. The AQuIRE Registry examined complication rates in 1,317 cases performed in 6 centers by 12 clinicians over a 19-month period. They found an overall complication rate of 1.44 % (95 % confidence interval, 0.87–2.24 %). Sustained hypoxia (0.3 %), pneumothorax (0.2 % if no concurrent transbronchial biopsy was performed), bleeding (0.2 %), and respiratory failure (0.2 %) were all seen. One death occurred in the cohort, resulting from bleeding following an endobronchial biopsy done during the procedure and not from the TBNA [18].

The complication rates for EBUS-TBNA in widespread clinical use are not well known but are also likely low. Asano and colleagues published the results of a nationwide survey of EBUS-TBNA in Japan, where the procedure is widely available, pooling data from 210 centers that did 7,345 cases over an 18-month period. They reported a complication rate of 1.23 % (95 % confidence interval, 0.97–1.48 %), one procedure-related death (from a cerebrovascular hemorrhage), and procedure-related infection rate of 0.19 %, including cases of mediastinitis, pneumonia, pericarditis, cyst infection, and sepsis [32]. The reported procedure-related infection in the Japanese study, which was not seen in the AQuIRE Registry data, was likely a result of the fact that the latter study limited complications to events occurring within 24 h of the procedure.

The possibility of inappropriate or inadequate staging by CP-EBUS when done by an inexperienced operator is another concern, however. The potential for erroneously upstaging or downstaging a patient with NSCLC has been cited by some as a reason to recommend that a minimum of 50 cases be proctored before a bronchoscopist is considered to have reached an appropriate level of competency with the procedure [33].

There are several major limitations to EBUS-TBNA which have critical clinical implications and important implications for the cytopathologist. Nondiagnostic aspirations are common and can occur for multiple reasons. Most studies of EBUS-TBNA classify a lymph node aspirate as nondiagnostic if it contains neither malignant cells nor lymphocytes. Rates of nondiagnostic EBUS-TBNA range from 4 % to 23 % across published series. These rates describe the final result of a patient's complete procedure, which most often involves multiple aspirations of a target lesion. When rapid on-site evaluation (ROSE) is employed, multiple aspirations of a target are often necessary before a diagnostic specimen is obtained; therefore, the nondiagnostic rate of individual aspiration attempts is lower. For this reason, when ROSE is not available, it is suggested that 3 aspirations be performed at each target to optimize yield [34, 35].

The transbronchial approach results in contamination of the cytologic specimen with bronchial cells; in one study of CP-EBUS-TBNA, bronchial cells were seen in up to 80 % of specimens [36]. A finding of only bronchial cells in the aspirated specimen is not uncommon with EBUS-TBNA. This occurs when the hollow bore needle picks up a bronchial plug as it passes through the airway wall, despite the presence of the stylet. The bronchial plug can occlude the needle tip, preventing successful aspiration of the target. Even if it is discharged by pushing out the stylet, it can be aspirated back into the needle after suction is applied. Certain characteristics of the tumor itself can contribute to a nondiagnostic finding. Necrotic tumors may contain few cells, for example.

One key to optimizing yield and to optimizing the efficiency of EBUS-TBNA lies with ROSE of the aspirated specimens. In a large meta-analysis, ROSE was shown to increase the sensitivity of EBUS-TBNA from 80 % to 88 % while decreasing procedure times [37]. Most (but not all) studies showing improved sensitivity and negative predictive values for EBUS-TBNA over mediastinoscopy used ROSE. Resource limitations are a reality in clinical medicine, and ROSE is not available in every institution, but the bronchoscopist who performs EBUS-TBNA should strongly advocate for it in order to optimize the benefits to patients.

## CP-EBUS-TBNA as Part of a Multidisciplinary, Multimodality Approach to Lung Cancer

With or without ROSE, the cytopathologist plays a critical role in the performance of the operator, providing feedback on the quality and quantity of samples obtained. Whether done by the bronchoscopist, bronchoscopy nurse, or cytopathologist on site, proper handling, triage, and processing of the aspirated sample is crucial to optimize the yield for immunohistochemical staining and full molecular analysis in the case of adenocarcinoma.

The negative predictive value of EBUS-TBNA is not 100 %, and false negatives do occur [38, 39]. Most studies classify EBUS-TBNA samples as negative or benign if they contain lymphocytes but no malignant cells. False negatives in nodal aspirates can occur due to true nodal sampling error, resulting from a needle pass missing microscopic lymph node invasion or due to limited sampling of a station with multiple nodes in which tumor invasion is present in only some. Nondiagnostic findings and false negatives present less of a clinical problem if EBUS-TBNA is employed as part of a sequential strategy. In patients where the suspicion of nodal involvement is high based on imaging, an EBUS-TBNA with a negative or nondiagnostic result should undergo confirmatory mediastinoscopy or other surgical sampling [36]. Confirmatory surgical sampling can be done as a separate procedure or as part of a combined procedure; at some institutions, EBUS-TBNA is performed immediately preceding a planned resection, with surgical intervention aborted if a patient is found to have mediastinal lymph node involvement. Most studies report a positive predictive value of 100 % for EBUS-TBNA, and therefore, confirmatory mediastinoscopy in patients with a positive EBUS-TBNA is not needed. In certain cases, a nonmalignant positive finding which drastically changes the level of clinical suspicion for malignancy, such as a finding of fungal infection, might lead to a reassessment of the likelihood of malignancy and therefore lead to an alternate approach. For patients in whom cancer remains a concern, however, the use of confirmatory surgical sampling after a negative or nondiagnostic EBUS-TBNA avoids a missed diagnosis.

Perhaps the most useful role for EBUS-TBNA is in patients with suspected N2 disease who will be receiving neoadjuvant chemotherapy in anticipation of later surgical resection. Such patients need diagnosis and pathological staging prior to therapy, following which they may require repeat pathological staging after chemotherapy. If mediastinoscopy were the only modality for staging available, the second mediastinoscopy would be complicated by the presence of scarring from the first. With EBUS-TBNA, initial confirmation of N2 disease can be done without surgery. If there is radiographic evidence of residual nodal disease after chemotherapy, then EBUS-TBNA can be performed a second time to confirm this. If there is radiographic evidence of a good response and surgery is planned, a mediastinoscopy can be done immediately prior to resection to confirm the clearance of nodal disease. This algorithm is shown in Fig. 2.1 [40].

It should be noted that the idea that EBUS-TBNA is superior to mediastinoscopy is not shared by all. In a recent review in the Annals of Thoracic Surgery, Shrager points out that in many of the studies comparing EBUS-TBNA to mediastinoscopy, EBUS was performed under general anesthesia, eliminating the theoretical benefits of a procedure performed under moderate sedation [41]. EBUS-TBNA has the potential for false negatives due to sampling error, and without confirmatory mediastinoscopy,

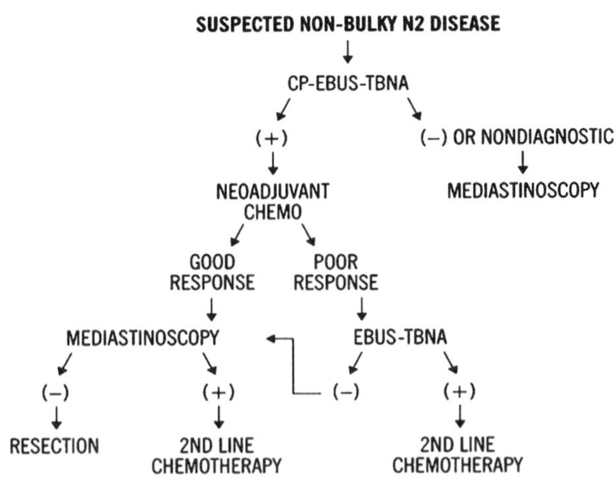


**Fig. 2.1** Treatment algorithm for suspected non-bulky N2 disease

the potential downside is great: missed N3 disease could lead to unnecessary surgery, whereas missed N2 disease could lead to a failure to prescribe beneficial neoadjuvant chemotherapy. When EBUS-TBNA is followed by confirmatory mediastinoscopy, the costs are additive. Shrager therefore advocates strongly for mediastinoscopy, not EBUS, as the procedure of choice in patients who have a low suspicion of mediastinal disease [41].

Quite rapidly, use of the convex probe for endobronchial ultrasound-guided transbronchial needle aspiration (EBUS-TBNA) has become the procedure of choice for sampling of mediastinal and airway-accessible central targets in patients with suspected lung cancer and other intrathoracic pathologies. Use of this technique has gained favor among both pulmonologists and surgeons. Unlike the blind Wang technique, the technique of EBUS-TBNA has not been confined to interventional pulmonologists, and many general pulmonogists who do few other interventional procedures have begun to perform the procedure. Given the importance of accurate staging in lung cancer, it is critical that this modality for sampling be handled with expert care.

## Pathologic Sampling of Peripheral Lesions

### *General Principles*

Peripheral lung nodules present different challenges for clinical decision-making and for pathologic sampling. Once a lung lesion is identified, multiple features are assessed to determine the likelihood of malignancy, including patient age, size of the nodule, smoking history, evidence of adenopathy, increasing nodule size on serial studies, and irregular lesion borders [42]. For solitary, peripheral nodules (SPN) for which there is a high suspicion of malignancy (estimated to be >60 %) [43], the option of primary resection should be considered. Although the ACCP Guidelines refer to this as a "diagnostic dilemma," this is not the case for some patients, where primary resection fulfills the criteria for "least" and "safest." A patient with suspected early-stage disease by PET-CT imaging who is a good candidate for surgical resection (calculated to have sufficient lung function to tolerate lobectomy or pneumonectomy, as dictated by the location of the primary tumor) should undergo VATS wedge resection of the tumor with frozen section analysis to definitively establish the diagnosis of malignancy, followed immediately by nodal staging and definitive resection if occult N2 or bulky N1 nodal disease is absent. In these patients, a biopsy of the primary tumor would be an unnecessary step in the majority of cases. In a high suspicion lesion, only a benign biopsy finding that led a very high degree of confidence that a false negative was unlikely should avert definitive resection. A finding of environmental fungal disease, such as histoplasmosis, coccidioidomycosis, or cryptococcosis, or a finding of tuberculosis, might satisfy these criteria, although the incidence of these findings in SPN is rare [42]. Rolston and colleagues [44], in a 3-year analysis of all of the patients referred to the University of Texas for suspected lung cancer, found that the diagnostic workup for suspected malignancy led to a finding of benign disease in only 6.7 % and a finding of infection mimicking lung cancer in only 1.3 %. The majority of the patients had an SPN on imaging, and they found no radiographic features which were necessarily predictive of either infection or neoplasm [44]. The possibility of a false-negative biopsy finding in a high suspicion patient should strongly favor an approach of definitive resection in these patients, contingent on having established good lung function [3, 43].

In other cases, uncertainty as to the nature of solitary peripheral nodule (SPN) or mass drives the need for pathologic sampling. Many pulmonary nodules are discovered incidentally on imaging done for other reasons. With the findings of the National Lung Screening Trial (NLST) showing a 20 % reduction in deaths from lung cancer among current or former heavy smokers who were screened with low-dose helical computed tomography (CT) versus those screened by chest X-ray, more individuals at risk for lung cancer will undergo CT imaging in the near future, and more pulmonary nodules of unclear clinical significance will be identified [45]. Given that the observed reduction in lung cancer mortality was invariably due to early accurate identification of malignant disease and subsequent early intervention, the diagnosis of the cancerous peripheral lung nodule is critical.

A total of 96.4 % of the positive screening results in the low-dose CT group in the NLST were *false positives*, however [45]. In the management of a patient with an uncharacterized SPN of unknown clinical significance, the clinician must determine based on the clinical context whether intervention is needed and, if so, what type. Some nodules, by virtue of their radiologic characteristics or stability over time, can be assumed to be benign, whereas some warrant immediate surgical resection. In between these extremes of inaction and complete surgical removal fall many pulmonary nodules and masses which require either radiologic monitoring or a biopsy to determine pathology, which in turn dictates the need for further intervention.

Clinical context is unique for every patient, however, and patient participation in the discussions related to these decisions is important. There are some patients for whom the idea of contemplating surgical resection without an established diagnosis is overwhelming, and pathologic sampling may be necessary to get them to the place where they can accept the imperative for potentially curative resection. In patients with an SPN where the suspicion of malignancy is low or intermediate, or in patients for whom surgical resection is not or may not be an option, or in patients with clear radiographic evidence of stage 4 disease where the primary lesion is the easiest and safest site to sample, multiple modalities are available. Bronchoscopic sampling (lavage, cytologic brushing, TBNA, and forceps biopsy), CT-guided needle sampling, bronchoscopic sampling with RP-EBUS guidance, and EMN bronchoscopy are options to be considered. The last three modalities will be discussed in detail.

## Radiographically Guided Needle Sampling of an SPN

Image-guided sampling of a thoracic target can be done with plain fluoroscopy, or with transthoracic ultrasound imaging if the lesion is near the pleural surface, or with CT guidance. CT-guided sampling allows for precise needle positioning, resulting in high yields and low morbidity, and is typically done by an experienced interventional radiologist. This procedure can be performed as an transthoracic fine-needle aspiration (TTNA), which is done with a smaller gauge needle (typically 20–22 g) and which yields a cytologic sample, or as a transthoracic needle biopsy (TTNB), most often done with a hollow larger-bore needle with a cutting mechanism following CT-guided insertion of a thinner localizing needle. TTNB is intended to yield a core histologic specimen which can demonstrate tissue architecture. Both can be done with or without ROSE, and the two procedures can be done in combination, usually TTNA followed by a TTNB. ROSE can be effectively used in a combination procedure to provide additional information beyond confirmation of a diagnosis. ROSE of an aspirate cytology specimen can confirm lesional tissue to guide the subsequent core biopsy, which can be sent in its entirety for pathologic processing, without "wasting" additional tissue for on-site fixation.

CT-guided sampling can be done with intermittent imaging with interval needle repositioning or with CT fluoroscopy with the radiologist tableside. Real-time CT fluoroscopic sampling is possible, with needle positioning done with active fluoroscopic imaging, although this can be technically difficult. Needle insertion is typically done with a breath hold, with cessation of tidal respiration rather than at deep inspiration. The challenges of CT-guided intrathoracic sampling include difficulties that arise as a result of a target size and location and accommodating respiratory motion. Although it would seem reasonable that a lesion adjacent to the pleura would be easier to access than a deeper, intraparenchymal lesion of the same size, this is often not the case. A needle passing through some lung tissue will result in an anchoring of the needle in place, and a deeper lesion can allow for more subtle directional changes on the way to the target that may not be possible with a lesion against the pleura as repositioning might necessitate repuncturing the pleura multiple times, thereby increasing the chance for complications.

If given a choice, needle insertion from the back with the patient prone is preferred over needle insertion with the patient supine for several reasons. First, patient anxiety is typically less if they are unable to see the long sampling needle. Second, it is generally recommended that patients recover post procedure with the biopsy site down, so that the weight of the lung rest on the puncture site, and it is easier for a patient to recover supine than prone.

The pleura is a fibrous membrane which, unlike the lung parenchyma, is innervated; crossing the pleura can cause pain. If the clinician does not cross the pleura in a rapid fashion but instead hesitates with the needle tenting the membrane, the resulting patient response can result in a laceration of the lung rather than a puncture, possibly resulting in pneumothorax. Emphysematous areas of lung adjacent to the entry site may also increase the risk of pneumothorax and should be avoided if possible. If a needle is inserted into the lung but misses the target lesion necessitating a second needlestick, it may be preferable to leave the first needle in place. This is because the first needle will tend to stabilize motion of the lung, aiding in the positioning of the second needle, and because of the possibility of pneumothorax following removal of the first needle. The patient will have this pneumothorax regardless with removal of the first needle, but better to have this complication after second (hopefully successful) sampling rather than before. One advantage of CT-guided biopsy performed by interventional radiology is that a chest tube, if needed, can be placed with imaging guidance by the radiologist obtaining the biopsy or aspiration. Sampling using a needle mechanism that employs a coaxial technique in which a single needle puncture is followed by multiple samplings over the finder needle has been thought to mitigate pneumothorax risk, although this potential benefit has not been seen in all studies [46].

## Performance Characteristics

TTNA has been shown to have good sensitivity for identifying malignancy in SPN. The 2007 ACCP Guidelines present an excellent review of the literature on the performance characteristics of transthoracic sampling for suspected lung cancer. No new relevant literature was identified in the 2013 ACCP Guidelines, which again presented the 2007 findings. In a meta-analysis of 46 studies, with nondiagnostic, nonspecific, and benign findings all considered to be negative, the pooled sensitivity of TTNA was 90 % (95 % CI, 88–91 %) with a range of 62–99 % [3]. These studies included TTNA performed under fluoroscopic guidance and CT guidance. In the presence of a nonspecific benign diagnosis following multiple passes and documented needle tip in the target, pathology follow-up demonstrated that approximately 90 % of lesions are benign [47]. False negatives do occur, however, therefore a nondiagnostic, nonspecific, or benign finding should prompt consideration of additional investigation, if the initial suspicion of cancer is high, as previously discussed. This could include re-sampling, resection, or close radiographic monitoring with careful attention to growth.

The performance characteristics of TTNA and TTNB have been compared in case series with variable results. Tuna and colleagues [48] retrospectively compared the yield in 105 patients who underwent CT-guided transthoracic lung biopsy, 83 by TTNB and 22 by TTNA. They reported finding a definitive diagnosis in 87 of 105 patients (83 %) overall, with 94 % of the diagnoses showing a malignancy. The sensitivity of TTNB was significantly higher, with a sensitivity of 92 % compared to a sensitivity of only 78 % for TTNA [49]. Ten percent of patients overall had a pneumothorax, and only 2 % had hemorrhage, with no significant difference in complications between TTNA and TTNB. Klein and colleagues [49] published a retrospective review of CT-guiding sampling performed on 127 lesions in 122 patients, with 87 samplings done as a TTNA and 99 sampling done as a cutting needle TTNB. Both procedures were performed using a coaxial technique with sampling needles placed through a 19-gauge needle placed in the lesion. TTNA was done with a 20-gauge Westcott needle (Becton Dickinson, Franklin Lakes, NJ) or a 22-gauge Chiba needle (Cook). TTNB was done with a 20-gauge ASAP automated cutting needle (Medi-Tech/Boston Scientific, Watertown, MA) or a 20-gauge Temno automated cutting needle (Bauer Medical, Clearwater, FL). The overall diagnostic yield for the study was 88 %. The sensitivity was 95 % for malignancy and 91 % for benign disease.

Although no significant difference was found for sensitivity between fine-needle aspiration and core biopsy of malignant lesions (92 % vs. 86 %), a statistically significant difference was found for benign lesions (44 % vs. 100 %). Pneumothorax rate in this study was high, occurring in 54 % of patients [49].

## Complications

Pneumothorax and hemorrhage are the most common complications of TTNA and TTNB. Richardson and colleagues [50] recently searched retrospectively over 5,000 cases of CT-guided thoracic samplings in the UK, reporting a pneumothorax rate of 20.5 %, with 3.1 % requiring chest drainage (3.1 %). Pneumothorax was similar in procedures done with a core cutting biopsy needle and those done as a FNA. Hemoptysis occurred in 5.3 % and death in 0.15 % of cases. Hiraki and colleagues [51] reported a much higher rate of pneumothorax in over 1,000 cases performed over a 9-year period in Japan using a 20-gauge coaxial cutting needle. They found an overall incidence of pneumothorax of 42.3 %, with 11.9 % needing a chest tube. In one of the largest series to date, Wiener and colleagues [52] reviewed over 15,000 CT-guided biopsies of pulmonary nodules identified in the 2006 State Ambulatory Surgery Databases and State Inpatient Databases for California, Florida, Michigan, and New York. 15.0 % of procedures (CI, 14.0 % to 16.0 %) were complicated by pneumothorax, and 6.6 % (CI, 6.0 % to 7.2 %) of patients required a chest tube. Bleeding was uncommon, with only 1.0 % (95 % CI, 0.9 % to 1.2 %) of procedures complicated by hemorrhage. Smokers and patients with chronic obstructive pulmonary disease were at higher risk for complications [52].

The risk factors predisposing to pneumothorax are variable across different studies. Some studies have shown pneumothorax rate to be independent of the size of the lesion and the size of the needle, whereas others have shown the opposite. Needle dwell time (the amount of time spent with the needle in the lung parenchyma), the need to cross a fissure, and the number of total punctures have been thought to correlate with the chance of pneumothorax. In the Japanese series, depth of the lesion, a lower lobe lesion, and needle trajectory <45° were associated with pneumothorax risk, and emphysema increased the risk of needing chest tube placement. Clinical features like prior lung or pleural surgery and the presence of pleural adhesions might be of some protective benefit [53].

## RP-EBUS

Convex probe EBUS evolved from radial probe EBUS, but they each now have a separate potential role to play in the management of patients with suspected thoracic malignancy. As noted above, the size of the CP-EBUS scope limits its reach in the segmental airways, so it plays little role in the diagnosis of most peripheral nodules. RP-EBUS has retained a useful role in the diagnosis and sampling of peripheral nodules, at least in the hands of experienced practitioners. The probe's small diameter (1.4 mm at the distal tip) allows for access to areas of the lung periphery beyond the wedge position of the bronchoscope. The high resolution with ability to delineate the layers of the bronchial wall allows for direct observation of bronchial wall invasion which could inform staging. Use of RP-EBUS to guide bronchoscopic sampling of peripheral lesions has been shown to improve the yield over standard bronchoscopy. Steinfort and colleagues published a meta-analysis of 16 studies with 1,420 patients. They found a specificity of 100 % (95 % CI 99–100) and a sensitivity of 73 % (95 % CI 70–76) for the detection of lung cancer. Yield was significantly better for lesions greater than 2 cm in size [54]. The rate of pneumothorax was very low, ranging from 0 % to 5.1 %, and the risk of bleeding was extremely low, with no patients experiencing bleeding which required an intervention. The 2013 ACCP Guidelines recommend consideration of RP-EBUS as an adjunct imaging tool for the bronchoscopic sampling of a suspicious SPN in patients where pathologic diagnosis is desired [3].

## Navigational Bronchoscopy

The search to improve diagnostic yield in the bronchoscopic sampling of SPNs has led to efforts to guide the bronchoscope and sampling tools through the tracheobronchial tree to the target lesion. These "navigational" systems employ 3-D reconstructions of the tracheobronchial tree from CT imaging, often with a virtual endobronchial view akin to the view seen through the bronchoscope, to produce a virtual roadmap to the lesion. One commercially available system, iLogic System (superDimension, Inc., Herzliya, Israel and Minnesota, MN), combines elements of virtual bronchoscopic reconstruction with real-time 3-D directional and positional mapping. Termed electromagnetic navigational bronchoscopy (ENB), this guidance system has been shown to improve the yield of diagnostic sampling over conventional bronchoscopy.

The technique of ENB was first reported in animal experiments in 2003 [55] and later described in humans in 2006 by the same researchers [56]. Leong and colleagues [57] have recently published an excellent review of ENB which describes both the iLogic System and the ENB procedure in detail. The system utilizes a software program and several pieces of novel hardware, including an extended working channel which functions as a guide sheath, an 8-way steerable probe with a miniaturized EM sensor at the distal tip, and a low frequency electromagnetic field generator and emitter.

A patient's CT imaging, which must be in the appropriate, standardized DICOM format (Digital Imaging and Communications in Medicine, Rosslyn, VA), is uploaded into the ENB software planning program prior to the procedure. The planning software converts the CT images into a multi-planar 3-D reconstruction and displays axial, coronal, sagittal, and 3-D views, and both the target lesion and a bronchial pathway to the lesion are plotted. At the time of the procedure, the patient is placed supine on the bronchoscopy table with an EM emitter, or location board, placed under the mattress. Additional location pads are placed on the patient's chest, and an EM field is generated which encompasses the patient's thorax.

An inspection bronchoscopy is performed with the EWC extending 8 mm from the distal end of the scope and the sensor probe, or location guide, deployed in the EWC. The location guide collects data on its position and orientation in the tracheobronchial tree 166 times per second to the ENB software program, and this information is superimposed on the virtual 3-D map (provided by the CT images) in real time. In the course of a full inspection bronchoscopy, the data collected automatically "registers" the patient's anatomy with the virtual 3-D reconstruction of the CT images. The two data sets are then aligned and presented as an overlay on the procedure screen. The highest allowable divergence between the two 3-D images is 5 mm; greater divergence should prompt re-registration. The aligned overlay of these two data sets is presented on the software's procedure display for real-time guidance through the tracheobronchial tree to the lesion. The display shows multiple views of the overlaid imaging, including the previously mapped route to the lesion and a head-on "tip view" showing the target as well as distance and direction to the target. Arrows in the tip view direct the operator to manipulate the steerable probe in the direction of the target as the probe is advanced. After reaching the target lesion with the probe and extended working channel, the location guide is removed and the working channel is left in place to allow introduction of tools for sampling. Fluoroscopy can be used to confirm positioning, as can RP-EBUS, deployed through the working channel after the LG is removed. ENB can also be used for the placement fiducial markers for subsequent interventions, including surgical resection or radiation.

## Performance Characteristics of ENB

ENB has been extensively studied since its development and has been consistently shown to improve the diagnostic yield of bronchoscopic sampling. Leong and colleagues [57] examined data from 12 studies of the performance of ENB, reporting diagnostic yields ranging from 59 to 77 %. Rates for pneumothorax were low, ranging from 0 to 10 %. There are multiple studies comparing the sensitivity and yield of ENB over conventional bronchoscopic biopsy techniques. In one of the larger single center series of 92 biopsies in 89 patients, Eberhardt and colleagues [58] reported an overall diagnostic yield of 67 %, with only 2 cases leading to pneumothorax. ENB has been used to guide SPN biopsy as well as lymph node biopsy. Gildea and colleagues prospectively studied 60 subjects undergoing ENB; they reported a navigational success rate (reaching the target lesion) of 100 %, with a yield of 74 % for SPN and 100 % for lymph nodes [59].

Multiple factors have been shown to affect yield. The procedure is technically challenging, and experience helps. Lamprecht and colleagues [60] looked at 112 cases comparing yield in the first 30 cases to the last 30, showing yields of 80 % and 87 % respectively. Larger lesions had a higher yield, with diagnoses obtained in 89 % of lesions greater than 2 cm compared to 75 % in lesions less than 2 cm. Location of the lesion did not appear to affect yield [60]. In one study, the presence of a "bronchus sign," an area of hypoattenuation on CT leading to or into an SPN, was the only variable on multivariate analysis which appeared to affect diagnostic yield of ENB [61].

## Comparison and Combination of Sampling Techniques

ENB is a newer technology than RP-EBUS, and its role in the management of SPNs is still being elucidated. Studies have shown that in expert hands, ENB increases the diagnostic sensitivity of bronchoscopic sampling over standard bronchoscopy. ENB requires equipment and software that represents a capital expense for the institution or operator; it requires time for data entry; and it requires expertise with the software and the hardware. As with all technological advances, it is remains to be seen whether the yield and complication rate seen in clinical studies can be duplicated in wider clinical use.

It is also obvious that all nodules are unique and each will have features that will alter the balance of risks and benefits in a way that may favor one diagnostic approach over another. Location with respect to the pleura, relationship to the airways and blood vessels, and relationship to emphysematous lung all will affect the expected sensitivity of a procedure and the potential for complications in an individual patient.

Comparing TTNA or TTNB with ENB, studies suggest that an ENB approach may offer the advantage of a lower complication rate at the expense of decreased sensitivity; an ENB approach would therefore increase the likelihood of requiring a second, alternate diagnostic intervention (subsequent CT-guided biopsy or VATS), increasing overall risk and increasing overall costs, in the subset of patients with nondiagnostic results on ENB. Researchers have used modeling to compare serial testing with ENB followed by CTGB or CTGB followed by ENB. The approach utilizing ENB as an initial modality could be more than twice as expensive, although the risk of complications would likely be lower than with the reverse serial strategy. Combining the two procedures in serial testing would have a combined sensitivity of 97 % [62].

Real-world utilization is likely to be dictated by clinical considerations, however not modeling. As noted, there are certainly features of individual tumors and individual patients which make one approach favorable over another and each case must be evaluated with an eye toward yield and risk specific to the clinical circumstances.

## References

1. Surveillance, Epidemiology, and End Results (SEER) Program of the National Cancer Institute, SEER Stat Fact Sheets: Lung and Bronchus Cancer
2. American College of Radiology: Lung Imaging Reporting and Data System. Available from: http://www.acr.org/Quality-Safety/Resources/LungRADS

3. Patricia Rivera M, Wahidi MM. Diagnosis and Management of Lung Cancer, 3rd ed: American college of chest Physicians Evidence-based clinical practice guidelines. Chest. 2013;143 (5 Suppl): e142S–e165S. doi:10.1378/chest.12-2353
4. Wang KP, Brower R, Haponik EF, Siegelman S. Flexible transbronchial needle aspiration for staging of bronchogenic carcinoma. Chest. 1983;84:571–6.
5. Wang KP, Terry PB. Transbronchial needle aspiration in the diagnosis and staging of bronchogenic carcinoma. Am Rev Respir Dis. 1983;127(3):344–7.
6. Holty J, Kuschner W, Gould M. Accuracy of transbronchial needle aspiration for mediastinal staging of non-small cell lung cancer: a meta-analysis. Thorax. 2005;60(11):949–55.
7. Feller-Kopman D, Yung RC-W, Burroughs F, Li QK. Cytology of endobronchial ultrasound-guided transbronchial needle aspiration. Cancer Cytopathol. 2009;117:482–90.
8. Hanna WC, Yasufuku K. Bronchoscopic staging of lung cancer. Ther Adv Respir Dis. 2013;7(2):111–8
9. Herth F, Becker HD, Ernst A. Conventional vs endobronchial ultrasound-guided transbronchial needle aspiration: a randomized trial. Chest. 2004;125(1):322–5.
10. Sheski FD, Mathur PN. Endobronchial ultrasound. Chest. 2008;133(1):264–70.
11. Wang Memoli JS, Nietert PJ, Silvestri GA. Meta-analysis of guided bronchoscopy for the evaluation of the pulmonary nodule. Chest. 2012;142(2):385–93.
12. Herth FJ, Krasnik M, Kahn N, et al. Combined endoscopic-endobronchial ultrasound-guided fine-needle aspiration of mediastinal lymph nodes through a single bronchoscope in 150 patients with suspected lung cancer. Chest. 2010;138(4):790–4. doi:10.1378/chest.09-2149.
13. Saji J, Kurimoto N, Morita K, Nakamura M, Inoue T, Nakamura H, Miyazawa T. Comparison of 21-gauge and 22-gauge needles for endobronchial ultrasound-guided transbronchial needle aspiration of mediastinal and hilar lymph nodes. J Bronchol Intervent Pulmonol. 2011; 18:239–46.
14. Yarmus LB, Akulian J, Lechtzin N, Yasin F, Kamdar B, Ernst A, Ost DE, Ray C, Greenhill SR, Jimenez CA, Filner J, Feller-Kopman D. American College of Chest Physicians Quality Improvement Registry, Education, and Evaluation (AQuIRE) Participants. Comparison of 21-gauge and 22-gauge aspiration needle in endobronchial ultrasound-guided transbronchial needle aspiration: results of the American College of Chest Physicians Quality Improvement Registry, Education, and Evaluation Registry. Chest. 2013;143(4):1036–43.
15. Herth FJ, Ernst A, Eberhardt R, Vilmann P, Dienemann H, Krasnik M. Endobronchial ultrasound-guided transbronchial needle aspiration of lymph nodes in the radiologically normal mediastinum. Eur Respir J. 2006;28(5):910–4.
16. Yarmus LB, Akulian JA, Gilbert C, Mathai SC, Sathiyamoorthy S, Sahetya S, Harris K, Gillespie C, Haas A, Feller-Kopman D, Sterman D, Lee HJ. Comparison of moderate versus deep sedation for endobronchial ultrasound transbronchial needle aspiration. Ann Am Thorac Soc. 2013;10(2):121–6.
17. Ost DE, Ernst A, Lei X, Feller-Kopman D, Eapen GA, Kovitz KL, Herth FJ, Simoff M, AQuIRE Bronchoscopy Registry. Diagnostic yield of endobronchial ultrasound-guided transbronchial needle aspiration: results of the AQuIRE Bronchoscopy Registry. Chest. 2011;140(6):1557–66.
18. Eapen GA, Shah AM, Lei X, Jimenez CA, Morice RC, Yarmus L, Filner J, Ray C, Michaud G, Greenhill SR, Sarkiss M, Casal R, Rice D, Ost DE. American College of Chest Physicians complications, consequences, and practice patterns of endobronchial ultrasound-guided transbronchial needle aspiration: results of the AQuIRE registry. Quality Improvement Registry, Education. Chest. 2013;143(4):1044–53.
19. Adams K, Shah PL, Edmonds L, Lim E. Test performance of endobronchial ultrasound and transbronchial needle aspiration biopsy for mediastinal staging in patients with lung cancer: systematic review and meta-analysis. Thorax. 2009;64(9):757–62.
20. Gu P, Zhao YZ, Jiang LY. Endobronchial ultrasound-guided transbronchial needle aspiration for staging of lung cancer: a systematic review and meta-analysis. Eur J Cancer. 2009;45: 1389–96.

21. Yasufuku K, Pierre A, Darling G, de Perrot M, Waddell T, Johnston M, da Cunha SG, Geddie W, Boerner S, Le LW, Keshavjee S. A prospective controlled trial of endobronchial ultrasound-guided transbronchial needle aspiration compared with mediastinoscopy for mediastinal lymph node staging of lung cancer. J Thorac Cardiovasc Surg. 2011;142(6):1393–400.
22. Detterbeck FC, Jantz MA, Wallace M, Vansteenkiste J, Silvestri GA. Invasive mediastinal staging of lung cancer: ACCP evidence-based clinical practice guidelines (2nd edition). Chest. 2007;132:202S–220S.
23. Harewood GC, Pascual J, Raimondo M, Woodward T, Johnson M, McComb B, Odell J, Jamil LH, Gill KR, Wallace MB. Economic analysis of combined endoscopic and endobronchial ultrasound in the evaluation of patients with suspected non-small cell lung cancer. Lung Cancer. 2010;67:366–71.
24. Kim K, Rice TW, Murthy SC, DeCamp MM, Pierce CD, Karchmer DP, Rybicki LA, Blackstone EH. Combined bronchoscopy, mediastinoscopy, and thoracotomy for lung cancer: Who benefits? J Thorac Cardiovasc Surg. 2004;127:850–6.
25. Wang KP, Mehta AC, Francis Turner Jr J. Flexible bronchoscopy. New York: Wiley; 2012. p. 35.
26. Eckardt SM, Kaul P. A40. Case reports in pleural disease. 2010: A1472. 10.1164/ajrccm-conference.2010.181.1_MeetingAbstracts.A1472
27. Smith JP, Selej M, Carlos WG, Diab K. D102. Case reports: interventional pulmonary and lung transplantation, 2013: A5812. 10.1164/ajrccm-conference.2013.187.1_MeetingAbstracts.A5812
28. Parker KL, Bizekis CS, Zervos MD. Severe mediastinal infection with abscess formation after endobronchial ultrasound-guided transbronchial needle aspiration. Ann Thorac Surg. 2010;89:1271–2.
29. Huang CT, Chen CY, Ho CC, Yu CJ. A rare constellation of empyema, lung abscess, and mediastinal abscess as a complication of endobronchial ultrasound-guided transbronchial needle aspiration. Eur J Cardiothorac Surg. 2011;40:264–5.
30. Navani N, et al. Endobronchial ultrasound–guided transbronchial needle aspiration prevents mediastinoscopies in the diagnosis of isolated mediastinal lymphadenopathy. Am J Respir Crit Care Med. 2012;186(3):255–260. doi: 10.1164/rccm.201203-0393OC
31. Aguilar-Lopez CA, Weir I, Winter S. D102. Case reports: interventional pulmonary and lung transplantation, 2013: A5809. 10.1164/ajrccm-conference.2013.187.1_MeetingAbstracts.A5809
32. Asano F, Aoe M, Ohsaki Y, Okada Y, Sasada S, Sato S, Suzuki E, Semba H, Fukuoka K, Fujino S, Ohmori K. Complications associated with endobronchial ultrasound-guided transbronchial needle aspiration: a nationwide survey by the Japan Society for Respiratory Endoscopy. Resp Res. 2013;14(50):1–8.
33. Erik Folch MD, Adnan Majid MD. FCCP point: are >50 supervised procedures required to develop competency in performing endobronchial ultrasound-guided transbronchial needle aspiration for mediastinal staging? Yes. Chest. 2013;143(4):888–91.
34. Lee HS, Lee GK, Lee HS, et al. Real-time endobronchial ultrasound-guided transbronchial needle aspiration in mediastinal staging of non-small cell lung cancer: how many aspirations per target lymph node station? Chest. 2008;134(2):368–74.
35. Diacon AH, Schuurmans MM, Theron J, et al. Transbronchial needle aspirates: how many passes per target site? Eur Respir J. 2007;29(1):112–6.
36. Alsharif M, Andrade RS, Groth SS, Stelow EB, Pambuccian SE. Endobronchial ultrasound-guided transbronchial fine-needle aspiration: the University of Minnesota experience, with emphasis on usefulness, adequacy assessment, and diagnostic difficulties. Am J Clin Pathol. 2008;130:434–43.
37. Micames CG, McCrory DC, Pavey DA, Jowell PS, Gress FG. Endoscopic ultrasound-guided fine-needle aspiration for non-small cell lung cancer staging: a systematic review and meta-analysis. Chest. 2007;131:539–48.
38. Zhang R, Mietchen C, Krüger M, Wiegmann B, Golpon H, Dettmer S, Haverich A, Zardo P. Endobronchial ultrasound guided fine needle aspiration versus transcervical mediastinoscopy in nodal staging of non small cell lung cancer: a prospective comparison study. J Cardiothorac Surg. 2012; 7:51.

39. Vincent BD, El-Bayoumi E, Hoffman B, Doelken P, DeRosimo J, Reed C, Silvestri GA. Real-time endobronchial ultrasound-guided transbronchial lymph node aspiration. Ann Thorac Surg. 2008;85(1):224–30.
40. Bulman W, Saqi A, Powell CA. Acquisition and processing of endobronchial ultrasound-guided transbronchial needle aspiration specimens in the era of targeted lung cancer chemotherapy. Am J Respir Crit Care Med. 2012;185(6): 606–611.
41. Shrager JB. Mediastinoscopy: still the gold standard. Ann Thorac Surg. 2010;89(6):S2084–9.
42. Cardillo G. The risk of malignancy is related to patient age, size of the nodule, smoking history, evidence of adenopathy, increasing nodule size on serial studies, and irregular lesion borders. Ann Thorac Surg. 2003;75(5):1607–11.
43. Ost DE, Gould MK. Decision making in patients with pulmonary nodules. Am J Respir Crit Care Med. 2012;185(4):363–72.
44. Rolston KV, Rodriguez S, Dholakia N, Whimbey E, Raad I. Pulmonary infections mimicking cancer: a retrospective, three-year review. Support Care Cancer. 1997;5(2):90–3.
45. National Lung Screening Trial Research Team, Aberle DR, Adams AM, Berg CD, Black WC, Clapp JD, Fagerstrom RM, Gareen IF, Gatsonis C, Marcus PM, Sicks JD. Reduced lung-cancer mortality with low-dose computed tomographic screening. N Engl J Med. 2011; 365:395–409
46. Mullan CP, Kelly BE, Ellis PK, Hughes S, Anderson N, McCluggage WG. CT-guided fine-needle aspiration of lung nodules: effect on outcome of using coaxial technique and Immediate cytological evaluation. Ulster Med J. 2004;73(1):32–6.
47. Gelbman BD, Cham MD, Kim W, Libby DM, Smith JP, Port JL, Altorki NK, Henschke CI, Yankelevitz DF. Radiographic and clinical characterization of false negative results from CT-guided needle biopsies of lung nodules. J Thorac Oncol. 2012;7(5):815–20.
48. Tuna T, Ozkaya S, Dirican A, Findik S, Gatici A, Erkan L. Diagnostic efficacy of computed tomography-guided transthoracic needle aspiration and biopsy in patients with pulmonary disease. OncoTargets Therapy. 2013;6:1553–7.
49. Klein JS, Salomon G, Stewart EA. Transthoracic needle biopsy with a coaxially placed 20-gauge automated cutting needle: results in 122 patients. Radiology. 1996;198(3):715–20.
50. Richardson CM, Pointon KS, Manhire AR, Macfarlane JT. Percutaneous lung biopsies: a survey of UK practice based on 5444 biopsies. Br J Radiol. 2002;75(897):731–5.
51. Hiraki T, Mimura H, Gobara H, Shibamoto K, Inoue D, Matsui Y, Kanazawa S. Incidence of and risk factors for pneumothorax and chest tube placement after ct fluoroscopy–guided percutaneous lung biopsy: retrospective analysis of the procedures conducted over a 9-year period. Am J Roentgenol. 2010;194:809–14.
52. Wiener RS, Schwartz LM, Woloshin S, Welch HG. Population-based risk for complications after transthoracic needle lung biopsy of a pulmonary nodule: an analysis of discharge records. Ann Intern Med. 2011;155(3):137–44.
53. Lorenz J, Blum M. Complications of percutaneous chest biopsy. Semin Intervent Radiol. 2006;23(2):188–93.
54. Steinfort DP, Khor YH, Manser RL, Inring RB. Radial probe endobronchial ultrasound for the diagnosis of peripheral lung cancer: systematic review and meta-analysis. Eur Rosp J. 2011;37(4):902–10.
55. Schwarz Y, Mehta AC, Ernst A, Herth F, Engel A, Besser D, Becker HD. Electromagnetic navigation during flexible bronchoscopy. Respiration. 2003;70(5):516–22.
56. Schwarz Y, Greif J, Becker HD, Ernst A, Mehta A. Real-time electromagnetic navigation bronchoscopy to peripheral lung lesions using overlaid CT images: the first human study. Chest. 2006;129(4):988–94.
57. Leong S, Ju H, Marshall H, Bowman R, Yang I, Ree AM, Saxon C, Fong KM. Electromagnetic navigation bronchoscopy: A descriptive analysis. J Thorac Dis. 2012;4(2):173–85.
58. Eberhardt R, Anantham D, Herth F, Feller-Kopman D, Ernst A. Electromagnetic navigation diagnostic bronchoscopy in peripheral lung lesions. Chest. 2007;131(6):1800–5.
59. Gildea TR, Mazzone PJ, Karnak D, Meziane M, Mehta AC. Electromagnetic navigation diagnostic bronchoscopy. A prospective study. Am J Respir Crit Care Med. 2006;174:982–9.

60. Lamprecht B, Porsch P, Wegleitner B, Strasser G, Kaiser B, Studnicka M. Electromagnetic navigation bronchoscopy (ENB): increasing diagnostic yield. Respir Med. 2012;106(5): 710–5.
61. Seijo LM, de Torres JP, Lozano MD, Bastarrika G, Alcaide AB, Lacunza MM, Zulueta JJ. Diagnostic yield of electromagnetic navigation bronchoscopy is highly dependent on the presence of a Bronchus sign on CT imaging: results from a prospective study. Chest. 2010;138(6):1316–21. doi:10.1378/chest.09-2708. Epub 2010 Apr 30.
62. Dale CR, Madtes DK, Fan VS, Gorden JA, Veenstra DL. Navigational bronchoscopy with biopsy versus ct-guided biopsy for the diagnosis of a solitary pulmonary nodule: a cost-consequences. Anal J Bronchol Interv Pulmonol. 2012;19(4):294–303.

# Chapter 3
# Adequacy and Tissue Preservation of Small Biopsy and Cytology Specimens

**John P. Crapanzano and Anjali Saqi**

## Introduction

Lung carcinoma remains the leading cause of mortality worldwide. It accounts for approximately 16,000 deaths annually [1], with nearly 70 % of patients presenting at an advanced stage. Several advances have been made in recent years, though. These comprise classification of non-small cell lung cancers (NSCLCs) in small biopsy and cytology specimens [2], identification of driver mutations, and treatment of lung carcinomas. For lung cancer, the recommendation is to subclassify NSCLCs on small specimens because the morphological subtype of NSCLC and molecular profile of lung adenocarcinoma impact therapy. Distinguishing lung adenocarcinoma from squamous cell carcinoma is important because of clinical observations—patients with squamous cell carcinomas are at increased risk for life-threatening hemorrhage when treated with bevacizumab, and patients with adenocarcinoma respond significantly better to pemetrexed than those with squamous cell carcinoma. Adenocarcinomas with an epidermal growth factor receptor (EGFR) mutation have better response to tyrosine kinase inhibitors as a first-line therapy, while those without the mutation have a better outcome with chemotherapy [3–9]. Similar benefits have been linked to treatment of anaplastic lymphoma kinase (ALK) rearranged lung adenocarcinomas [9].

J.P. Crapanzano, M.D.
Department of Pathology and Cell Biology,
Columbia University Medical Center, New York-Presbyterian Hospital,
New York, NY, USA

A. Saqi, M.D., M.B.A. (✉)
Department of Pathology and Cell Biology,
Columbia University Medical Center, New York-Presbyterian Hospital,
630 West 168th Street, VC14-215, New York, NY 10032, USA
e-mail: aas177@cumc.columbia.edu

 
A.L. Moreira, A. Saqi (eds.), *Diagnosing Non-small Cell Carcinoma in Small Biopsy and Cytology*, DOI 10.1007/978-1-4939-1607-8_3

Moreover, there has been a shift to perform minimally invasive procedures, where the goal is to obtain the necessary information for diagnosis, and possibly staging, with the least risk to the patient. There are multiple available sampling methods, particularly for (suspected) lung cancer [10], whether primary or metastatic, to obtain needle core biopsy and/or fine-needle aspiration (FNA). Usually performed under image guidance, the modalities include directed sampling with computed tomography (CT), endobronchial ultrasound (EBUS), endoscopic ultrasound (EUS), and electromagnetic navigational bronchoscopy, with each offering its advantages.

Based on this paradigm shift in the treatment of lung cancer, it is appropriate that standardized criteria have been proposed that apply to pathological diagnosis in small biopsies and cytology specimens in the new International Association for the Study of Lung Cancer/American Thoracic Society/European Respiratory Society (IASLC/ATS/ERS) classification of lung cancer [2], molecular testing guidelines have been outlined [11], and diagnostic tests have been developed.

There is a practice gap with limited data on acquisition, triage, processing, and management of small specimens, however [12, 13] (Fig. 3.1). In today's era of personalized medicine, pathologists find themselves not only shifting away from the diagnosis of NSCLC-not otherwise specified (NOS), but also challenged by decreasing sample size and increasing information required for patient care. Adequacy requires material to subclassify NSCLC via routine stains [hematoxylin and eosin (H&E),

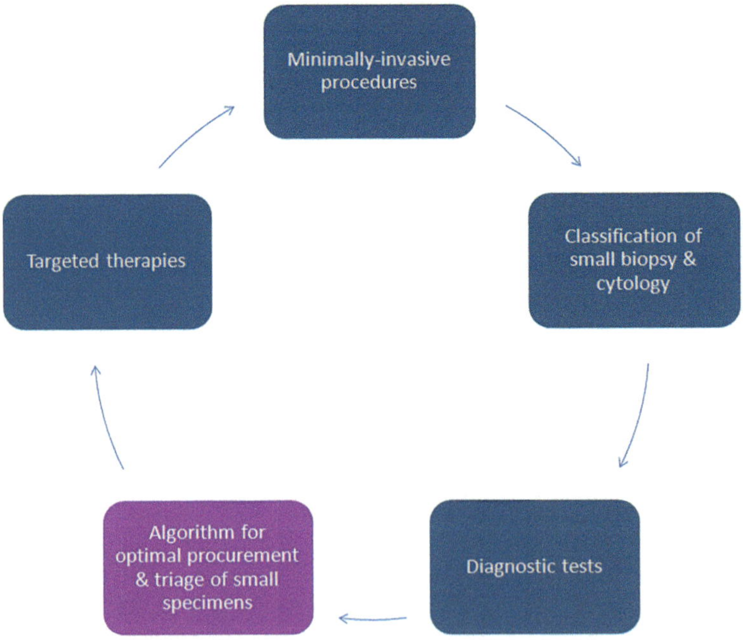


**Fig. 3.1** Practice gap. Currently, there is no standardized algorithm for optimal procurement, processing, and triaging of small specimens

Diff-Quik, and/or Papanicolaou], immunohistochemical (IHC) stains, and/or mucicarmine stain and for patients presenting with advanced stage lung adenocarcinomas, sufficient tissue for the identification of underlying driver mutations, which is the current standard of care for assigning treatment.

Since diagnoses are based more frequently on small biopsy and/or cytology specimens, which sometimes represent the only sample, it is of utmost importance to obtain and manage specimens in a manner that provides all of the pertinent information necessary for appropriate therapy. This chapter outlines methods to optimize small biopsy and cytology acquisition and preservation.

## Cytology Specimens and Core Biopsies

There is ongoing debate centering on which specimen type, an aspirate or a core biopsy, is the better method for providing sufficient tissue. The method, FNA or needle core biopsy, chosen is influenced by several issues, including the preference and comfort of the radiologist and/or pathologist [14], the procedure being performed (e.g., only FNAs are performed with EBUS), availability of on-site evaluation by a cytologist, risk to the patient (e.g., underlying lung pathology, such as emphysema/bullous disease), and nature of the lesion (e.g., size, location, consistency).

There are various types of cytology specimens available for diagnosis, including FNAs and exfoliative specimens such as pleural effusions, bronchoalveolar lavages, and bronchial brushings. Of these, FNAs offer the highest sensitivity (80–95 %) and specificity (98–100 %) in diagnosing malignancies [15–17]. Data strongly support that subtyping of NSCLC on cytological specimens is possible and accurate [18] particularly when cytomorphology is combined with IHC stains [19]. When compared, FNAs are equivalent to core biopsies at definitively and specifically classifying NSCLC [20] and have similar rates of yielding sufficient material for molecular testing [19, 21, 22]. Recent studies have reported that not only are cytology specimens, including FNAs, effusions, and exfoliative specimens, suitable for EGFR and Kirsten rat sarcoma (KRAS) testing [19, 21], but there is also complete concordance of molecular testing results between FNA specimens and their histological counterparts, including resections and cores [23]. For heterogeneous lesions, FNAs may outperform cores because of their strength to sample different aspects of the lesion with a single pass [24].

Core biopsies are an alternative source of diagnostic tissue. Recently, the performance of cores has been advocated by pathologists who are unavailable for rapid on-site assessment of FNAs and/or who sign-out mostly surgical pathology [14]. Some have reported that optimal results are obtained when the two modalities are performed concurrently [20]. Others follow a FNA with a core, if necessary [24], or commonly irrespective of a diagnostic result at the time of ROSE due to clinicians' requests [25]. In scenarios where both FNA and core biopsies are performed, comparison of the two is recommended because the two modalities may provide complementary information to render a specific and concordant diagnosis [26].

Overall, there is no consensus on the method of choice—FNA and/or core biopsy—and ultimate determination may rest upon institutional establishment of adequacy protocols and rates of success with each modality.

## Rapid On-Site Evaluation: Fine-Needle Aspirations

### *Advantages*

Rapid on-site evaluation (ROSE) involves a cytology staff member, either a (cyto)-pathologist or cytotechnologist, providing real-time evaluation of the specimen during the procedure and communicating the findings to the clinician (e.g., pulmonologist, interventional radiologist, surgeon, or endosonographer). Correlation with the history and imaging provides an integrated approach to the diagnosis (Table 3.1).

Traditionally, providing a preliminary assessment was sufficient. Now, in light of the added importance and responsibility for the cytologist to properly triage the specimen, it is intuitive that the individual performing ROSE has experience in cytomorphology interpretation, be knowledgeable about ancillary tests necessary for various diagnoses, ensures that sufficient tissue is allocated for potential ancillary tests (e.g., immunohistochemistry and/or molecular testing for carcinomas, microbiological cultures in cases of inflammation or granulomas, or flow cytometry for lymphoma assessment), and be informed about methods of specimen fixation/preservation required for each test. Proper decision-making and specimen submission at the time of the procedure can directly affect patient care. Recent data strongly support that aspirates performed with ROSE optimize the use of the aspiration procedure [27, 28] by improving diagnostic yield [29] and aiding in the procurement of additional material for potential necessary special studies [29–40].

**Table 3.1** Advantages of ROSE

| |
|---|
| Proper triage |
| Ensures sufficient tissue for diagnosis |
| Specimen procured for ancillary studies |
| Expedites clinical decisions |
| Enables scheduling of additional imaging/appointment(s) during single visit |
| Improves diagnostic accuracy |
| Sensitivity |
| Specificity |
| Positive predictive value |
| Enhances efficiency and cost-effectiveness of patient care |
| Reduces repeat procedures |
| Minimizes complication rate of procedure |

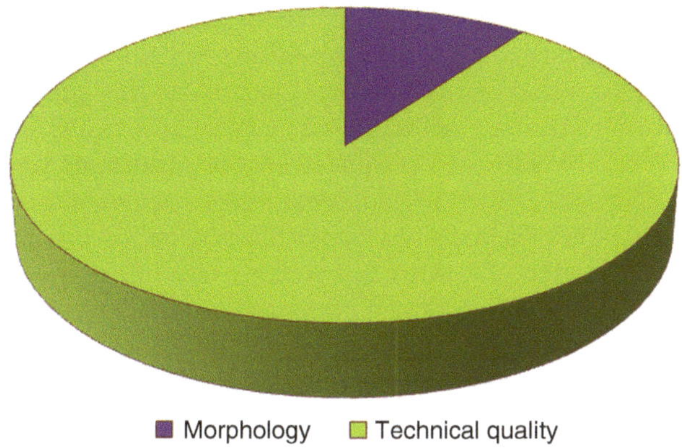


**Fig. 3.2** Role of specimen preparation in diagnostic interpretation. Technical quality, which includes smear preparation and staining, plays a significant role in the final interpretation. When performed appropriately, the morphology is well preserved, and interpretations at time of ROSE and final diagnosis are not compromised

There is also value added to a well-prepared specimen—one without poor preservation or preparation—which expedites final examination. When the technical quality of a specimen is maximized, final interpretation is not compromised (Fig. 3.2). High-quality preparations limit intradepartmental consults and time consumed interpreting slides with limited cellularity, poor preparation, or artifacts and shift focus on diagnostic dilemmas. In cases where the same pathologist performs ROSE and issues the final report, time may not be "wasted" [13] as on-site assessment provides an opportunity to obtain the clinical history and preview of a fraction of the slides.

ROSE of lung nodule aspirates is effective at discriminating malignant versus nonmalignant lesions, such as sarcoidosis [41], and having a cytopathologist present is associated with a significantly greater accuracy in diagnosis of malignancy [32–34, 37, 39]. ROSE increases sensitivity and specificity [42] and the predictive value of a negative test. Moreover, it increases the likelihood of attaining a higher rate of positive diagnoses [34], when present, and decreases unsatisfactory results [37]. While the average reported non-diagnostic rate of FNAs is 20 % when on-site evaluation is not utilized [27], a diagnostic rate of 98 % has been achieved in a study of over 5,600 FNAs with ROSE [27]. Diagnoses rendered at time of ROSE are highly accurate and usually concordant with the final interpretation [43, 44]. In the same study with >5,600 FNAs, the on-site interpretation was in agreement with the final diagnosis in 85 % of cases; there was disagreement in 2.7 % of cases and deferment to the final diagnosis in 12 %.

The high concordance of on-site immediate interpretation and final diagnosis allows for reliable decision-making that can enhance efficiency and cost-effectiveness of patient care [27]. With a preliminary diagnosis, clinical decisions can be expedited [27, 45–49] and scheduling for additional imaging, appointment with a specialist, or surgical procedure can be initiated. The procedure can be terminated as soon as diagnostic material is obtained. By doing so, fewer needle passes [34, 50, 51] than those predetermined in the absence of ROSE [51] are performed at fewer sites, thereby decreasing the time a patient is under sedation, reducing the complication rate [52], and increasing the safety of the procedure. Next, ROSE results in a decrease in the number of repeat [37] or additional procedures necessary for a diagnosis [50], which has downstream effects. Assuming non-diagnostic FNAs are repeated, direct institutional charges can be significant. The diagnostic value and cost-effectiveness of ROSE was evaluated in 5,688 FNAs [27]. In the absence of ROSE, the estimated calculated cost of performing repeat FNAs of non-diagnostic specimens resulted in additional direct institutional charges of $2,022,626 over 5 years. These savings are significant despite the professional service fee of on-site interpretation [27]. Also, this does not take into account indirect costs to the patient, such as time off work and prolonged hospital stays. ROSE has downstream effects on the facility as well. Specifically, with shorter procedures times and fewer re-biopsies, utilization of procedure rooms and imaging facilities [53] is optimized.

## *Disadvantages*

ROSE is not always feasible, either by a pathologist or cytotechnologist, due to limited resources of the facility. For a pathologist, ROSE results in time consumption, workflow disruption, and little reimbursement, i.e., high cost for time spent at the procedure [29, 53, 54] (Table 3.2). From a pathologist's economic standpoint, time is spent better signing out cases in the office than performing immediate, on-site evaluation of FNA specimens [53]. Compared with routine surgical pathology, compensation schedules for intraprocedural FNA consultations by pathologists are insufficient [40, 53]. Moreover, relative value units for signing out cases in the office outweigh those generated during a single ROSE. The time and overall benefit are not calculated in the measurement of productivity. In light of this suboptimal compensation and often prolonged procedure times [54], some institutions defer ROSE to cytotechnologists or forego ROSE and place the entire specimen in a liquid-based cytological container [55]. Despite the extra expense for the on-site cytology service [56], reports document that on-site analysis, specifically for trans-bronchial FNA, is cost-effective [56, 57].

**Table 3.2** Disadvantages of ROSE

| |
|---|
| Time consumption |
| Prolonged procedure time |
| Travel time |
| Workflow disruption |
| Low reimbursement |
| Relative value units disproportionate to time and effort |
| Possibility of diagnostic misinterpretation |
| Sampling error |
| Scant cellularity |
| Need for consultation or ancillary studies |
| Challenging diagnosis |

Though infrequent [49], another drawback of ROSE includes diagnostic misinterpretation, both false positive and false negative [58, 59]. In the majority of cases with differing on-site immediate diagnosis and final diagnosis, the reason is sampling error, i.e., only normal-appearing tissue evident on Diff-Quik stained smears and diagnostic cells present in the remaining specimen. In one report, the diagnostic yield (determining tissue adequacy) of ROSE in cases with high suspicion for lung cancer was 77.1 % (101 of 131) but increased to 93.9 % upon final cytological analysis following review of the remaining material processed in the laboratory [60]. This suggests that the lesional tissue was sampled but not identified during ROSE; training in procurement and triage can improve the on-site yield in such instances. Additional reasons for discrepancy include scant cellularity, need for intradepartmental consultation or ancillary studies, intraobserver variability, and challenging diagnosis [49].

## ROSE: Lymph Node Assessment with Endobronchial Ultrasound

When sampling a lymph node for staging, it is important to determine if the sample is adequate or not, especially when it lacks metastatic tumor or granulomatous inflammation [29, 31]. In the absence of lesional cells, the presence or absence of lymphocytes and/or pigmented (anthracotic) macrophages to confirm localization of the needle within the target and assessment of the quantity of lymphocytes impacts the negative predictive value, which is reportedly variable [13].

Currently, there are no strict guidelines to determine adequacy of a negative lymph node sample [58], and evaluation of the amount of lymphocytes can be subjective [13]. For instance, a focally dense collection may be deemed adequate, but a similar number of lymphocytes scattered throughout the slide and diluted by blood and bronchial cells may be considered scant [13].

Criteria for objective evaluation have been proposed (Table 3.3) [29, 61, 62]. While some have suggested that a certain number of lymphocytes per high-power field and/or the presence of clusters of pigmented macrophages are good predictors of final adequacy assessment of a benign lymph node [29, 62], others report that the occurrence of moderate to abundant numbers of lymphocytes and/or pigmented macrophages is indicative of adequate lymph node sampling in most cases [31, 59]. One proposed system uses a scale (unsatisfactory=0 lymphocytes; less than optimal=<40 lymphocytes/high power field (HPF); satisfactory=>40 lymphocytes/HPF in most cellular areas) [61], and a high false-negative rate was associated with unsatisfactory and less than optimal lymphocytes, demonstrating that adequacy impacts the false-negative rate. Another semiquantitative scoring system for evaluating lymphocytes (0=<40 lymphocytes; 1=41–200 lymphocytes; 2 = >200 nonconfluent lymphocytes; 3=confluent sheets of lymphocytes or germinal centers; [29] true negatives had scores of 2 or 3) also confirmed that true negatives were associated with greater numbers of lymphocytes. These criteria require time to count lymphocytes, which can be cumbersome, can delay the procedure, and can

**Table 3.3** Proposed systems for evaluation of lymph nodes in the absence of pathology

| | | | | | |
|---|---|---|---|---|---|
| Karunamurthy et al. [61] | Unsatisfactory | Less than optimal | Satisfactory | Interpretation | |
| | Number of lymphocytes/high-power field (HPF) | | | | |
| | 0 | <40/HPF | ≥40/HPF | Higher false negativity in unsatisfactory and less than optimal cases. Fibrosis/hyalinization due to Hodgkin lymphoma or treatment related changes have lower cellular yield | |
| Alsharif et al. [29] | 0 | 1 | 2 | 3 | |
| | Number of lymphocytes | | | | |
| | <40 | 41–200 | >200 | Confluent sheets or germinal centers | True negatives have scores of 2 or 3 |
| Nayak et al. [62] | Inadequate | Adequate[a] | Adequate[a] | | |
| | Number of lymphocytes/low power field (LFP) (×100) | | | | |
| | Either "adequate" category is not satisfied | Germinal center fragments | >5 fields with > 100/LPF and <2 groups of bronchial cells/LPF | | If not adequate, re-aspirate lymph node or aspirate another lymph node |

[a]Satisfaction of either category is considered "adequate"

thus be a drawback. Also, presence of pigmented macrophages has to be interpreted with caution, as they can be derived inadvertently from non-lesional adjacent lung.

The presence of bronchial cells in transbronchial aspirations of lymph nodes has no bearing on adequacy. However, excess incidental ciliated bronchial cells, reactive bronchial cells lacking cilia, or dysplastic bronchial cells may pose difficult differential diagnostic problems; they may obscure the presence of scant malignant cells and/or mimic carcinoma [29, 58, 62]. Air-drying artifact and poor fixation/preservation may also cause difficulty with interpretation since atypical bronchial epithelium and reserve cell hyperplasia may be present as tight cohesive clusters with apparent nuclear molding and without apparent cilia, thus mimicking small cell carcinoma [29]. Performing IHC on cell block material may be helpful in such cases [29]. Additionally, presence of granulomas in a sampled lymph node does not necessarily exclude malignancy since they may coexist with metastatic carcinoma.

## ROSE: Touch Preparations of Core Biopsies

While ROSE is typically utilized for FNAs, touch preparations of core biopsies for on-site assessment of adequacy and preliminary diagnoses are also frequently employed. As with ROSE of FNAs, radiologists prefer ROSE on touch preparations of core biopsies to ensure adequate sampling of the lesion and triage of the specimen [14].

Performing on-site touch preparations of CT-guided core biopsies has been associated with greater diagnostic accuracy [63] and is comparable to that of frozen section diagnosis [64–66]. Touch preparations are sensitive (96 %) in detecting malignant thoracic lesions and predicting malignancy (98 % of cases) [67]. Diagnostic accuracies of touch preparations and core biopsies are both high (92.3–94 % and 93–94 %, respectively), but the combination of touch preparation with core biopsy improves the diagnostic accuracy to 96.4–98 % [67, 68]. Similarly, it has been observed in a study of touch preparations of thoracic lesions that the combined evaluation of touch preparations and core biopsies has a higher NPV (90 %) than that of touch preparations (83 %) or core biopsies (79 %) alone [67]. This stresses the value in a collective interpretation of both preparations.

The number of biopsies procured has been reported to be higher in patients with negative or inadequate touch preparation diagnoses compared to those with positive or suspicious touch preparation diagnoses (2.9 versus 3.7, respectively) [67]. These data suggest that positive touch preparations indicate a true positive, and no further biopsy attempts are necessary, but further biopsy or diagnostic evaluation should be considered if the touch preparation is negative. Negative results may represent true negatives, as is evident in cases of organizing pneumonia in which the fibroblastic tissue is not readily evident on touch preparations [69], or false negatives, stemming from suboptimal on-site specimen processing [70], sampling of adjacent normal tissue [67], scant cellularity, suboptimal needle position, surrounding or superimposed inflammation, severe necrosis, mucinous nature of the tumor, or coexisting tuberculosis [68].

There is debate about the role of touch preparations. There is concern of lesional cell transfer onto the touch preparation, leaving behind non-lesional tissue on the core biopsy [63]. This may deem a specimen adequate on-site but inadequate for ancillary studies. Assessment of a touch preparation differs from that of a FNA. The transfer (touch) onto a slide is unlike that of a smear of a FNA [14]. This may result in examination of fewer cells, cellular distortion, and air-drying artifact [14]. Clues to diagnosis, such as dyscohesion of cells associated with lymphocytes, may be muted on a touch preparation, and excessive manipulation of the core may cause crush artifact raising concern for possible small cell carcinoma. Care in processing can minimize these artifacts.

## Alternatives to ROSE

### *Telepathology/Telecytology*

Laboratories may find it challenging to provide ROSE due to high volume, insufficient staffing, time constraints, and distance issues. Telecytology (TC), a relatively recent means to view slides remotely in real time, addresses these issues while allowing the pathologist to be involved in the evaluation process. Telepathology (TP) has been shown to be a valuable tool for frozen section diagnosis with high diagnostic accuracy [71–74]. While TC still lags behind TP in validation and use [75], it has value in off-site assessment of multiple organs [36, 76–83] and lymph nodes sampled under EUS, EBUS, and CT guidance [36, 78, 82] without significant difference in agreement between TC and ROSE [83]. Concordance between TC and conventional ROSE has also been reported in adequacy assessment, assignment of preliminary diagnostic categories (non-diagnostic, benign, atypical, suspicious, malignant), correlation with final diagnoses [36, 77–81], and average number of passes performed [78]. Although sample size was small, one study showed an 89 % sensitivity of both ROSE and TC; however, ROSE showed a higher specificity compared to TC (93 % versus 87 %, respectively) [83].

There are three main available methods of image transmission for TC and TP including (1) static image capture, (2) dynamic live video (real time), and (3) whole slide image (WSI) [75, 84]. For both the static and dynamic systems, a team approach that involves a skilled on-site operator experienced in cytology is essential. Briefly, static image capture, consisting of a microscope with an attached digital camera and internet access for file transmission, offers low cost, wide applicability, and access. Limitations include selective and narrow scope of image review and inability to view on multifocal planes [75, 84]. With the dynamic system, comprising a microscope with an attached camera capable of generating video, the operator at the originating site controls the microscope, and the pathologist situated remotely views the slide passively [84]. Robotic systems are also available with capability of complete and unbiased slide review as well changes in magnification and focusing by the interpreting pathologist. WSI captures the entire slide content and permits slide review in a manner similar to that of a glass slide under a microscope [75, 84]. Disadvantages include increased time for entire slide scan and suboptimal depth of field views [75, 84].

TC has been shown to be a more effective use of a pathologist's time on the clinical service, with a reported average time of 30 min saved per procedure [78]. Although the actual time spent reviewing a case via TC versus conventional on-site assessment may be similar and not statistically significant [36, 78], the potential time saved in a given day for a pathologist working on a busy FNA service can be significantly reduced by eliminating time spent traveling to and from the procedure site and downtime either during prepping or in between passes. In a high-volume FNA service, the time saved for cytopathologists could potentially be measured in hours.

Loss of personal contact and communication between the cytopathologist and clinician/radiologist performing the FNA is a noteworthy concern. Although this issue is not addressed in much of the TC literature, one study noted that clinician satisfaction has not been negatively impacted by using TC over in-person assessment and that no issues related to TC have been identified by them [78]. Others specifically report that even with TC, interaction with the endoscopist is not sacrificed and that TC allows for mass communication/teaching beyond any distance and advances communication so that pathologists can reach out to more clinicians, thereby improving patient care [81].

TC also allows the cytopathologist to actively participate in making decisions about proper triage for ancillary studies [78], including IHC, flow cytometry, molecular testing, and cultures; however, successful triaging requires that the on-site operator, whether a cytotechnologist, cytology fellow, or pathology resident, be knowledgeable of various preservation media and technically skilled in the preparation of slides that allows for necessary material to be saved for such ancillary tests. Comparison of rates of adequate material for ancillary tests, specifically IHC and molecular testing for lung cancer, in FNAs with in-person ROSE versus TC ROSE has not yet been addressed and is an issue that is worth investigating.

## Tissue Preservation

Several fixatives and transport media are available for cytology specimens. For EGFR molecular testing, guidelines provided by the College of American Pathologists, the International Association for the Study of Lung Cancer, and the Association for Molecular Pathology recommend using formalin-fixed (10 % neutral buffered), alcohol-fixed (70 % ethanol), fresh, or frozen specimens following validation [11]. Cytology specimens initially placed in other solutions (i.e., saline, RPMI) can be transferred to formalin or CytoLyt subsequently. Fixation for 6 to 12 hours is recommended for small specimens [11].

## *Formalin*

As stated above and discussed in the following section on cell blocks, formalin-fixed paraffin-embedded (FFPE) tissue is currently recommended for ancillary tests such as IHC stains and molecular assays [2, 11, 85, 86]. Typically, formalin is the fixative in which IHC stains and most molecular assays are optimized and validated, and FFPE material has potential to yield multiple tissue sections that are suitable for these ancillary studies [38, 87–90].

## *Liquid-Based Preparations*

Liquid-based preparations (LBPs) offer a standardized alternative to conventional smear preparation and fixation for FNAs and exfoliative specimens, including respiratory specimens and effusions. The current FDA-approved liquid-based preparations (LBPs) in use are ThinPrep®/CytoLyt (Cytyc Corp, Marlborough, MA) and SurePath™ (Becton Dickinson) [91]. The specimen is placed in an alcohol-based solution (e.g., CytoLyt), which serves as a fixative and transport medium. An automated system in the laboratory creates slides, which are stained with Papanicolaou stain, with an even distribution of cells and without loss of cells. Additionally, the process and solution minimize contamination by blood, inflammation, and debris.

There are several additional advantages of LBPs (Table 3.4). They preserve cells at room temperature in the fixative solution for extended periods of time (3 weeks in CytoRich and 3 months in PreservCyt) [91]. CytoLyt solution appears to be superior to CytoRich Red in terms of the yield of suitable DNA [92]. Cell blocks for ancillary tests [55] can be prepared from the unused cells in solution. Even without cell blocks, ancillary tests, such as IHC [93–95] and molecular analysis [92, 96–100], can be performed on LBPs. In fact, the percentage of malignant cells on FNA specimens assessed on ThinPrep® has been found to be significantly high [101]. EGFR and KRAS mutation analyses have been successfully carried on lung carcinomas preserved in CytoLyt [96–98] and have shown comparable results between FNA samples and histological tissues [98]. Potential advantages of utilizing LBP for molecular techniques include (1) homogeneous cell distribution, which is helpful in determining percentage of malignant cells in a specimen dominated by benign or normal cells, and (2) preparation of multiple slides, which spares the original routinely stained slides/smears [92].

**Table 3.4** Utility of liquid-based preparation

| |
|---|
| Standardizes slide preparation |
| Simplifies fixation |
| Offers material for cell block ancillary tests |
| Preserves cells for extended periods |

The disadvantages to liquid-based preparations include additional costs of equipment and supplies. Since these specimens are fixed in alcohol rather than formalin, the typical preservative used for biopsies, a laboratory may need to conduct tests to validate the results of ancillary studies. Also, it precludes analysis by flow cytometry [91]. Due to automation, ROSE cannot be performed.

As this slide preparation technique is different from conventional smears, there is a learning curve for interpretation of liquid-based cytology. Features evident on LBP include disruption of architectural pattern, shrunken cell and nuclear size, loss of background material such as necrosis, and loss/reduction of extracellular elements such as mucus [91]. For the most part, LBPs allow for accurate diagnosis of lung cancer with most cytological features that are typically observed in direct smears being preserved, thus allowing accurate cell typing, especially when used in conjunction with CBs [91]. Two entities frequently encountered in pulmonary and mediastinal cytology specimens that pose diagnostic challenges are small cell carcinoma, which appears as dyshesive cells with subtle nuclear molding, and granulomas, which may also have disassociated cells.

## *Alternative Tissue Preservation Methods*

While formalin- and alcohol-based fixatives are recommended for procuring nucleic acid from tissue for molecular testing of NSCLC [11], other fixatives such as heavy metal fixatives (e.g., B5, acid zinc formalin, Zenker, B plus) and acidic solutions (e.g., decalcifying solution, Bouin) should be avoided [11] because they have an adverse effect on the quality of DNA obtained and interfere with subsequent molecular test results [102–104].

Recently, the use of Whatman FTA cards for storing cytological samples and for molecular testing was investigated [105]. These FTA cards are comprised of paper that is infused with reagents that lyse cells, thus liberating DNA that attaches to the matrix of the card and is left stable at room temperature [105]. Results of EGFR and KRAS mutational analyses conducted on NSCLC using this method are similar to those from cell blocks.

Using fresh cells obtained at the time of diagnosis ensures quality material for molecular analyses and may provide better than formalin-fixed tissue for such tests [106]; however, studies that have utilized fresh cells rely mainly on cryopreservation for storage of the material, which may be expensive and necessitate extra storage space [106].

## Cell Blocks

Cell blocks serve as an adjunct to smears and liquid-based preparations. They can be used for cytological diagnoses and ancillary testing, including in the evaluation of lung carcinoma, and be prepared from FNAs, bronchial washings, bronchial

**Table 3.5** Value of cell blocks

| |
|---|
| Provide formalin-fixed paraffin-embedded tissue for ancillary studies |
| Highlight architecture |
| Concentrate specimen |
| Allow long-term specimen preservation |

brushings received in liquid media, bronchoalveolar lavages, or effusions. They are advantageous for numerous reasons (Table 3.5). Most importantly they provide (1) increased diagnostic yield [35, 88, 89, 107–109]; (2) architectural detail on cell clusters and tissue fragments [38, 87–89] similar to histological specimens; (3) H&E stained slides, which are familiar to all pathologists [87]; (4) a concentration of diagnostic cells in a limited field for easier microscopic evaluation [88, 89]; (5) material in FFPE tissue that can yield multiple tissue sections suitable for these ancillary studies [38, 87–90]; (6) easy assimilation into existing validated methods for IHC stains and molecular testing [11, 110] that provide results similar to those obtained on paraffin-embedded histological sections [111]; and (7) a source of long-term specimen preservation for supply of archival DNA for future diagnostics/research [112] and retrospective studies [11, 12, 88].

Although alcohol and alcohol-based fixatives are comparable, if not better, than formalin for molecular assays requiring nucleic acid extraction, 10 % neutral buffered formalin is the fixative in which most molecular assays have been optimized [11], and use of other preparations deviates from standard protocols of histological tissue [113]. Ancillary studies can be performed on direct smears and liquid-based preparations, but cell blocks are preferred for several reasons. First, current expert consensus opinion communicated by the College of American Pathologists, the International Association for the Study of Lung Cancer, the Association for Molecular for Molecular Pathology, the American Thoracic Society, and the European Respiratory Society advocates using cell blocks for ancillary testing [2, 11, 85, 86]. Although IHC stains performed on direct smears or liquid-based specimens show results concordant with those obtained on histological sections [114] and using these preparations avoids having a patient undergo a second procedure, cell blocks are more suitable due to minimal background/aberrant staining [86], consistency in classic staining patterns [115], no need for additional validation studies, and lack of large sheets or clusters sometimes seen in smears, which may not provide material feasible for IHC stains [38]. Especially in instances of limited or scantily cellular slides, the use of smears and liquid-based preparations may result in the use of diagnostic material, which can have subsequent medicolegal implications [113]. Cell block sections also allow for correlation between morphological features and immunostaining expression, a valuable feature particularly in cases of scant isolated cells and well-differentiated lung adenocarcinoma, which may show overlapping cytomorphological features with adjacent reactive pneumocytes [38].

Moreover, cell blocks play a valuable role in molecular diagnostics. The results of EGFR and KRAS molecular testing performed on cell blocks of FNAs are reported to be 100 % concordant with their histological counterparts [23]. Cell blocks allow for assessment of the tumor volume and percentage to determine if the sample is adequate for molecular testing [11, 110]. Determining the ratio of tumor to total cellularity may be difficult with a liquid-based preparation, such as ThinPrep®, and has the potential to lead to interpretive errors when the ratio is low. For cytological samples of lung carcinoma, cell blocks are preferred over smears for EGFR and ALK testing [11].

A cell block consists of a cohesive tissue pellet formed from dyshesive cells, small tissue fragments, and intermixed blood or fixative/preservative comprising a cytology specimen. The pellet is formed by centrifuging the specimen, removing the liquid supernatant, and collecting the concentrated pellet. If the pellet is not well formed, one of several agents (agar, plasma thrombin, gelatin) [13] or methods is used to congeal and/or collect the specimen [116]. Following this step, the tissue is embedded in paraffin and processed like a biopsy. This process requires technical expertise and can be challenging.

Currently, there is no standardized means to process cell blocks, and there are greater than 10 different methods in use [117]. A survey demonstrated that approximately 40 % of respondents are either unsatisfied or only sometimes satisfied with the quality of their cell blocks with scant cellularity being the leading underlying reason [117]. Valid comparison of the efficacy of various methods is difficult due to the lack of uniform methodology and vast differences in technical detail [87] even within a single method.

Two of the most common methods use plasma thrombin and HistoGel to collate the specimen. Greater cellularity is reported with plasma thrombin blocks, but cellular preservation and architecture scored higher with HistoGel-prepared blocks [116, 118, 119]. For scant specimens, the collodion bag technique has been suggested as a high cellular yield method for preparation of cell blocks [87, 118]. Also, an automated cell block preparing system, Cellient (Hologic), is available. Cellient demonstrates 50 [120]–80 % [121] concordance with immunostains performed on paraffin-embedded and formalin-fixed tissue and yields high-quality DNA [121]. Drawbacks include purchase of the system and consumables.

Another method for cell block preparation from FNAs involves placing excess material onto a glass slide, allowing it to clot for a few minutes, and placing it directly into 10 % formalin for processing in order to preserve and process the material in a manner similar to histological specimens. With this method, suction to create a bloody aspirate may be helpful since blood serves as a clotting agent to form a cell block without addition of other substances. This should follow after a diagnosis has been established on a non-bloody pass. An alternative method, the so-called tissue coagulum clot method [90], is similar but involves placing the material onto filter paper and once the coagulum is completely congealed, wrapping the filter paper and submitting in a formalin container for further processing. This method is reported to show higher diagnostic rates compared to rinsing the aspirate needle in saline for subsequent centrifugation and cell block preparation [90].

## References

1. Siegel R, Naishadham D, Jemal A. Cancer statistics, 2013. CA Cancer J Clin. 2013;63: 11–30.
2. Travis WD, Brambilla E, Noguchi M, et al. International association for the study of lung cancer/american thoracic society/european respiratory society international multidisciplinary classification of lung adenocarcinoma. J Thorac Oncol. 2011;6:244–85.
3. Travis WD, Rekhtman N, Riley GJ, et al. Pathologic diagnosis of advanced lung cancer based on small biopsies and cytology: a paradigm shift. J Thorac Oncol. 2010;5:411–4.
4. Ciuleanu T, Brodowicz T, Zielinski C, et al. Maintenance pemetrexed plus best supportive care versus placebo plus best supportive care for non-small-cell lung cancer: a randomised, double-blind, phase 3 study. Lancet. 2009;374:1432–40.
5. Johnson DH, Fehrenbacher L, Novotny WF, et al. Randomized phase II trial comparing bevacizumab plus carboplatin and paclitaxel with carboplatin and paclitaxel alone in previously untreated locally advanced or metastatic non-small-cell lung cancer. J Clin Oncol. 2004;22:2184–91.
6. Mok TS, Wu YL, Thongprasert S, et al. Gefitinib or carboplatin-paclitaxel in pulmonary adenocarcinoma. N Engl J Med. 2009;361:947–57.
7. Scagliotti G, Hanna N, Fossella F, et al. The differential efficacy of pemetrexed according to NSCLC histology: a review of two Phase III studies. Oncologist. 2009;14:253–63.
8. Scagliotti GV, Parikh P, von Pawel J, et al. Phase III study comparing cisplatin plus gemcitabine with cisplatin plus pemetrexed in chemotherapy-naive patients with advanced-stage non-small-cell lung cancer. J Clin Oncol. 2008;26:3543–51.
9. Chen Z, Akbay EA. Mikse OR, et al. Clin Cancer Res: Co-clinical trials demonstrate superiority of crizotinib to chemotherapy in ALK-rearranged non-small cell lung cancer and predict strategies to overcome resistance; 2013.
10. Rivera MP, Mehta AC. Initial diagnosis of lung cancer: ACCP evidence-based clinical practice guidelines (2nd edition). Chest. 2007;132:131S–48.
11. Lindeman NI, Cagle PT, Beasley MB, et al. Molecular testing guideline for selection of lung cancer patients for EGFR and ALK tyrosine kinase inhibitors: guideline from the College of American Pathologists, International Association for the Study of Lung Cancer, and Association for Molecular Pathology. Arch Pathol Lab Med. 2013;137:828–60.
12. Bulman W, Saqi A, Powell CA. Acquisition and processing of endobronchial ultrasound-guided transbronchial needle aspiration specimens in the era of targeted lung cancer chemotherapy. Am J Respir Crit Care Med. 2012;185:606–11.
13. Yasufuku K, Fleury FJ. Cytological specimens obtained by endobronchial ultrasound-guided transbronchial needle aspiration: sample handling and role of rapid on-site evaluation. Ann Pathol. 2012;32(e35–46):421–32.
14. Cobb CJ. FNA or core needle biopsy? Why not both? CAP Today. Northfield, IL: Bob McGonnagle; 2007.
15. Todd TR, Weisbrod G, Tao LC, et al. Aspiration needle biopsy of thoracic lesions. Ann Thorac Surg. 1981;32:154–61.
16. Sagel SS, Ferguson TB, Forrest JV, Roper CL, Weldon CS, Clark RE. Percutaneous transthoracic aspiration needle biopsy. Ann Thorac Surg. 1978;26:399–405.
17. Jackson R, Coffin LH, DeMeules JE, Miller DB, Dietrich P, Fairbank J. Percutaneous needle biopsy of pulmonary lesions. Am J Surg. 1980;139:586–90.
18. Vazquez MF, Koizumi JH, Henschke CI, Yankelevitz DF. Reliability of cytologic diagnosis of early lung cancer. Cancer. 2007;111:252–8.
19. Rekhtman N, Brandt SM, Sigel CS, et al. Suitability of thoracic cytology for new therapeutic paradigms in non-small cell lung carcinoma: high accuracy of tumor subtyping and feasibility of EGFR and KRAS molecular testing. J Thorac Oncol. 2011;6:451–8.
20. Sigel CS, Moreira AL, Travis WD, et al. Subtyping of non-small cell lung carcinoma: a comparison of small biopsy and cytology specimens. J Thorac Oncol. 2011;6:1849–56.

21. Billah S, Stewart J, Staerkel G, Chen S, Gong Y, Guo M. EGFR and KRAS mutations in lung carcinoma: molecular testing by using cytology specimens. Cancer Cytopathol. 2011;119:111–7.
22. Coley SM, Crapanzano JP, Saqi A. Optimizing lung carcinoma diagnosis: FNA, core, or both. United States and Canadian Academy of Pathology 101st Annual Meeting. Vancouver, BC, Canada: Mod Pathol, 2012:475A.
23. Heymann JJ, Bulman WA, Maxfield RA, Powell CA, Halmos B, Sonett J, Beaubier NT, Crapanzano JP, Mansukhani MM, Saqi A. Molecular testing guidelines for lung adenocarcinoma: utility of cell blocks and concordance between fine needle aspiration cytology and histology samples. CytoJournal. 2014;11:12.
24. Fischer AH, Cibas ES, Howell LP, et al. Role of cytology in the management of non-small-cell lung cancer. J Clin Oncol. 2011;29:3331–2. author reply 3332–3333.
25. Griffin AC, Schwartz LE, Baloch ZW. Utility of on-site evaluation of endobronchial ultrasound-guided transbronchial needle aspiration specimens. CytoJournal. 2011;8:20.
26. Travis WD, Brambilla E, Noguchi M, et al. Diagnosis of lung cancer in small biopsies and cytology: implications of the 2011 International Association for the Study of Lung Cancer/American Thoracic Society/European Respiratory Society classification. Arch Pathol Lab Med. 2013;137:668–84.
27. Nasuti JF, Gupta PK, Baloch ZW. Diagnostic value and cost-effectiveness of on-site evaluation of fine-needle aspiration specimens: review of 5,688 cases. Diagn Cytopathol. 2002;27:1–4.
28. Nakajima T, Yasufuku K. How I do it–optimal methodology for multidirectional analysis of endobronchial ultrasound-guided transbronchial needle aspiration samples. J Thorac Oncol. 2011;6:203–6.
29. Alsharif M, Andrade RS, Groth SS, Stelow EB, Pambuccian SE. Endobronchial ultrasound-guided transbronchial fine-needle aspiration: the University of Minnesota experience, with emphasis on usefulness, adequacy assessment, and diagnostic difficulties. Am J Clin Pathol. 2008;130:434–43.
30. Khazai L, Kundu UR, Jacob B, et al. Endobronchial ultrasound-guided transbronchial needle aspiration biopsy is useful evaluating mediastinal lymphadenopathy in a cancer center. CytoJournal. 2011;8:10.
31. Feller-Kopman D, Yung RC, Burroughs F, Li QK. Cytology of endobronchial ultrasound-guided transbronchial needle aspiration: a retrospective study with histology correlation. Cancer. 2009;117:482–90.
32. Austin JH, Cohen MB. Value of having a cytopathologist present during percutaneous fine-needle aspiration biopsy of lung: report of 55 cancer patients and metaanalysis of the literature. AJR Am J Roentgenol. 1993;160:175–7.
33. Campisi P, Accinelli G, De Angelis C, Pacchioni D. Bussolati G [On-site evaluation and triage for endoscopic ultrasound-guided fine needle aspiration cytology. The Turin experience]. Minerva Med. 2007;98:395–400.
34. Davenport RD. Rapid on-site evaluation of transbronchial aspirates. Chest. 1990;98:59–61.
35. Esterbrook G, Anathhanam S, Plant PK. Adequacy of endobronchial ultrasound transbronchial needle aspiration samples in the subtyping of non-small cell lung cancer. Lung Cancer. 2013;80:30–4.
36. Khurana KK, Kovalovsky A, Wang D, Lenox R. Feasibility of dynamic telecytopathology for rapid on-site evaluation of endobronchial ultrasound-guided transbronchial fine needle aspiration. Telemed J E Health. 2013;19:265–71.
37. Klapman JB, Logrono R, Dye CE, Waxman I. Clinical impact of on-site cytopathology interpretation on endoscopic ultrasound-guided fine needle aspiration. Am J Gastroenterol. 2003;98:1289–94.
38. Loukeris K, Vazquez MF, Sica G, et al. Cytological cell blocks: Predictors of squamous cell carcinoma and adenocarcinoma subtypes. Diagn Cytopathol. 2012;40:380–7.
39. Tournoy KG, Praet MM, Van Maele G, Van Meerbeeck JP. Esophageal endoscopic ultrasound with fine-needle aspiration with an on-site cytopathologist: high accuracy for the diagnosis of mediastinal lymphadenopathy. Chest. 2005;128:3004–9.

40. Jhala NC, Jhala DN, Chhieng DC, Eloubeidi MA, Eltoum IA. Endoscopic ultrasound-guided fine-needle aspiration. A cytopathologist's perspective Am J Clin Pathol. 2003;120:351–67.
41. Plit ML, Havryk AP, Hodgson A, et al. Rapid cytological analysis of endobronchial ultrasound-guided aspirates in sarcoidosis. Eur Respir J. 2013;42(5):1302–8.
42. Fassina A, Corradin M, Zardo D, Cappellesso R, Corbetti F, Fassan M. Role and accuracy of rapid on-site evaluation of CT-guided fine needle aspiration cytology of lung nodules. Cytopathology. 2011;22:306–12.
43. Woon C, Bardales RH, Stanley MW, Stelow EB. Rapid assessment of fine needle aspiration and the final diagnosis–how often and why the diagnoses are changed. CytoJournal. 2006;3:25.
44. Nakajima T, Yasufuku K, Saegusa F, et al. Rapid on-site cytologic evaluation during endobronchial ultrasound-guided transbronchial needle aspiration for nodal staging in patients with lung cancer. Ann Thorac Surg. 2013;95:1695–9.
45. Cha I, Goates JJ. Fine-needle aspiration of lymph nodes: use of flow cytometry immunophenotyping. Pathology (Phila). 1996;4:337–64.
46. Ducatman BS, Hogan CL, Wang HH. A triage system for processing fine needle aspiration cytology specimens. Acta Cytol. 1989;33:797–9.
47. Dunphy CH, Ramos R. Combining fine-needle aspiration and flow cytometric immunophenotyping in evaluation of nodal and extranodal sites for possible lymphoma: a retrospective review. Diagn Cytopathol. 1997;16:200–6.
48. Nasuti JF, Yu G, Boudousquie A, Gupta P. Diagnostic value of lymph node fine needle aspiration cytology: an institutional experience of 387 cases observed over a 5-year period. Cytopathology. 2000;11:18–31.
49. Eloubeidi MA, Tamhane A, Jhala N, et al. Agreement between rapid onsite and final cytologic interpretations of EUS-guided FNA specimens: implications for the endosonographer and patient management. Am J Gastroenterol. 2006;101:2841–7.
50. Oki M, Saka H, Kitagawa C, et al. Rapid on-site cytologic evaluation during endobronchial ultrasound-guided transbronchial needle aspiration for diagnosing lung cancer: a randomized study. Respiration. 2013;85:486–92.
51. Schmidt RL, Kordy MA, Howard K, Layfield LJ, Hall BJ, Adler DG. Risk-benefit analysis of sampling methods for fine-needle aspiration cytology: a mathematical modeling approach. Am J Clin Pathol. 2013;139:336–44.
52. Trisolini R, Cancellieri A, Tinelli C, et al. Rapid on-site evaluation of transbronchial aspirates in the diagnosis of hilar and mediastinal adenopathy: a randomized trial. Chest. 2011;139: 395–401.
53. Layfield LJ, Bentz JS, Gopez EV. Immediate on-site interpretation of fine-needle aspiration smears: a cost and compensation analysis. Cancer. 2001;93:319–22.
54. O'Malley ME, Weir MM, Hahn PF, Misdraji J, Wood BJ, Mueller PR. US-guided fine-needle aspiration biopsy of thyroid nodules: adequacy of cytologic material and procedure time with and without immediate cytologic analysis. Radiology. 2002;222:383–7.
55. Wallace WA, Monaghan HM, Salter DM, Gibbons MA, Skwarski KM. Endobronchial ultrasound-guided fine-needle aspiration and liquid-based thin-layer cytology. J Clin Pathol. 2007;60:388–91.
56. Diacon AH, Schuurmans MM, Theron J, et al. Utility of rapid on-site evaluation of transbronchial needle aspirates. Respiration. 2005;72:182–8.
57. Baram D, Garcia RB, Richman PS. Impact of rapid on-site cytologic evaluation during transbronchial needle aspiration. Chest. 2005;128:869–75.
58. Monaco SE, Schuchert MJ, Khalbuss WE. Diagnostic difficulties and pitfalls in rapid on-site evaluation of endobronchial ultrasound guided fine needle aspiration. CytoJournal. 2010;7:9.
59. Natu S, Hoffman J, Siddiqui M, Hobday C, Shrimankar J, Harrison R. The role of endobronchial ultrasound guided transbronchial needle aspiration cytology in the investigation of mediastinal lymphadenopathy and masses, the North Tees experience. J Clin Pathol. 2010;63:445–51.
60. Joseph M, Jones T, Lutterbie Y, et al. Rapid on-site pathologic evaluation does not increase the efficacy of endobronchial ultrasonographic biopsy for mediastinal staging. Ann Thorac Surg. 2013;96:403–10.

61. Karunamurthy A, Cai G, Dacic S, Khalbuss WE, Pantanowitz L, Monaco SE. Evaluation of endobronchial ultrasound-guided fine-needle aspirations (EBUS-FNA): correlation with adequacy and histologic follow-up. Cancer Cytopathol. 2014;122(1):23–32.
62. Nayak A, Sugrue C, Koenig S, Wasserman PG, Hoda S, Morgenstern NJ. Endobronchial ultrasound-guided transbronchial needle aspirate (EBUS-TBNA): a proposal for on-site adequacy criteria. Diagn Cytopathol. 2012;40:128–37.
63. Tsou MH, Tsai SF, Chan KY, et al. CT-guided needle biopsy: value of on-site cytopathologic evaluation of core specimen touch preparations. J Vasc Interv Radiol. 2009;20:71–6.
64. Guarda LA. Intraoperative cytologic diagnosis: evaluation of 370 consecutive intraoperative cytologies. Diagn Cytopathol. 1990;6:235–42.
65. Khalid A, Ul HA. Touch impression cytology versus frozen section as intraoperative consultation diagnosis. Int J Pathol. 2004;2:63–70.
66. Mair S, Lash RH, Suskin D, Mendelsohn G. Intraoperative surgical specimen evaluation: frozen section analysis, cytologic examination, or both? A comparative study of 206 cases. Am J Clin Pathol. 1991;96:8–14.
67. Liao WY, Jerng JS, Chen KY, Chang YL, Yang PC, Kuo SH. Value of imprint cytology for ultrasound-guided transthoracic core biopsy. Eur Respir J. 2004;24:905–9.
68. Chang YC, Yu CJ, Lee WJ, et al. Imprint cytology improves accuracy of computed tomography-guided percutaneous transthoracic needle biopsy. Eur Respir J. 2008;31:54–61.
69. Saqi A, Coley SM, Crapanzano JP. Granulomatous inflammation and organizing pneumonia: Role of computed tomography-guided lung fine needle aspirations, touch preparations and core biopsies in the evaluation of common non-neoplastic diagnoses. CytoJournal. 2014;11.
70. Krishnan K, Dalal S, Nayar R, Keswani RN, Keefer L, Komanduri S. Rapid on-site evaluation of endoscopic ultrasound core biopsy specimens has excellent specificity and positive predictive value for gastrointestinal lesions. Dig Dis Sci. 2013;58:2007–12.
71. Baak JP, van Diest PJ, Meijer GA. Experience with a dynamic inexpensive video-conferencing system for frozen section telepathology. Anal Cell Pathol. 2000;21:169–75.
72. Evans AJ, Chetty R, Clarke BA, et al. Primary frozen section diagnosis by robotic microscopy and virtual slide telepathology: the University Health Network experience. Hum Pathol. 2009;40:1070–81.
73. Frierson Jr HF, Galgano MT. Frozen-section diagnosis by wireless telepathology and ultra portable computer: use in pathology resident/faculty consultation. Hum Pathol. 2007;38:1330–4.
74. Liang WY, Hsu CY, Lai CR, Ho DM, Chiang IJ. Low-cost telepathology system for intraoperative frozen-section consultation: our experience and review of the literature. Hum Pathol. 2008;39:56–62.
75. Khurana KK. Telecytology and its evolving role in cytopathology. Diagn Cytopathol. 2012;40:498–502.
76. Wotruba AL, Stewart 3rd J, Scheberl T, Selvaggi SM. Added value, decreased cost: the evolving role of the cytotechnologist for preliminary screening and triage of thyroid aspirates. Diagn Cytopathol. 2011;39:896–9.
77. Alsharif M, Carlo-Demovich J, Massey C, et al. Telecytopathology for immediate evaluation of fine-needle aspiration specimens. Cancer Cytopathol. 2010;118:119–26.
78. Heimann A, Maini G, Hwang S, Shroyer KR, Singh M. Use of telecytology for the immediate assessment of CT guided and endoscopic FNA cytology: diagnostic accuracy, advantages, and pitfalls. Diagn Cytopathol. 2012;40:575–81.
79. Kerr SE, Bellizzi AM, Stelow EB, Frierson Jr HF, Policarpio-Nicolas ML. Initial assessment of fine-needle aspiration specimens by telepathology: validation for use in pathology resident-faculty consultations. Am J Clin Pathol. 2008;130:409–13.
80. Khurana KK, Kovalovsky A, Masrani D. Feasibility of telecytopathology for rapid preliminary diagnosis of ultrasound-guided fine needle aspiration of axillary lymph nodes in a remote breast care center. J Pathol Inform. 2012;3:36.
81. Kim B, Chhieng DC, Crowe DR, et al. Dynamic telecytopathology of on site rapid cytology diagnoses for pancreatic carcinoma. CytoJournal. 2006;3:27.
82. Marotti JD, Johncox V, Ng D, Gonzalez JL, Padmanabhan V. Implementation of telecytology for immediate assessment of endoscopic ultrasound-guided fine-needle aspirations compared

to conventional on-site evaluation: analysis of 240 consecutive cases. Acta Cytol. 2012;56:548–53.
83. Buxbaum JL, Eloubeidi MA, Lane CJ, et al. Dynamic telecytology compares favorably to rapid onsite evaluation of endoscopic ultrasound fine needle aspirates. Dig Dis Sci. 2012;57:3092–7.
84. Collins BT. Telepathology in cytopathology: challenges and opportunities. Acta Cytol. 2013;57:221–32.
85. Cagle PT, Allen TC, Dacic S, et al. Revolution in lung cancer: new challenges for the surgical pathologist. Arch Pathol Lab Med. 2011;135:110–6.
86. Khan S, Omar T, Michelow P. Effectiveness of the cell block technique in diagnostic cytopathology. J Cytol. 2012;29:177–82.
87. Kalhor N, Wistuba II. Perfecting the fine-needle aspirate cell block. Cancer Cytopathol. 2013;121:109–10.
88. Shivakumarswamy U, Arakeri SU, Karigowdar MH, Yelikar B. Diagnostic utility of the cell block method versus the conventional smear study in pleural fluid cytology. J Cytol. 2012;29:11–5.
89. Thapar M, Mishra RK, Sharma A, Goyal V, Goyal V. Critical analysis of cell block versus smear examination in effusions. J Cytol. 2009;26:60–4.
90. Yung RC, Otell S, Illei P, et al. Improvement of cellularity on cell block preparations using the so-called tissue coagulum clot method during endobronchial ultrasound-guided transbronchial fine-needle aspiration. Cancer Cytopathol. 2012;120:185–95.
91. Hoda RS. Non-gynecologic cytology on liquid-based preparations: A morphologic review of facts and artifacts. Diagn Cytopathol. 2007;35:621–34.
92. Dejmek A, Zendehrokh N, Tomaszewska M, Edsjo A. Preparation of DNA from cytological material: effects of fixation, staining, and mounting medium on DNA yield and quality. Cancer Cytopathol. 2013;121:344–53.
93. Fadda G, Rossi ED, Mule A, Miraglia A, Vecchio FM, Capelli A. Diagnostic efficacy of immunocytochemistry on fine needle aspiration biopsies processed by thin-layer cytology. Acta Cytol. 2006;50:129–35.
94. Malle D, Valeri RM, Pazaitou-Panajiotou K, Kiziridou A, Vainas I, Destouni C. Use of a thin-layer technique in thyroid fine needle aspiration. Acta Cytol. 2006;50:23–7.
95. Dabbs DJ, Abendroth CS, Grenko RT, Wang X, Radcliffe GE. Immunocytochemistry on the Thinprep processor. Diagn Cytopathol. 1997;17:388–92.
96. Malapelle U, de Rosa N, Bellevicine C, et al. EGFR mutations detection on liquid-based cytology: is microscopy still necessary? J Clin Pathol. 2012;65:561–4.
97. Malapelle U, de Rosa N, Rocco D, et al. EGFR and KRAS mutations detection on lung cancer liquid-based cytology: a pilot study. J Clin Pathol. 2012;65:87–91.
98. Petriella D, Galetta D, Rubini V, et al. Molecular profiling of thin-prep FNA samples in assisting clinical management of non-small-cell lung cancer. Mol Biotechnol. 2013;54:913–9.
99. Pollett A, Bedard YC, Li SQ, Rohan T, Kandel R. Correlation of p53 mutations in ThinPrep-processed fine needle breast aspirates with surgically resected breast cancers. Mod Pathol. 2000;13:1173–9.
100. Tisserand P, Fouquet C, Marck V, et al. ThinPrep-processed fine-needle samples of breast are effective material for RNA- and DNA-based molecular diagnosis: application to p53 mutation analysis. Cancer. 2003;99:223–32.
101. Ernst LM, Rimm DL. Quantitative examination of mechanophysical tumor cell enrichment in fine-needle aspiration specimens. Cancer. 2002;96:275–9.
102. Baloglu G, Haholu A, Kucukodaci Z, Yilmaz I, Yildirim S, Baloglu H. The effects of tissue fixation alternatives on DNA content: a study on normal colon tissue. Appl Immunohistochem Mol Morphol. 2008;16:485–92.
103. Guillou L, Coindre J, Gallagher G, et al. Detection of the synovial sarcoma translocation t(X;18) (SYT;SSX) in paraffin-embedded tissues using reverse transcriptase-polymerase chain reaction: a reliable and powerful diagnostic tool for pathologists. A molecular analysis of 221 mesenchymal tumors fixed in different fixatives. Hum Pathol. 2001;32:105–12.

104. Moreira AL, Thornton RH. Personalized medicine for non-small-cell lung cancer: implications of recent advances in tissue acquisition for molecular and histologic testing. Clin Lung Cancer. 2012;13:334–9.
105. da Cunha SG, Liu N, Tsao MS, Kamel-Reid S, Chin K, Geddie WR. Detection of EGFR and KRAS mutations in fine-needle aspirates stored on Whatman FTA cards: is this the tool for biobanking cytological samples in the molecular era? Cancer Cytopathol. 2010;118:450–6.
106. da Cunha SG, Saieg MA, Geddie W, Leighl N. EGFR gene status in cytological samples of nonsmall cell lung carcinoma: controversies and opportunities. Cancer Cytopathol. 2011;119:80–91.
107. Sanz-Santos J, Serra P, Andreo F, Llatjos M, Castella E, Monso E. Contribution of cell blocks obtained through endobronchial ultrasound-guided transbronchial needle aspiration to the diagnosis of lung cancer. BMC Cancer. 2012;12:34.
108. Collins GR, Thomas J, Joshi N, Zhang S. The diagnostic value of cell block as an adjunct to liquid-based cytology of bronchial washing specimens in the diagnosis and subclassification of pulmonary neoplasms. Cancer Cytopathol. 2012;120:134–41.
109. Dekker A, Bupp PA. Cytology of serous effusions. An investigation into the usefulness of cell blocks versus smears Am J Clin Pathol. 1978;70:855–60.
110. Dumur CI, Idowu MO, Powers CN. Targeting tyrosine kinases in cancer: the converging roles of cytopathology and molecular pathology in the era of genomic medicine. Cancer Cytopathol. 2013;121:61–71.
111. Shidham VB, Lindholm PF, Kajdacsy-Balla A, Chang CC, Komorowski R. Methods of cytologic smear preparation and fixation. Effect on the immunoreactivity of commonly used anticytokeratin antibody AE1/AE3. Acta Cytol. 2000;44:1015–22.
112. Caraway NP. Strategies to diagnose lymphoproliferative disorders by fine-needle aspiration by using ancillary studies. Cancer. 2005;105:432–42.
113. Jurado J, Saqi A. Maxfield R, et al. Ann Thorac Surg: The Efficacy of Endobronchial Ultrasound-Guided Transbronchial Needle Aspiration for Molecular Testing in Lung Adenocarcinoma; 2013.
114. Kalhor N, Zander DS, Liu J. TTF-1 and p63 for distinguishing pulmonary small-cell carcinoma from poorly differentiated squamous cell carcinoma in previously pap-stained cytologic material. Mod Pathol. 2006;19:1117–23.
115. Fetsch PA, Simsir A, Brosky K, Abati A. Comparison of three commonly used cytologic preparations in effusion immunocytochemistry. Diagn Cytopathol. 2002;26:61–6.
116. Benkovich VC, Khalbuss W, Pantanowitz L, Palekar A, Monaco S. Comparison of cell block preparation using HistoGel and Plasma Thrombin techniques. Journal of the American Society of Cytopathology. 2012;1:S114–5.
117. Crapanzano JP, Heymann JJ, Monaco S, Nassar A, Saqi A. The state of cell block variation and satisfaction in the era of molecular diagnostics and personalized medicine. CytoJournal. 2014;11:7.
118. Balassanian R, Ono JC, Wool GD, Olejnik-Nave J, Mah MM, Sweeney BJ, Ljung BM, Pitman MB. A superior technique for cell block preparation for fine needle aspiration. Mod Pathol. 2013;26:83A.
119. Nigro K, Tynski Z, Wasman J, Abdul-Karim F, Wang N. Comparison of cell block preparation methods for nongynecologic ThinPrep specimens. Diagn Cytopathol. 2007;35:640–3.
120. Wagner DG, Russell DK, Benson JM, Schneider AE, Hoda RS, Bonfiglio TA. Cellient automated cell block versus traditional cell block preparation: a comparison of morphologic features and immunohistochemical staining. Diagn Cytopathol. 2011;39:730–6.
121. van Hemel BM, Suurmeijer AJ. Effective application of the methanol-based PreservCyt() fixative and the Cellient() automated cell block processor to diagnostic cytopathology, immunocytochemistry, and molecular biology. Diagn Cytopathol. 2013;41:734–41.

# Chapter 4
# Optimization and Triage of Small Specimens

**Anjali Saqi and John P. Crapanzano**

## Introduction

Lung cancer is the leading cause of cancer-related deaths worldwide [1]. Significant advances in identifying the underlying mechanisms, detecting mutations, and developing treatments have been made, however. Previously, distinguishing small cell carcinomas from non-small cell lung cancers (NSCLCs) was sufficient, and the latter were managed based on stage. More recently, it has been recognized that the histologic subtype of NSCLC is important in the selection of therapy, which affects both efficacy and safety [2]. Also, a subset of patients with key driver mutations benefit from targeted treatments. Following these observations, there has been a shift to subclassify NSCLCs and test for driver mutations in lung adenocarcinomas.

Significant focus has centered on small specimens—biopsies and cytology [3]. This is largely because greater numbers of small specimens are being procured with minimally invasive procedures with image guidance, including with computed tomography (CT), endobronchial ultrasound (EBUS), endoscopic ultrasound (EUS), and electromagnetic navigational bronchoscopy. Especially for patients who present at advanced stages, are poor surgical candidates, have nonsurgical diseases (lymphoma, granuloma) [4], are undergoing restaging, and/or develop fibrosis following prior surgery [4], small specimens often represent the only tissue amenable or attainable.

A. Saqi, M.D., M.B.A. (✉)
Department of Pathology and Cell Biology,
Columbia University Medical Center, New York-Presbyterian Hospital,
630 West 168th Street, VC14-215, New York, NY 10032, USA
e-mail: aas177@cumc.columbia.edu

J.P. Crapanzano, M.D.
Department of Pathology and Cell Biology,
Columbia University Medical Center, New York-Presbyterian Hospital,
New York, NY, USA



A.L. Moreira, A. Saqi (eds.), *Diagnosing Non-small Cell Carcinoma in Small Biopsy and Cytology*, DOI 10.1007/978-1-4939-1607-8_4

Therefore, it is of utmost importance to triage the tissue appropriately. A poorly managed specimen may deter an accurate diagnosis and lack sufficient material for ancillary studies to determine treatment.

Currently, there is a gap in practice, as there are limited data available for the management of small specimens [5, 6]. In the past, not much significance was placed on triaging small biopsy or cytology. With a shift in treatment based upon the histology and molecular profile of NSCLCs, triaging small biopsy and cytology, which comprise the vast majority or only diagnostic tissue, has become critical. Sufficient tissue for ancillary studies, including immunohistochemical (IHC) stains and/or molecular tests, is necessary. This is challenging because the size of the tissue obtained by minimally invasive procedures is much smaller than that attained by traditional methods, such as mediastinoscopy, video-assisted thoracoscopic surgery, and thoracotomy, yet the information required has increased substantially.

Surgical biopsies are typically placed in formalin at the time of acquisition and processed in the laboratory; there is little variability, and formalin fixation and hematoxylin and eosin (H&E) stain are standard. The same does not hold true for cytology specimens, especially fine needle aspirations (FNAs), however. FNAs are prepared and fixed in one or more of several ways—both following the procedure and in the laboratory. There are various stains [Diff-Quik, Papanicolaou, H&E, and ultrafast Papanicolaou], slide preparations [smear, cytospin, ThinPrep® (Cytyc Corp, Boxborough, MA), and SurePath™ (Becton Dickinson)], cell block processing methods (>10 homebrew and automated) [7], and fixatives/preservatives [saline, alcohol-based, formalin, Roswell Park Memorial Institute (RPMI) culture media, Hanks, and CytoRich (Becton Dickinson)]. In addition, there is no uniform protocol for triaging specimens. All of these factors result in inconsistent results across laboratories.

To obtain optimal results, a standardized protocol needs to be implemented in the laboratory. For FNAs, it is important to triage at the time of the procedure. Ideally, this involves immediate assessment to confirm specimen adequacy, which entails not only establishing the presence of diagnostic material but also ensuring that it is sufficient for ancillary studies when necessary.

This chapter outlines techniques to optimally triage and prepare small specimens, including biopsies and FNAs, for diagnosis and ancillary studies.

## Algorithm: FNA with Rapid On-Site Evaluation (ROSE)

There is no standardized algorithm for processing FNA specimens, and few methods have been outlined [5, 8]. With a combination of the following algorithm and ROSE [5], sufficient cytological material for molecular testing was successfully attained in >90 % of cases reflexively tested lung adenocarcinomas [9].

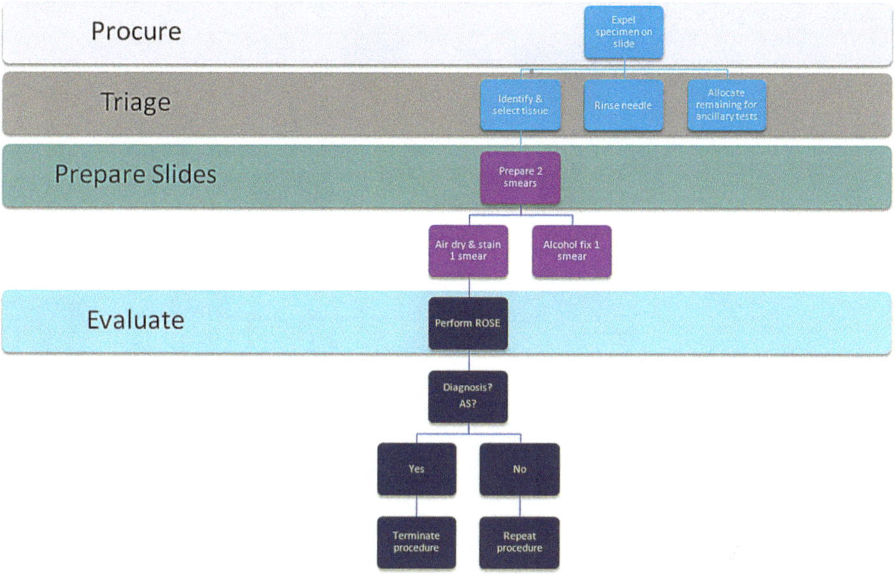


**Fig. 4.1** Algorithm for procuring fine needle aspirations with rapid on-site evaluation (ROSE): The algorithm for optimizing FNAs with ROSE is divided into 3 main categories: (1) specimen procurement and triage, (2) slide preparation, and (3) tissue evaluation for diagnoses and assessment of adequacy for ancillary studies (AS), if necessary. First, select diagnostic tissue for slide preparation. This is best accomplished by expelling the material in the needle and hub onto a slide and identifying tissue particles. These are usually tan white but may vary depending on the nature of the lesion (e.g., mucoid material in cases of a mucinous carcinoma). The sample may be scant and allow for preparation of only smear(s). Alternatively, the sample may be bloody and contain clots. In samples with clots, gently pressing the clot between two slides distinguishes lesional tissue from blood. Second, prepare two slides from the tissue particles selected. Perform ROSE to determine if there is diagnostic tissue and if additional material is needed for ancillary studies. Repeat these steps in cases of insufficient tissue. Meanwhile, to capture all possible cells, rinse the needle within a liquid media (e.g., alcohol, saline, RPMI). In cases of smaller length needles, like the ones used for CT-guided FNAs, the media/preservative in the transport vial can be drawn into the syringe and then flushed back and rinsed into the vial multiple times. For longer needles, like the ones used for EBUS-FNAs, pass approximately 0.5 to 1 ml of sterile saline through the proximal end of the needle and into the vial containing the media/preservative. In instances where only blood is seen under microscopic examination, an additional smear can be prepared from the unused material. Otherwise, the remainder of expelled and unused specimen is placed in the appropriate fixative for ancillary studies, if necessary and indicated

1. For each FNA pass, expel the specimen onto a single slide with a syringe (Fig. 4.1).

    a. In case the material cannot be expelled due to clotting, use a stylet to dislodge the specimen.

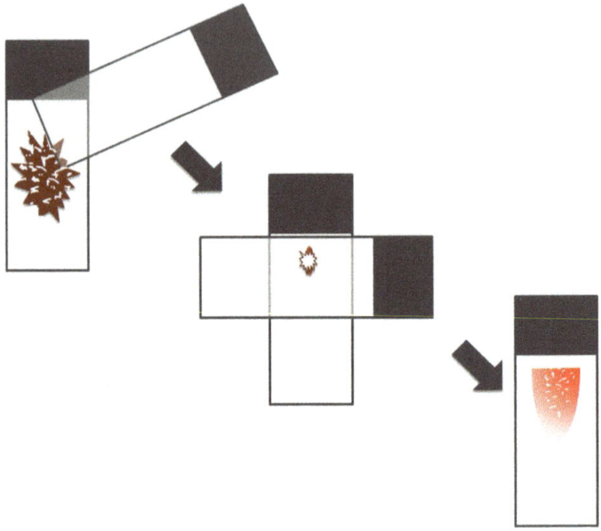

**Fig. 4.2** Smear preparation: With the corner of a slide, select a tissue particle(s). Place the tissue on a clean slide and smear holding the second slide perpendicularly

2. Identify diagnostic tissue particles, often tan or white specs, and select [10–12] with the corner of a second slide.
   a. In case of significant clot formation, tissue particles can be identified by gently pressing the specimen in between two slides.
3. Prepare two smears from the selected tissue particles for each pass [10] (Fig. 4.2).
   a. Air-dry one smear and stain with Diff-Quik, or similar method, for ROSE.
   b. Fix one smear in alcohol for Papanicolaou staining in the laboratory.
4. Flush the needle and/or syringe to remove any remaining cells.
   a. In cases of CT-guided aspirations, the needle and syringe are rinsed in CytoLyt (or other preservatives used by the laboratory).
   b. In cases of EBUS and/or EUS FNAs, approximately 0.5 to 1 ml of saline is passed through the needle into CytoLyt (or other preservatives used by the laboratory).
5. Place the remaining specimen in media appropriate for ancillary studies and/or cell block preparation.
   a. One technique for making cell blocks involves allowing the specimen to clot on the expelled slide for a few minutes and then placing it into formalin. (Partial) Clotting simplifies cell block processing.
   b. Separating diagnostic material/more cellular passes from non-diagnostic ones (e.g., containing mostly blood) prevents specimen dilution and improves cellular yield of cell blocks.

6. Perform ROSE.
   a. Is there sufficient material for diagnosis?
      i. If not, repeat steps 1–5.
   b. If so, and there is a need for ancillary studies, determine whether there is sufficient material.
      i. If no, perform dedicated passes for ancillary studies.
      ii. If yes, the procedure is terminated.

## Maximizing Efficiency of ROSE

Some of the time challenges of ROSE can be overcome by implementing the following steps that increase efficiency: (1) arrangement with the interventionist to notify pathology staff with the appropriate lead time (i.e., after the patient has been consented and prepped and the lesion has been identified/localized) necessary to travel to the procedure site and set up in advance of when the specimen will be procured—a mutual coordination effort increases efficiency and minimizes perpetuation of late arrivals of the cytologist and unnecessary advance requests for ROSE by the interventionists, (2) completed requisition with pertinent clinical history and labels prepared for identifying the specimen vial(s), (3) microscopes deployed in all procedure rooms and clinics that routinely request ROSE, (4) fully stocked FNA baskets and cart that are restocked following each FNA to ensure all necessary items, such as needles, syringes, CytoLyt, 95 % alcohol, Diff-Quik stain, RPMI, sterile saline syringes, etc., are readily available, and (5) ROSE forms in all FNA baskets and FNA cart.

## FNA Without ROSE

An experienced cytotechnologist or pathologist is qualified to render an accurate, immediate interpretation [13]. Yet, due to workload, time and cost constraints, as well as limited diagnostic accuracy [14, 15], yield [14, 16–18], or adequacy [17, 19] at a facility, some forgo ROSE.

There are several steps that can be undertaken in the absence of ROSE to ensure that diagnostic material is sampled and optimally processed. First, even the best preparations cannot overcome inadequate sampling. In some instances, as described for EUS FNAs, utilizing the fanning technique, which involves sampling different areas with multiple back and forth motions [20], increases cellular yield and samples from different areas. This is advantageous in cases of heterogeneity of lesional tissue. Second, performing three aspirates per site [21] and a dedicated pass(es) for cell block preparation [20] and/or ancillary studies can enhance the cellular yield.

Even in the presence of adequate tissue, slides of suboptimal technical quality can compromise diagnosis. Though an experienced cytologist makes smear preparation appear effortless, smearing requires skill. Liquid-based preparations, like ThinPrep® and SurePath™, offer a standardized alternative for slide preparation. For the interventionist, the process involves placing the aspirate in an alcohol-based solution (e.g., CytoLyt or SurePath™ vial), which serves as a fixative and transport medium. Slides are prepared in the laboratory with an automated processor. This eliminates the need for non-experienced personnel to prepare smears, possibly poorly, and reduces the number of slides for diagnosis. These factors in turn decrease the amount of time spent examining slide(s) for each case and result in fewer issues with fixation/preservation [22]. Also, a combination of a liquid-based slide and cell block preparation from the fixative standardizes processing. Similar adequacy rates between conventionally processed aspirates [22] and those placed directly into CytoLyt—especially with an experienced aspirator—and high-quality specimens without on-site support at the time of the procedure [23] have been reported. For hemorrhagic thyroid aspirates, preparing only cell blocks correlates with slide reduction [24]. These methods neither ensure nor are substitutes for sample adequacy, however.

## Optimization and Triage

Optimizing a specimen requires appropriate handling and triaging. Even in the presence of abundant tissue, poor preparation and allocation can preclude a definitive diagnosis and ancillary studies. When performing ROSE, particularly for aspirations or core biopsies of lung and difficult-to-access lesions, it is of utmost importance to approach the triage of each pass as though that is the only specimen that will be procured. Complications, such as pneumothorax and obscuring hemorrhage, may preclude the opportunity to obtain additional material necessary for ancillary tests, resulting in the need for a repeat procedure.

## Optimizing Slide Preparation: Fine Needle Aspirations

There are several explanations for not having sufficient tissue for ancillary studies. One of the more common reasons is "wasting" tissue by making excessive smears—those beyond what is required to make a diagnosis [9] (Fig. 4.3). At the time of ROSE, whenever possible, only two smears should be prepared—one air-dried for Diff-Quik staining and the second fixed in alcohol for Papanicolaou staining—with the remaining material, if any, allocated for cell block or other ancillary studies. Also, avoiding thick smears serves two purposes: first, it allows for easier visualization of diagnostic cells, and second, an even and thin preparation minimizes the tissue expended on smears. Placing excessive material and clots in solution reduces the likelihood of additional passes for ancillary studies. Lastly, smearing by placing slides perpendicular, rather than parallel, to each other creates smears with

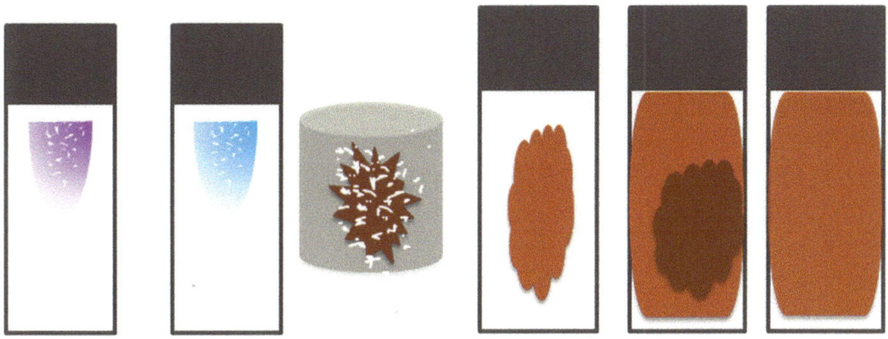


**Fig. 4.3** Optimal and suboptimal utilization of tissue: Optimal utilization involves preparation of smears (stained with Diff-Quik and Papanicolaou stains) from selected tissue particles with excess placed in media for potential ancillary studies. Suboptimally prepared specimens consist of numerous slides that are thick and bloody, contain clots, and encompass almost the entire surface of the slides. This obscures cellular detail, hinders accurate interpretation of slides, and risks having inadequate material for ancillary studies

concentration of specimen at the top and thin distribution below for easy visualization. Application of excessive pressure, which can create artifacts, may hinder interpretation and/or lead to misdiagnosis.

## Optimizing Slide Preparation: Touch Preparations

There is debate about performing touch preparations of core biopsies. If performed, touch preparations require handling with care [25]. Provided that core biopsies are typically thin and delicate, they dry rapidly, and significant manipulation can cause them to fragment. Touching the core once or twice to a slide by lifting it with a needle from the sheath or while it is still in the needle sheath and then placing it into formalin (or the appropriate media) minimizes excessive handling and yields optimal results (Fig. 4.4). If the touch preparation has abundant material, it can be smeared with a second slide to yield a thin and even distribution of cells.

Preparing a Papanicolaou-stained touch preparation can be challenging. Even if touched rapidly and placed in alcohol immediately, the slide may have air-drying artifact. One approach to minimizing this is to hydrate the slide with a few drops of normal saline, which is available in syringes, for a few minutes. Subsequently, placing a slide hydrated in this manner in alcohol salvages the nuclear features. This technique can also be applied to FNA smears when there is a delay in alcohol fixation.

At times, core biopsies consist of minute and thin fragments. If the laboratory is proficient at making cell blocks, the possibility of processing the cores using the same methodology as that employed for FNAs may prevent inadvertent loss of tissue during multiple transfer steps involved in routine core biopsy handling in histology.

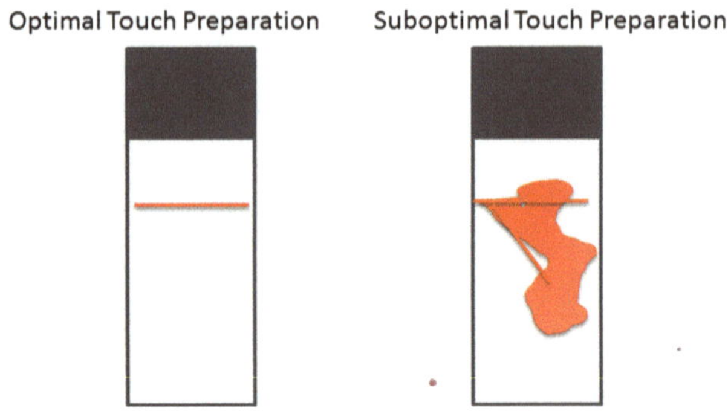


**Fig. 4.4** Optimal and suboptimal touch preparations: Optimal touch preparations involve gently touching the core to the slide once or twice. If it adheres to the slide, lift the core with a needle and place it in the appropriate media for fixation or transport. A smear can be prepared from a touch preparation when there is excessive tissue or liquid component. Suboptimal touch preparations: smearing or rubbing the core onto a slide can result in crush artifact and transfer of a significant portion of lesional cells onto the slide that can hinder final interpretation and compromise the core

## Triage: Carcinomas

For carcinomas, smears should have material to render a diagnosis of small cell carcinoma or NSCLC; the remainder of the specimen, if any, should be allocated for cell block preparation for subtyping (Fig. 4.5). It has been noted, especially in instances of poorly differentiated NSCLCs, that IHC and/or special stains (e.g., mucicarmine) are necessary to establish the histologic subtype [26, 27]. For NSCLCs, notably those presenting at advanced stages, an effort should be made to preserve as much tissue as possible for molecular analysis [28] when any proportion of adenocarcinoma is present or cannot entirely be excluded.

## Optimizing: Processing Core Biopsies and Cell Blocks for Carcinomas

There are several measures that can be undertaken to ensure that there is sufficient material in core biopsies and cell blocks and that the tissue is not exhausted (Table 4.1). The clinician obtaining the biopsy can play a significant role by performing a gross examination of the biopsy. It is important to determine if the core represents a solid piece of tan white tissue, which is typical of carcinomas, or not. Sometimes the "cores" consist of mostly red blood cell clot, mucus, liquefied necrotic inflammatory tissue, or bronchial cell contamination [9]. Similar findings can be observed in FNA samples. Both situations necessitate additional tissue, and typically, the greater the number of cores obtained, the greater the likelihood of having sufficient tissue for ancillary testing. Currently, there are no guidelines dictating the minimum number. However, if feasible and accessible without significant risk to the

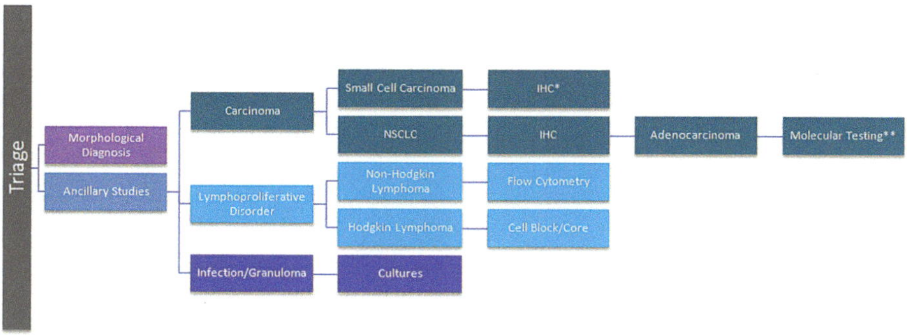


**Fig. 4.5** Algorithm for triage of small specimens. NSCLC, non-small cell lung carcinoma; IHC, immunohistochemistry; (*asterisk*) Perform immunohistochemistry to confirm diagnosis, if necessary; (*double asterisk*) Perform molecular testing on carcinomas with adenocarcinoma or when a component of adenocarcinoma cannot entirely be excluded

**Table 4.1** Core biopsy and cell block management in the laboratory

**Create >1 block when possible**

| Core biopsies | Cell blocks (Fine Needle Aspirates and Exfoliatives) |
|---|---|
| Divide cores/fragments into multiple blocks | Separate passes with scant diagnostic tissue from those non-diagnostic passes (e.g. mostly blood) |

**Minimize tissue loss**

| | ROSE | No ROSE |
|---|---|---|
| Avoid excessive trimming of paraffin block | • Order blank slides for ancillary studies upfront | • Cut blanks and/or save intervening levels upfront<br>• Following H&E evaluation and at time of IHC order, request blanks |

**Limit single section per slide**

More slides are available for ancillary testing

patient, 1 to 6 cores (from 18- to 20-gauge core needles) have yielded sufficient tissue for mutational analysis [7, 29–31] By placing fewer fragments and/or cores [32] (1 to 3) in a single histology cassette, inadvertent trimming of one block leaves the other(s) available for ancillary testing, if necessary. The consequences of excessive facing of the block should also be communicated to the histotechnologists cutting the blocks.

## Optimizing: Immunohistochemistry for Carcinomas

When using immunohistochemistry in the distinction between adenocarcinoma and squamous cell carcinoma, a limited panel should be performed in a stepwise fashion to ensure that tissue remains for molecular diagnosis in case of lung adenocarcinoma. If sufficient tumor tissue/cells are available, then a minimal set of two IHC stains, i.e., TTF-1 and p63, can be utilized; however, if the amount of tumor is limited, then the initial work-up can begin with a TTF-1 stain alone [33] (Fig. 4.6).

## Optimizing: Molecular Testing for Carcinomas

For patients presenting with advanced stage (IV) lung adenocarcinomas who are suitable for therapy, testing for epidermal growth factor receptor (EGFR) and anaplastic lymphoma kinase (ALK) is standard of care and should be ordered at the time of diagnosis [34]. Even in the presence of an EGFR mutation or ALK rearrangement, patients have relatively short life expectancies [34], so obtaining sufficient tissue and appropriately triaging it without delay or having to perform a repeat procedure is important. Similarly, when EBUS is being performed for simultaneous staging and diagnosis of NSCLC, the sample has to be managed especially carefully. Dedicated passes improve the yield of the specimen [35]. For various reasons, including the inability of the patient to tolerate the procedure, risk of a pneumothorax, difficulty reaching the target, or lack of time or willingness, obtaining an additional pass may be difficult [35].

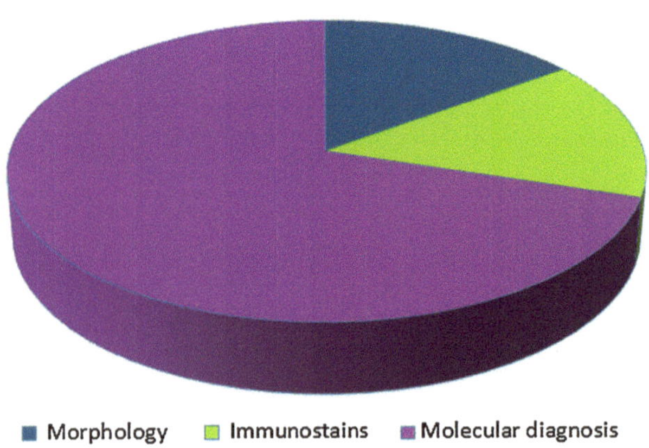


**Fig. 4.6** Triage of NSCLC: The most important step in optimizing a specimen involves appropriate triage. Especially in a case of an advanced, poorly differentiated NSCLC, selecting tissue particles for smear preparation permits allocation of the majority of specimen for ancillary studies. A limited panel of immunohistochemical stains leaves adequate tissue for molecular testing, when indicated

The minimum number of cells necessary for molecular testing is variable. The threshold depends on the absolute number of tumor cells, ratio of tumor cells to adjacent nucleated nonneoplastic cells, the molecular technique utilized, and resources available to enrich the sample with microdissection (i.e., manual or laser capture). EGFR mutation has been detected in as few as 50 cells [6]. Per recently published guidelines, it is recommended that for EGFR mutation testing performed using a polymerase chain reaction (PCR)-based method, laboratories use a test that detects mutations in specimens with at least 50 % tumor; however, a test capable of identifying as little as 10 % tumor in a sample is ideal [34]. With the use of next-generation sequencing, the minimum cell number threshold will likely fall.

Recently published guidelines suggest that results of molecular testing should be available within 10 days of receiving the specimen in the molecular pathology laboratory. Reflex testing is an option. By instituting such a protocol in collaboration with clinical colleagues, molecular testing results can be expedited. Its drawbacks include performing additional FNAs or core biopsies, testing patients that present with earlier stage localized cancers or those who may not be candidates for tyrosine kinase inhibitors (e.g., presentation at advanced stages and seeking palliative care only) [34], and conducting molecular testing when a larger resection is expected.

In staging procedures for previously diagnosed adenocarcinomas with IHC and molecular testing, the presence of tumor cells may be sufficient [6], especially if a patient cannot tolerate additional biopsies/aspirates.

## Triage: Lymphoproliferative Disorders

There is controversy about diagnosing lymphoma based on FNAs [6], as they do not allow for assessment of architecture [36] and obtaining tissue in cases of nodular sclerosing Hodgkin lymphoma [36] can be difficult. However, FNAs confirm recurrence in patients with a history of lymphoma and provide tissue to determine the cause of the underlying lymphadenopathy without having the patient undergo an invasive procedure in the absence of a neoplastic process.

The key to diagnosing lymphoproliferative disorders by FNA is through a multiparameter approach [37]. When used in conjunction with ancillary studies, FNA shows a relatively high sensitivity and specificity in the diagnosis of lymphoma [37–39], including both primary and recurrent Hodgkin lymphoma [40–42]. In particular, EBUS-TBNA is useful in the diagnosis of lymphoma in patients with mediastinal lymphadenopathy [39, 43, 44] with sensitivity, specificity, positive predictive value, and negative predictive values of 90.9 %, 100 %, 100 %, and 92.9 %, respectively, being reported [39].

If there is a clinical and/or morphological suspicion for non-Hodgkin lymphoma (NHL), additional aspirates and/or cores should be obtained for flow cytometry [41, 42, 50–53] and placed directly into RMPI, which appears to be the best storage media for maintaining viability [38] and preserving cells for flow cytometry [38, 45]. Other transport/storage media, including saline, Hanks' Balanced Salt Solution, and Dulbecco's Modified Eagle's Medium storage media, are also available, and some institutions routinely collect samples in these media, especially in the absence of ROSE, so flow cytometry can be performed, if necessary. (Flow cytometry cannot be performed on alcohol- or formalin-fixed tissues.) Two to three dedicated passes for flow cytometry [46] have been recommended in cases suspicious for lymphoma or in the absence of ROSE. Adequacy can also be ascertained by examining the fluid (RPMI or saline) for clarity or cloudiness. In the absence of a significantly bloody specimen, the latter is an indicator of cellularity. A similar method of assessment and dedicated passes can be applied to core biopsies, which can be divided between RPMI and saline.

If sufficient material is available, cell block preparation allows for numerous IHC stains. When Hodgkin lymphoma is suspected and material is limited, then making a cell block as opposed to submitting for flow cytometry studies should be considered, since immunohistochemistry is more helpful in such cases. FISH and PCR analyses, which are routinely performed on formalin-fixed paraffin-embedded tissue from surgical biopsies [47], can be performed on cell block sections, smears, CytoLyt- or alcohol-fixed slides, and cytospins [37, 44, 48, 49].

## Triage: Infectious Processes and Granulomas

Small biopsies and FNAs play an important role in the diagnosis of nonneoplastic processes, including granulomas and infections. In fact, EBUS is used frequently for diagnosing sarcoidosis [50]. In cases with suspected infectious etiology or granulomas, a sample should be sent for microbiological cultures to exclude the presence of organisms. Also, material should be reserved to perform special stains in the laboratory.

## Optimizing: Navigational Bronchoscopy FNAs and Cores

With navigational bronchoscopy, a sample can be acquired either with aspiration or forceps/core biopsy. There are limited published data on which method has greater cellular yield. One study reported that catheter aspiration correlated with greater success relative to biopsy [51], possibly because its back and forth motion accesses target cells that may not be amenable to forceps biopsy. In practice, when both modalities are performed, preference is given to aspiration first, as it results in a less bloody sample that does not dilute the cells of interest, followed by biopsy.

## Cytological Preparations

Familiarity with the various cytological preparations is important because each is unique and offers different yet complementary information valuable in rendering a diagnosis.

## Diff-Quik Stain

The Diff-Quik (or similar) stain is ideal for ROSE, because it can be performed rapidly on smears and utilizes only three solutions. It is useful for the assessment of diagnostic tissue, including the origin of cells—lymphoid (mostly single cells) or epithelial (mostly cohesive clusters)—and subtyping epithelial cells as either squamous or glandular based on the cytoplasmic characteristics. Keratinizing squamous cells typically have dense, blue, and homogeneous cytoplasm, whereas the cytoplasm of glandular cells is often vacuolated or foamy. In addition, Diff-Quik stain highlights mucus and metachromatic stroma, which are key features associated with certain neoplasms, such as mucinous/colloid carcinomas and hamartomas [52], respectively.

Allowing the tissue to dry completely is a key factor in preparing a Diff-Quik smear. Staining a partially dried slide masks cellular detail, limits evaluation of adequacy, and possibly leads to misinterpretation.

## Papanicolaou Stain

A Papanicolaou stain is typically performed in the laboratory on alcohol-fixed slides. It offers nuclear detail—membrane irregularities, chromatin pattern, intranuclear invaginations—important for establishing a diagnosis of malignancy, especially well-differentiated neoplasms that lack significant pleomorphism. It also demonstrates the speckled or "salt and pepper" chromatin pattern associated with neuroendocrine differentiation. Most importantly, the Papanicolaou stain highlights keratinizing squamous cells, which have orange/pink cytoplasm. This is a specific finding and precludes the need for immunostain(s) to make the distinction between squamous and glandular origin [53].

Unlike a Diff-Quik slide that has to be dried completely prior to staining, a slide for Papanicolaou staining has to be placed in alcohol immediately. Any delay in fixation results in air-drying artifacts (e.g., cellular enlargement and loss of nuclear detail) that challenge interpretation and possibly prevent a definitive diagnosis. Also, air-drying artifact can lead to misdiagnosis because the cells can undertake an orange hue, mimicking squamous differentiation. Spray fixation is an alternative to placing the slide in a jar of alcohol. Though this provides fixation, at times, the spray has a tendency to aggregate cells in distinct colonies rather than form an even distribution.

## Liquid-Based Preparations

Traditionally, a combination of well-prepared and fixed Diff-Quik- and Papanicolaou-stained smears has been the most commonly used method for evaluating cytological specimens. Smearing requires technical skill, which is not always available and/or optimal, however. For these reasons and to limit obscuring blood, inflammation, and debris, liquid-based preparations offer a standardized alternative for slide preparation.

The two most commonly used methods include ThinPrep® and SurePath™. At the time of collection, the specimen is placed in an alcohol-based solution (e.g., CytoLyt), which serves as a fixative and transport medium. This fixative can be used for FNAs and other exfoliative specimens, including fluids, brushings, and lavages. In the laboratory, an automated processor homogenizes the specimen and prepares a slide with uniform distribution of cells and without loss of cells while minimizing obscuring background blood, inflammation, and debris. The slides are then stained with Papanicolaou stain. Provided that there is sufficient sample, additional slides with similar content can be prepared for ancillary studies. Because of automation, liquid-based preparations cannot be used for ROSE.

## References


1. Jemal A, Siegel R, Xu J, Ward E. Cancer statistics, 2010. CA Cancer J Clin. 2010;60:277–300.
2. Langer CJ, Besse B, Gualberto A, Brambilla E, Soria JC. The evolving role of histology in the management of advanced non-small-cell lung cancer. J Clin Oncol. 2010;28:5311–20.
3. Travis WD, Brambilla E, Noguchi M, et al. International Association for the Study of Lung Cancer/American Thoracic Society/European Respiratory Society: international multidisciplinary classification of lung adenocarcinoma: executive summary. Proc Am Thorac Soc. 2011;8:381–5.
4. Monaco SE, Schuchert MJ, Khalbuss WE. Diagnostic difficulties and pitfalls in rapid on-site evaluation of endobronchial ultrasound guided fine needle aspiration. CytoJournal. 2010;7:9.
5. Bulman W, Saqi A, Powell CA. Acquisition and processing of endobronchial ultrasound-guided transbronchial needle aspiration specimens in the era of targeted lung cancer chemotherapy. Am J Respir Crit Care Med. 2012;185:606–11.
6. Yasufuku K, Fleury FJ. Cytological specimens obtained by endobronchial ultrasound-guided transbronchial needle aspiration: sample handling and role of rapid on-site evaluation. Ann Pathol. 2012;32(e35–46):421–32.
7. Crapanzano JP, Heymann JJ, Monaco S, Nassar A, Saqi A. The state of cell block variation and satisfaction in the era of molecular diagnostics and personalized medicine. CytoJournal. 2014;11:7.
8. Yasufuku K, Pierre A, Darling G, et al. A prospective controlled trial of endobronchial ultrasound-guided transbronchial needle aspiration compared with mediastinoscopy for mediastinal lymph node staging of lung cancer. J Thorac Cardiovasc Surg. 2011;142:1393–1400 e1391.
9. Jurado J, Saqi A. Maxfield R, et al. Ann Thorac Surg: The Efficacy of Endobronchial Ultrasound-Guided Transbronchial Needle Aspiration for Molecular Testing in Lung Adenocarcinoma; 2013.
10. Giri D, Vazquez MF. "Pick and smear" tissue concentration technique for bloody aspirates. Acta Cytol. 2001;45:889–90.

11. Kumar N, Jain S. Tissue concentration and preservation of morphology in bloody aspirates. Acta Cytol. 2004;48:456–7.
12. Tong TR, Chan O. A method of processing bloody aspirates in fine needle aspiration cytology. Acta Cytol. 2002;46:1168.
13. Nasuti JF, Gupta PK, Baloch ZW. Diagnostic value and cost-effectiveness of on-site evaluation of fine-needle aspiration specimens: review of 5,688 cases. Diagn Cytopathol. 2002;27:1–4.
14. Griffin AC, Schwartz LE, Baloch ZW. Utility of on-site evaluation of endobronchial ultrasound-guided transbronchial needle aspiration specimens. CytoJournal. 2011;8:20.
15. Oki M, Saka H, Kitagawa C, et al. Rapid on-site cytologic evaluation during endobronchial ultrasound-guided transbronchial needle aspiration for diagnosing lung cancer: a randomized study. Respiration. 2013;85:486–92.
16. Trisolini R, Cancellieri A, Tinelli C, et al. Rapid on-site evaluation of transbronchial aspirates in the diagnosis of hilar and mediastinal adenopathy: a randomized trial. Chest. 2011;139:395–401.
17. Yarmus L, Van der Kloot T, Lechtzin N, Napier M, Dressel D, Feller-Kopman D. A randomized prospective trial of the utility of rapid on-site evaluation of transbronchial needle aspirate specimens. J Bronchol Interv Pulmonol. 2011;18:121–7.
18. Joseph M, Jones T, Lutterbie Y, et al. Rapid on-site pathologic evaluation does not increase the efficacy of endobronchial ultrasonographic biopsy for mediastinal staging. Ann Thorac Surg. 2013;96:403–10.
19. O'Malley ME, Weir MM, Hahn PF, Misdraji J, Wood BJ, Mueller PR. US-guided fine-needle aspiration biopsy of thyroid nodules: adequacy of cytologic material and procedure time with and without immediate cytologic analysis. Radiology. 2002;222:383–7.
20. Ramesh J, Varadarajulu S. How can we get the best results with endoscopic ultrasound-guided fine needle aspiration? Clin Endosc. 2012;45:132–7.
21. Diacon AH, Schuurmans MM, Theron J, et al. Transbronchial needle aspirates: how many passes per target site? Eur Respir J. 2007;29:112–6.
22. Natu S, Hoffman J, Siddiqui M, Hobday C, Shrimankar J, Harrison R. The role of endobronchial ultrasound guided transbronchial needle aspiration cytology in the investigation of mediastinal lymphadenopathy and masses, the North Tees experience. J Clin Pathol. 2010;63:445–51.
23. Wallace WA, Monaghan HM, Salter DM, Gibbons MA, Skwarski KM. Endobronchial ultrasound-guided fine-needle aspiration and liquid-based thin-layer cytology. J Clin Pathol. 2007;60:388–91.
24. Qiu L, Crapanzano JP, Saqi A, Vidhun R, Vazquez MF. Cell block alone as an ideal preparatory method for hemorrhagic thyroid nodule aspirates procured without onsite cytologists. Acta Cytol. 2008;52:139–44.
25. Tsou MH, Tsai SF, Chan KY, et al. CT-guided needle biopsy: value of on-site cytopathologic evaluation of core specimen touch preparations. J Vasc Interv Radiol. 2009;20:71–6.
26. Vazquez MF, Koizumi JH, Henschke CI, Yankelevitz DF. Reliability of cytologic diagnosis of early lung cancer. Cancer. 2007;111:252–8.
27. Rekhtman N, Brandt SM, Sigel CS, et al. Suitability of thoracic cytology for new therapeutic paradigms in non-small cell lung carcinoma: high accuracy of tumor subtyping and feasibility of EGFR and KRAS molecular testing. J Thorac Oncol. 2011;6:451–8.
28. Cagle PT, Allen TC, Dacic S, et al. Revolution in lung cancer: new challenges for the surgical pathologist. Arch Pathol Lab Med. 2011;135:110–6.
29. Ferretti GR, Busser B, de Fraipont F, et al. Adequacy of CT-guided biopsies with histomolecular subtyping of pulmonary adenocarcinomas: influence of ATS/ERS/IASLC guidelines. Lung Cancer. 2013;82:69–75.
30. Hasanovic A, Ang D, Moreira AL, Zakowski MF. Use of mutation specific antibodies to detect EGFR status in small biopsy and cytology specimens of lung adenocarcinoma. Lung Cancer. 2012;77:299–305.
31. Chen CM, Chang JW, Cheung YC, et al. Computed tomography-guided core-needle biopsy specimens demonstrate epidermal growth factor receptor mutations in patients with non-small-cell lung cancer. Acta Radiol. 2008;49:991–4.

32. Travis WD, Brambilla E, Noguchi M, et al. Diagnosis of lung adenocarcinoma in resected specimens: implications of the 2011 International Association for the Study of Lung Cancer/ American Thoracic Society/European Respiratory Society classification. Arch Pathol Lab Med. 2013;137:685–705.
33. Travis WD, Rekhtman N. Pathological diagnosis and classification of lung cancer in small biopsies and cytology: strategic management of tissue for molecular testing. Semin Respir Crit Care Med. 2011;32:22–31.
34. Lindeman NI, Cagle PT, Beasley MB, et al. Molecular testing guideline for selection of lung cancer patients for EGFR and ALK tyrosine kinase inhibitors: guideline from the College of American Pathologists, International Association for the Study of Lung Cancer, and Association for Molecular Pathology. Arch Pathol Lab Med. 2013;137:828–60.
35. Khan S, Omar T, Michelow P. Effectiveness of the cell block technique in diagnostic cytopathology. J Cytol. 2012;29:177–82.
36. Steinfort DP, Conron M, Tsui A, et al. Endobronchial ultrasound-guided transbronchial needle aspiration for the evaluation of suspected lymphoma. J Thorac Oncol. 2010;5:804–9.
37. Caraway NP. Strategies to diagnose lymphoproliferative disorders by fine-needle aspiration by using ancillary studies. Cancer. 2005;105:432–42.
38. Shetuni B, Lakey M, Kulesza P. Optimal specimen processing of fine needle aspirates of non-Hodgkin lymphoma. Diagn Cytopathol. 2012;40:984–6.
39. Kennedy MP, Jimenez CA, Bruzzi JF, et al. Endobronchial ultrasound-guided transbronchial needle aspiration in the diagnosis of lymphoma. Thorax. 2008;63:360–5.
40. Fulciniti F, Vetrani A, Zeppa P, et al. Hodgkin's disease: diagnostic accuracy of fine needle aspiration; a report based on 62 consecutive cases. Cytopathology. 1994;5:226–33.
41. Jimenez-Heffernan JA, Vicandi B, Lopez-Ferrer P, Hardisson D, Viguer JM. Value of fine needle aspiration cytology in the initial diagnosis of Hodgkin's disease. Analysis of 188 cases with an emphasis on diagnostic pitfalls. Acta Cytol. 2001;45:300–6.
42. Moreland WS, Geisinger KR. Utility and outcomes of fine-needle aspiration biopsy in Hodgkin's disease. Diagn Cytopathol. 2002;26:278–82.
43. Yasuda I, Goto N, Tsurumi H, et al. Endoscopic ultrasound-guided fine needle aspiration biopsy for diagnosis of lymphoproliferative disorders: feasibility of immunohistological, flow cytometric, and cytogenetic assessments. Am J Gastroenterol. 2012;107:397–404.
44. Ko HM, da Cunha SG. Darling G, et al. Diagn Cytopathol: Diagnosis and subclassification of lymphomas and non-neoplastic lesions involving mediastinal lymph nodes using endobronchial ultrasound-guided transbronchial needle aspiration; 2011.
45. Jhala NC, Jhala DN, Chhieng DC, Eloubeidi MA, Eltoum IA. Endoscopic ultrasound-guided fine-needle aspiration. A cytopathologist's perspective. Am J Clin Pathol. 2003;120:351–67.
46. Al-Haddad M. Introduction to endoscopic ultrasound fine needle aspiration (EUS-FNA) sample preparation. In: Medicine IUSo, editor. Sampling techniques, cytology vs. histology & case studies. Natick, MA: Boston Scientific Corporation; 2012.
47. Ochs RC, Bagg A. Molecular genetic characterization of lymphoma: application to cytology diagnosis. Diagn Cytopathol. 2012;40:542–55.
48. Katz RL. Cytologic diagnosis of leukemia and lymphoma. Values and limitations. Clin Lab Med. 1991;11:469–99.
49. Tani EM, Christensson B, Porwit A, Skoog L. Immunocytochemical analysis and cytomorphologic diagnosis on fine needle aspirates of lymphoproliferative disease. Acta Cytol. 1988;32: 209–15.
50. Tournoy KG, Bolly A, Aerts JG, et al. The value of endoscopic ultrasound after bronchoscopy to diagnose thoracic sarcoidosis. Eur Respir J. 2010;35:1329–35.
51. Eberhardt R, Morgan RK, Ernst A, Beyer T, Herth FJ. Comparison of suction catheter versus forceps biopsy for sampling of solitary pulmonary nodules guided by electromagnetic navigational bronchoscopy. Respiration. 2010;79:54–60.
52. Saqi A, Shaham D, Scognamiglio T, et al. Incidence and cytological features of pulmonary hamartomas indeterminate on CT scan. Cytopathology. 2008;19:185–91.
53. Sigel CS, Moreira AL, Travis WD, et al. Subtyping of non-small cell lung carcinoma: a comparison of small biopsy and cytology specimens. J Thorac Oncol. 2011;6:1849–56.

# Chapter 5
# Ancillary Immunohistochemical Techniques for the Subclassification of Non-small Cell Lung Cancer

**Daisuke Nonaka**

Approximately 70 % of NSCLC are unresectable at first presentation due to advanced stage of disease, and molecular testing and therapeutic decision are often based on diagnoses rendered from small biopsy and/or cytologic samples. The subclassification of NSCLC was, until recently, only morphology based in conjunction with mucin stains if necessary; however, the morphological features may be subtle or absent in small specimens, particularly in poorly differentiated tumors. Consequently NSCLC-not otherwise specified (NOS) became one of the most common diagnoses in small specimens [1], which accounts for approximately 20–30 % of lung cancers [1, 2].

In the past, the specific subclassification of NSCLC was regarded as being irrelevant since all subtypes were considered to have the same prognosis and were treated in a similar fashion. However, the subtyping of NSCLC has assumed increasing importance due to recent advances in targeted, molecular-based therapy. Although gene expression profiling and micro-RNA have been studied to assist distinguishing between adenocarcinoma and squamous cell carcinoma, immunohistochemistry is the most practical and cost-effective method [3]. Indeed, immunohistochemistry is an integral part of diagnosing and subclassifying a tumor, and it is particularly useful when dealing with poorly differentiated tumors and metastatic tumors. The appropriate use of immunohistochemistry lowers the rate of NSCLC-NOS and interobserver variability in small samples [4–6]. A variety of markers have been investigated for efficacy in distinguishing between adenocarcinoma and squamous cell carcinoma of the lung. Details of each marker are described under a subsection of each NSCLC subtype. Tables 5.1 and 5.2 list data on the

D. Nonaka, M.D. (✉)
Department of Histopathology, The Christie Hospital,
Wilmslow Road, Manchester M20 4BX, United Kingdom
e-mail: dnonaka@msn.com



A.L. Moreira, A. Saqi (eds.), *Diagnosing Non-small Cell Carcinoma in Small Biopsy and Cytology*, DOI 10.1007/978-1-4939-1607-8_5

**Table 5.1** Adenomarkers (in the context of adeno vs. squamous)

| | | TTF-1 | Napsin A | CK7 | Surfactant A protein |
|---|---|---|---|---|---|
| Overall[a] | Sensitivity | 76 | 77.8 | 97 | 61.8 |
| | Specificity | 95.9 | 98.1 | 68.8 | 97 |
| Biopsy and cytology[b] | Sensitivity | 76.1 | 69.1 | 100 | 80.6 |
| | Specificity | 94.2 | 96.1 | 52 | 100 |

[a]Overall indicates data extracted from studies based on TMA, whole sections from resection, biopsies, and cytology
[b]Biopsy and cytology refers to data originated from biopsy- and cytology-based studies [2, 5–64]

**Table 5.2** Squamous markers (in the context of adeno vs. squamous)

| | | p40 | p63 | CK5/6 | Desmocollin 3 | 34βE12 |
|---|---|---|---|---|---|---|
| Overall[a] | Sensitivity | 93.3 | 94.5 | 86.4 | 82.3 | 87.2 |
| | Specificity | 98 | 78.1 | 95 | 99.3 | 56.5 |
| Biopsy and cytology[b] | Sensitivity | 90.9 | 94.2 | 87.6 | 89.5 | 94.6 |
| | Specificity | 96.6 | 78.8 | 91.2 | 100 | 72.3 |

[a]Overall indicates data extracted from studies based on TMA, whole sections from resection, biopsies, and cytology
[b]Biopsy and cytology refers to data originated from biopsy- and cytology-based studies [2, 5–64]

sensitivity and specificity of each marker, extracted from published series. Since none of the markers is completely specific for a particular tumor histotype and each marker has different sensitivity and specificity, a panel of stains needs to be used to overcome and compensate for their deficits. Knowledge on the tissue distribution pattern of each marker and its sensitivity and specificity would be helpful when selecting markers for a particular case. Indiscriminate use of immunohistochemistry should be avoided since this may deplete the tissue for further molecular analysis of the tumor [65]. In order to preserve tissue for this purpose, a minimalistic approach is discussed at the end of the chapter.

## Squamous Cell Carcinoma

A majority of squamous cell carcinomas do not pose a diagnostic problem, but poorly differentiated tumors can be challenging since intercellular bridges and keratinization, hallmark features of these tumors, may not be identifiable. Pulmonary squamous cell carcinoma frequently expresses high molecular weight cytokeratins (HMW-CKs) and p63, both of which are generally regarded as markers for stratified epithelium. There are a variety of commercially available HMW-CKs. In lung tumor pathology, the most frequently investigated and commonly used markers are 34βE12 and CK5/6, and less frequently CK14.

**34βE12** is a monoclonal antibody that reacts with HMW-CKs 1, 5, 10, and 14. It is a sensitive marker for squamous cell carcinoma (88–100 %), with homogeneously strong and diffuse staining expected in the vast majority of tumors, but its specificity is variable (33–94 %) [2, 4–6, 31, 50, 52, 55]. In adenocarcinomas, diffuse 34βE12 staining is also common (up to 82 %); therefore, it is not recommended as the first line of immunohistochemistry to distinguish between squamous cell carcinoma and adenocarcinoma [5].

34βE12 may be useful to distinguish squamous cell carcinoma from small cell carcinoma since the latter is negative for this marker, while p63 expression is not uncommonly seen in small cell carcinoma (reported incidence as high as 76.9 %) [8] though generally weak and focal staining [66]. It should be noted that p40 is negative in small cell carcinoma [66].

CK5 and CK14 are expressed in the basal layer of the stratified squamous epithelia; therefore, they are often used as markers for squamous cell carcinoma [67].

**Anti-CK5/6** antibody reacts with CK5 and CK6 and, hence, recognizes basal cells of squamous epithelia and mesothelium, but is not reactive with simple epithelium or their tumors such as adenocarcinoma. As a marker for squamous cell carcinoma, CK5/6 is slightly less sensitive than or comparable to 34βE12, with reported sensitivity ranging from 53 to 100 % (Fig. 5.1) [2, 4–6, 26, 28, 31, 39, 40, 43, 46, 55, 59, 68], and the extent of its expression can be focal or weak in approximately 10 % of squamous cell carcinomas [55]. An inverse association is generally found between tumor grade and CK5/6 expression; hence, higher-grade tumors show decreased CK5/6 expression [69]. It has been reported that 20 % of poorly differentiated tumors

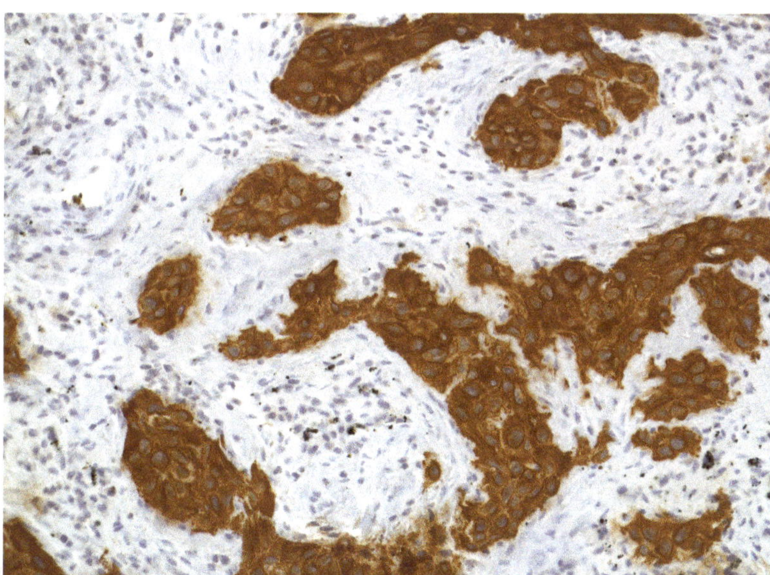

**Fig. 5.1** CK5/6 cytoplasm staining in poorly differentiated squamous cell carcinoma

had less than 10 % of CK5/6 reactivity [5]. Approximately 20 % of adenocarcinomas express CK5/6 (reported frequency from 0 to 27 %), but its expression is usually focal and weak [2, 5, 6, 22, 26, 28, 31, 46, 55, 59].

Of note, CK5/6 is expressed by approximately 80 % of malignant mesotheliomas and useful to distinguish between adenocarcinoma and mesothelioma when used in a panel of immunohistochemistry markers [68, 70].

The utility of **CK14** for the diagnosis of pulmonary squamous cell carcinoma has not been fully explored. The majority of squamous cell carcinoma is positive for CK14, with reported sensitivity from 77 to 92 % [14, 17, 44, 61]. However, a subset of adenocarcinoma (0–25 %) also expresses CK14 [14, 44, 61, 71]. One study reported that reactivity was similar regardless of tumor grade [14].

Desmosomes, which are intercellular junctions whose primary function is cell adhesion, contain three major component protein groups, including the desmosomal cadherins which comprise desmogleins (DSG1–4) and desmocollins (DSC1–3).

**Desmocollin 3 (DSC3)** is a component of the transmembrane core of desmosomes, and it is present in the lower portion of squamous epithelium [72]. It shows membranous staining. DSC3 has been described as a squamous marker with high sensitivity and specificity [35, 58]. DSC3 is expressed in 72–84 % of squamous cell carcinoma, while its expression is rarely seen in adenocarcinoma with reported incidence being 0–0.75 %; hence, it provides high specificity [35, 55, 71]. However, its sensitivity to poorly differentiated tumors drops to 52 % [55]. Overall, p63 and CK5/6 provide better sensitivity, and DSC3 is not likely to have an additional effect on sensitivity over CK5/6 or p63 in the vast majority of cases.

**Desmoglein 3 (DSG3)** is a calcium-binding transmembrane glycoprotein component of desmosomes, similar to DSC3, and positive immunoreaction occurs as a membranous staining.

Using gene expression profiling, DSG3 was found to be highly expressed in squamous cell carcinomas compared with adenocarcinomas [73]. The study also reported that DSG3 was more frequently expressed by immunohistochemistry in squamous cell carcinoma (79.5 %) than adenocarcinoma (54.8 %), but DSG3 was also expressed in typical carcinoid (93 %), atypical carcinoid (82.8 %), large cell neuroendocrine carcinoma (56 %), and small cell carcinoma (32.3 %). However, other studies demonstrated higher sensitivity with fairly high specificity. DSG3 is expressed in the majority of squamous cell carcinomas (92.8–98.5 %) [74, 75]. It is rarely expressed in adenocarcinomas (2–7 %) of the lung or other types including carcinoid tumors, large cell neuroendocrine carcinoma, or small cell carcinoma [71, 74, 75]. Hence, it seems to have high sensitivity and specificity comparable to DSC3 although further studies are needed.

**p63:** The human *p63* gene, a homolog of the *p53* tumor suppressor gene, contains two promoters that generate two classes of proteins: the full-length protein TAp63, which contains the N-terminal transactivation (TA) domain, and N-terminal truncated protein isoform ΔNp63, which lacks this transactivation domain [76]. The ΔNp63 is thought to function as a transcription factor for the stratified epithelium. The commonly used clone 4A4 recognizes both TAp63 and ΔNp63, while p40 only recognizes ΔNp63 [41, 77]. p63 expression using clone 4A4 is seen in basal cells and myoepithelial cells of glands of various organs as well as cells of stratified epithelium such as squamous, transitional, and thymic epithelium, and in the squamous and transitional epithelium, more intense expression is observed in the lower portion of the epithelium, particularly basal and parabasal cells [78]. Likewise p63 is expressed in squamous cell carcinomas, urothelial carcinomas, and thymomas as well as basal cell components of a number of benign and malignant tumors including basal cell carcinoma of the skin, various skin adnexal tumors [79], and salivary gland-type tumors such as adenoid cystic carcinoma, mucoepidermoid carcinoma, and myoepithelioma [78, 79]. In addition to the tumors with squamous, urothelial, and basal cell elements, p63 expression, by using 4A4, has been reported in a number of other tumors, including adenocarcinomas of the lung, colon, breast, and ovary, epithelioid trophoblastic tumor, choriocarcinoma, rhabdomyosarcoma, and B cell lymphomas [78]. It is believed that p63 expression in these tumors using clone 4A4 is most likely attributed to TA isoform expression [41].

p63 expression is seen in the vast majority of squamous cell carcinomas, with reported sensitivity ranging from 82 to 100 % (Fig. 5.2) [2, 4–6, 8, 9, 12, 26, 28, 31, 39–41, 46, 49, 55, 59–61], and it is a highly stable marker regardless of the grade of differentiation [5]. p63 expression can be seen in a subset of lung adenocarcinoma with reported frequency ranging from 0 to 48.4 % (Fig. 5.3) [2, 5, 8, 9, 12, 41, 46, 49, 55, 59]. p63 reaction has also been reported in small cell carcinoma, large cell neuroendocrine carcinoma, atypical carcinoid tumor, and typical carcinoid tumor [8]. Its expression in adenocarcinoma is generally focal (usually 25–30 % of the tumor) and

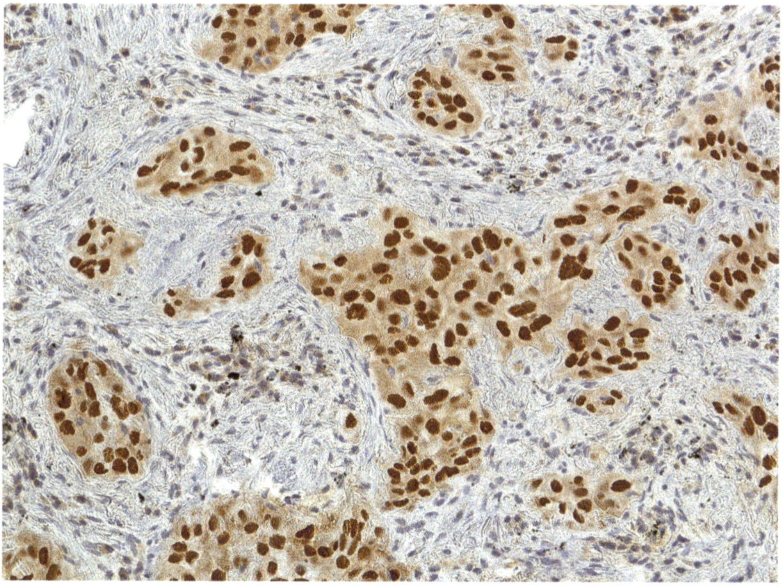

**Fig. 5.2** p63 nuclear staining in poorly differentiated squamous cell carcinoma

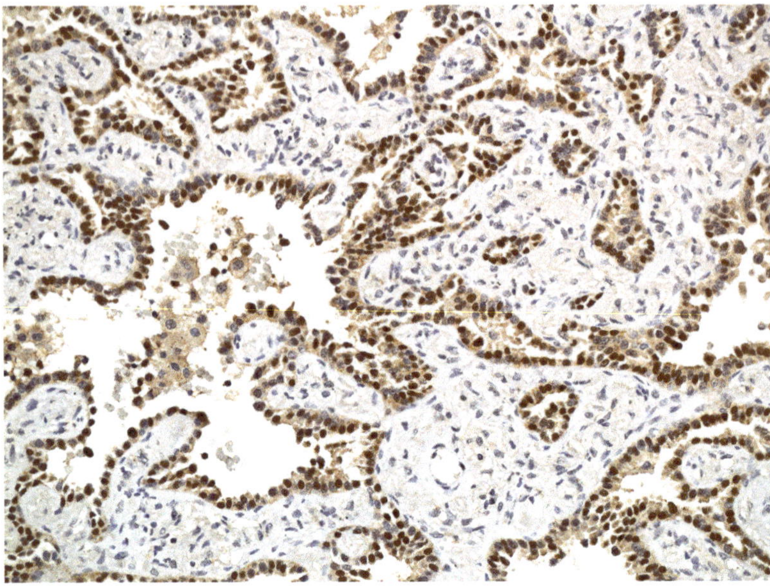

**Fig. 5.3** p63 nuclear staining in well-differentiated adenocarcinoma

weak in resected tumors, and diffuse and strong p63 expression at the level typical for squamous cell carcinoma is an exceptional occurrence in adenocarcinoma. One study showed that the positive predictive value of p63 staining alone for diagnosing squamous cell carcinoma was only 53 % when no quantitative thresholds were placed, but it went to up to 100 % when positive staining was defined as labeling of at least 40 % of tumor cells in the context of negative expression of TTF-1 and Napsin A [9]. However, when dealing with small tumor volume in biopsy or cytology samples, focality of p63 expression may not be appreciated, and any positive reaction can be potentially interpreted as evidence of squamous differentiation. In this scenario, any TTF-1 or Napsin A reaction allows poorly differentiated tumors to be diagnosed as adenocarcinoma or adenosquamous carcinoma [4].

According to a recent study, ALK mutated adenocarcinoma often shows p63 expression [64]. In the study, nine out of ten ALK mutated adenocarcinomas co-expressed p63 and TTF-1.

**p40:** Recent studies have demonstrated p40 provides very high sensitivity and specificity for squamous differentiation [41, 77, 80]. It is available as both monoclonal and polyclonal antibodies. All the published studies utilized polyclonal antibodies since the monoclonal antibody has become available only recently, which offers less technical problems. Reported sensitivity of p40 for the diagnosis of squamous cell carcinoma is 100 % and specificity ranges from 83 to 100 % (Fig. 5.4) [41, 49, 77, 80].

p40 expression is generally absent in adenocarcinoma. Rare cases of adenocarcinoma (up to 3 %) may contain scattered p40 positive tumor cells [77]. One study demonstrated that if reactivity of <5 % was disregarded, the specificity became 100 % for p40.

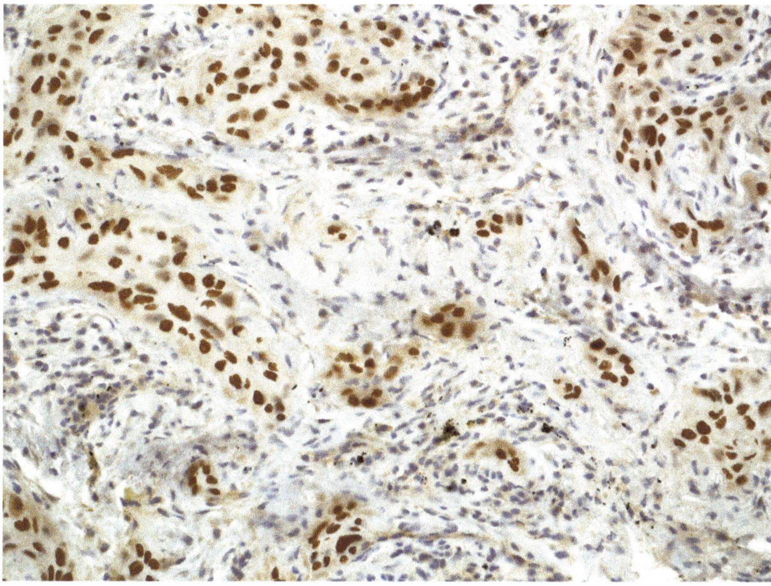

**Fig. 5.4** p40 nuclear staining in poorly differentiated squamous cell carcinoma

A recent study using TMAs showed p40 expression in 36/317 adenocarcinomas [71], which is markedly skewed from data from the majority of studies published in the literature.

As mentioned in the p63 section, ALK mutated adenocarcinoma often shows p63 expression, but in tumors with features of morphologically unequivocal adenocarcinoma, p40 expression was negative [71].

## Adenocarcinoma

Well-differentiated adenocarcinoma generally does not require immunohistochemistry and special stains to confirm the diagnosis. Immunohistochemistry is often required in poorly differentiated tumors, particularly those with solid growth, so-called squamoid morphology. Additionally immunohistochemistry may be needed for confirmation of lung origin. A number of studies have confirmed the efficacy of TTF-1 and Napsin A in the diagnosis of pulmonary adenocarcinoma over other antibodies [81, 82].

**TTF-1**, thyroid transcription factor-1, also known as Nkx2.1 or thyroid-specific enhancer binding protein, is a homeobox transcription factor of the *NK-2* gene family, and its locus is found on chromosome 14q13. TTF-1 is expressed in the lungs, thyroid gland, and ventral forebrain [83]. In the lungs, TTF-1 regulates surfactant apoproteins A, B, and C and Clara cell secretory protein in type II pneumocytes and Clara cells; therefore, these cells are positive for TTF-1 [84]. The majority of adenocarcinomas show differentiation toward these cells, and approximately 75–80 % of

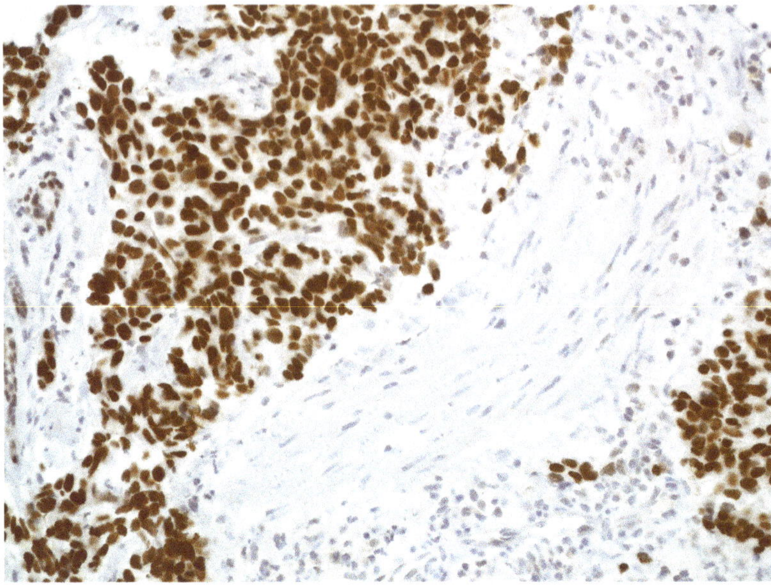

**Fig. 5.5** TTF-1 nuclear staining in poorly differentiated adenocarcinoma

pulmonary adenocarcinomas express TTF-1 (Fig. 5.5). 8G7G3/1 and SPT24 monoclonal antibodies are commonly used. Both antibodies show similar sensitivity; however, the specificity of SPT24 is reportedly lower. The majority of pulmonary adenocarcinomas are positive for TTF-1 by using both clones. One study compared both clones and reported sensitivity being 72.4 % for SPT24 and 65.4 % for 8G7G3/1 [34]. The SPT24 clone, however, detects more primary lung tumors of various histologic subtypes, including squamous cell carcinomas, large cell carcinoma, and carcinoid tumors, than clone 8G7G3/1 [34]. A recent study using SPT24 has shown statistical differences between tumor differentiation and positivity: 98 % in well differentiated, 94.2 % in moderately differentiated, and 72.4 % in poorly differentiated [55]. A small proportion of carcinomas from prostate, stomach, salivary gland, and colon are positive for both antibodies, with similar intensity and distribution [34]. It should be noted that the majority of pulmonary and extrapulmonary small cell carcinoma expresses TTF-1. Likewise TTF-1 expression is not uncommonly seen in pulmonary or extrapulmonary large cell neuroendocrine carcinoma [82].

**Napsin A**, also known as aspartyl protease 4, is predominantly expressed in alveolar type II pneumocytes where it is involved in the processing of the prosurfactant B protein [85]. Napsin A expression is also commonly seen in intra-alveolar macrophages, which is believed to be a result of phagocytosis [81]. Localization of the positive reaction is cytoplasm with granular staining quality.

For Napsin A, both polyclonal and monoclonal (TMU-Ad02, IP64, KCG1.1, MRQ60) antibodies are available. It has been reported that the monoclonal antibody shows greater specificity for lung adenocarcinoma. Napsin A expression is seen in 58–91 % of lung adenocarcinoma by monoclonal antibody (Fig. 5.6) and 81 % by polyclonal antibody [36, 81]. In a combined review of 11 studies, 627 (75 %) of 836

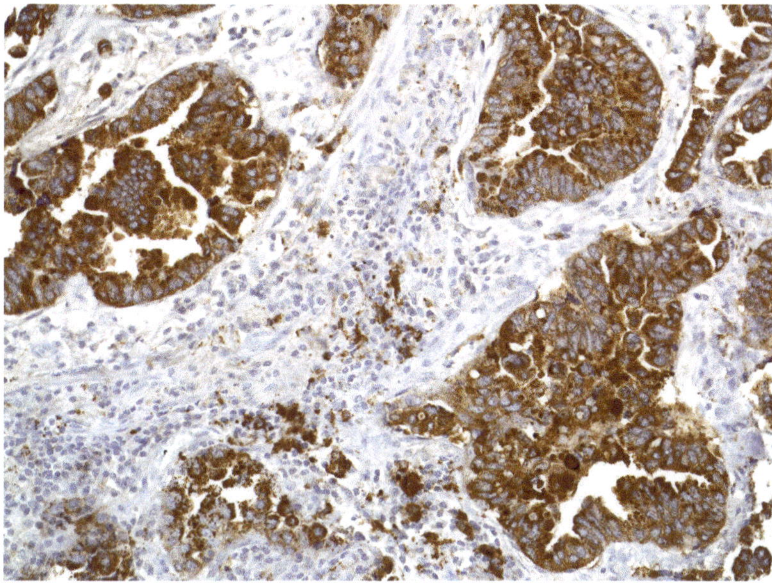

**Fig. 5.6** Napsin A granular cytoplasmic staining in adenocarcinoma of the lung

lung adenocarcinomas were reported to be Napsin A positive, whereas 623 (74.4 %) of 837 exhibited TTF-1 positivity [81]. These results indicate that the sensitivity of Napsin A for lung adenocarcinomas is comparable with that of TTF-1. This marker is negative in small cell carcinoma and carcinoid tumor contrary to TTF-1. There are rare adenocarcinomas where TTF-1 is positive but Napsin A negative or vice versa, which may indicate the importance of including the two markers for the diagnosis of pulmonary adenocarcinoma in difficult cases [51, 62].

Napsin A expression is also commonly seen in carcinomas of the kidney (45 and 67 % each by monoclonal and polyclonal) and thyroid gland (50 % each by monoclonal and polyclonal). While its expression is only rarely seen in carcinomas of other organs such as liver and endometrium by monoclonal antibody, Napsin A positive reaction using the polyclonal antibody is seen in a variety of adenocarcinomas, such as those from the colon, pancreas, esophagus, and stomach, as well as urothelial carcinomas [36, 81]. Napsin A is not expressed in pulmonary squamous cell carcinoma. Alleged Napsin A expression in squamous cell carcinoma is believed to represent expression in hyperplastic type II pneumocytes and intra-alveolar macrophages, both of which are sometimes seen entrapped within the tumor (Fig. 5.7) [81].

**CK7** is an intermediate-sized and basic keratin and expressed in bronchial and alveolar epithelium, while CK20 is not expressed in respiratory epithelium. Lung adenocarcinoma typical shows CK7+/CK20– pattern. This may be helpful for supporting a diagnosis of primary lung malignancies, especially in cases with negative TTF-1. However, a subset of the tumors show an aberrant expression pattern. CK7 status has been thought to be useful to distinguish between lung adenocarcinoma and squamous cell carcinoma since CK7 is more frequently expressed in adenocarcinomas than in squamous cell carcinomas. In a typical scenario, CK7 is positive in

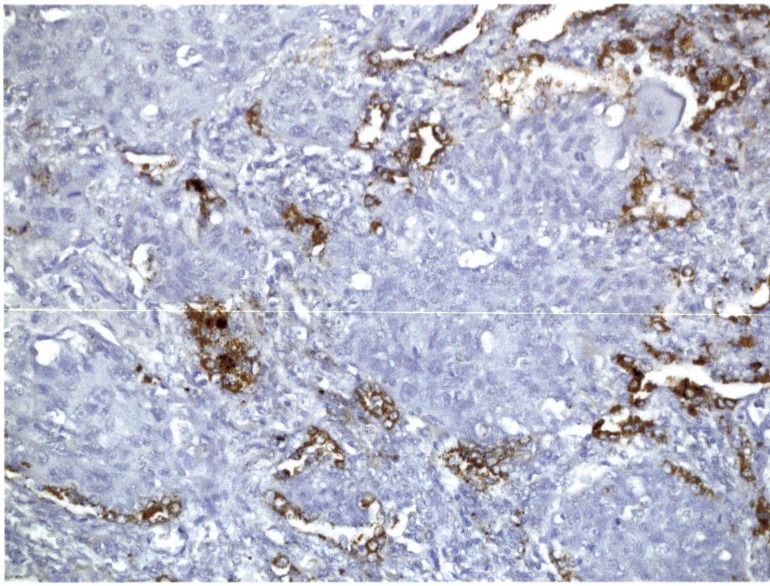

**Fig. 5.7** Napsin A expression seen in type II pneumocytes/intra-alveolar pneumocytes entrapped in poorly differentiated squamous cell carcinoma

adenocarcinoma and negative in squamous cell carcinoma. This finding might be helpful when dealing with TTF-1 negative poorly differentiated carcinoma since CK7 reaction tends to be retained in poorly differentiated adenocarcinoma, which is occasionally TTF-1 negative. However, this marker solely is not specific enough to stand as an adenocarcinoma marker. Indeed, 95 % of adenocarcinoma is positive for CK7, and 20 % of lung squamous cell carcinoma is also positive for CK7 [58]. These findings lead to the conclusion that CK7 should not be used to differentiate between adenocarcinoma and squamous cell carcinoma [4].

There are several antibodies specific for Clara cells and type II pneumocytes, which have been tested in pulmonary adenocarcinomas. As expected, they are expressed predominantly in well-differentiated adenocarcinoma but not in poorly differentiated carcinoma; therefore, they are not particularly useful in the setting of poorly differentiated tumors.

**Surfactant protein-A (Sp-A)** is expressed in Clara cells and type II pneumocytes of the lung parenchyma, and its gene expression is regulated by TTF-1 [86]. It is a marker for tumors differentiating into cells of such lineage and has high specificity, but sensitivity is low, and as expected it is usually negative in poorly differentiated adenocarcinomas. The monoclonal antibody PE10 detected Sp-A in 24–74 % of lung adenocarcinomas by using clone PE10, which is now out of production [62, 87–89]. No expression was seen in squamous cell carcinoma by using clone PE10 [62] or clone 32E12 [71].

**Surfactant protein-B (Sp-B)** is also detected in type II pneumocytes and Clara cells. Likewise, Sp-B is generally expressed by well-differentiated tumors but much more infrequently by poorly differentiated tumors. The reported specificity ranges from 80 to100%, but its sensitivity is 38–61 % [27, 29, 56].

**DC-LAMP (CD208)** and **CC-10 (Clara cell protein 10)** also stain differentiated pulmonary adenocarcinomas with Clara cell differentiation, but they are usually negative in poorly differentiated adenocarcinomas where immunohistochemistry is usually needed for histotyping; therefore, the usage of these markers is limited to more academic purposes [89].

## Large Cell Carcinoma

The entity represents poorly differentiated carcinoma where the tumor lacks morphological features of squamous cell carcinoma, adenocarcinoma, or small cell carcinoma. As such, the diagnosis requires thorough sampling of the resected tumor, and its definitive diagnosis is not made based on a small biopsy or cytologic material. It is a morphologically defined entity; however, it is known that a proportion of large cell carcinoma, not otherwise specified, expresses lineage markers for either squamous cell or adenocarcinoma [35]. A recent study showed that approximately 80 % of this group of tumor can be classified as variants of adenocarcinoma (60 %) or squamous cell carcinoma (20 %), when defined by TTF-1+/p40– for adenocarcinoma variant, TTF-1-/p40+ for squamous cell carcinoma variant, TTF-1+/p40+ for adenosquamous carcinoma variant, and TTF-1-/p40– for null type [90]. Interestingly, molecular alterations characteristic of adenocarcinoma occurred in tumors with immunoprofiles of adenocarcinoma or marker null but not in tumors with squamous immunoprofiles. Whether such tumors should be classified to adenocarcinoma or squamous cell carcinoma solely by immunohistochemistry is arguable from the point of histology-based classification [91], but the abovementioned molecular findings support some therapeutic relevance for immunohistochemistry-based classifications.

**Basaloid carcinoma** expresses squamous-lineage markers such as HMW-CKs and p63 [44, 52]. Basaloid carcinoma shares morphological features with small cell carcinoma and large cell neuroendocrine carcinoma, and this may cause great diagnostic difficulties, particularly when dealing with a small biopsy or fine-needle biopsy specimens. Focal expression of neuroendocrine markers further complicates the diagnostic dilemma [92]. Basaloid carcinoma is negative for TTF-1 and almost invariably positive for 34βE12, while high-grade neuroendocrine carcinoma often expresses TTF-1 but it is negative for 34βE12.

**Lymphoepithelioma-like carcinoma** is a distinct clinicopathologic entity with characteristic morphological features, and similar to the more familiar nasopharyngeal counter, most of the cases reported in Asians are associated with Epstein-Barr virus (EBV) [93]. Evidence of EBV can be demonstrated by both immunohistochemistry and in situ hybridization. Detection of EBER-1 RNA by in situ hybridization method is very sensitive. Immunohistochemistry with antibodies to latent membrane protein 1 (LMP1) is less sensitive and often results in heterogeneous staining reaction. The tumors in Caucasians are less frequently associated with EBV [93].

## Sarcomatoid Carcinoma

Multiple keratin antibodies can demonstrate the epithelial lineage of spindle and pleomorphic cell components in many of the cases. AE1/3, CAM 5.2, CK18, and CK7 are positive more frequently than epithelial membrane antigen (EMA), carcinoembryonic antigen (CEA), CD15, and Ber-EP4. Keratin antibodies may also highlight the epithelial component of carcinosarcoma. Positive epithelial markers are not required for diagnosis if components of differentiated carcinoma such as adenocarcinoma or squamous cell carcinoma are present. Sarcomatoid carcinoma that is negative for any of the epithelial markers is difficult to separate from sarcoma. Alternatively, expression of epithelial markers, particularly, low molecular weight cytokeratins in the sarcoma, has a weak and focal staining quality [94]. Conversely, a true strong CK expression is also seen in certain sarcomas with epithelioid morphology, such as synovial sarcoma, epithelioid hemangioendothelioma, and epithelioid sarcoma.

Vimentin is usually diffusely positive in sarcomatoid carcinoma, and it may support the morphological interpretation of sarcomatoid carcinoma since it is infrequently expressed in squamous cell carcinoma and adenocarcinoma, with usually focal staining extent [46].

Muscle markers and S100 protein stain rhabdomyosarcoma and chondrosarcoma, respectively, when present in either carcinosarcoma or pulmonary blastoma.

CK7 is positive in approximately 60–70 % of spindle or giant cell component of sarcomatoid carcinoma. The frequency is higher in sarcomatoid carcinoma associated with adenocarcinoma than tumors associated with squamous cell carcinoma (80 % vs. 16 %) [95]. Only a subset of sarcomatoid carcinoma expresses TTF-1 (55 %), which is useful in supporting the pulmonary origin of these tumors, and its expression is usually focal [95]. Approximately 80 % of sarcomatoid carcinoma is accompanied by better differentiated carcinoma component, such as squamous cell carcinoma or adenocarcinoma [95]. If a tumor presents as a solitary lung tumor with no history of tumors in other anatomic location, and a tumor expresses epithelial markers such as cytokeratins, or a tumor is associated with better differentiated component, the diagnosis of sarcomatoid carcinoma can be rendered with confidence, but in the absence of these features, the diagnosis can be challenging, with differential diagnosis lying between sarcomatoid carcinoma and sarcoma, either primary or metastatic, or when pleura is diffusely involved, sarcomatoid mesothelioma. Synovial sarcoma, which is the most common primary lung sarcoma, can be ruled out by examining the characteristic translocation t(X;18)(p11;q11) by FISH or RT-PCR. However, for the majority of cases, solid diagnosis cannot be rendered by histology and immunohistochemistry alone, and clinical and radiographical correlations are necessary for disease management.

Differentiation from sarcomatoid mesothelioma is challenging since both share morphological and immunohistochemical similarities, and requires a panel of immunohistochemical stains. Mesothelial markers, such as calretinin, CK5/6, and WT1, are less frequently expressed in sarcomatoid mesothelioma, and sarcomatoid component of biphasic mesothelioma and their reactions are generally weaker than epithelioid component, while these markers are commonly expressed in spindle cell component of sarcomatoid carcinoma and sarcoma [96]. Approximately 85 % of sarcomatoid mesothelioma expresses D2-40 to variable extent, while only 25 % of sarcomatoid carcinoma shows weak D2-40 expression [96]; therefore, D2-40 may be useful in this differential context. However, identification of epithelial component may be the only clue for the correct diagnosis of sarcomatoid carcinoma.

## Salivary Gland-Type Carcinoma

In general, the diagnosis of salivary gland-type tumor is based on conventional morphological features, and immunohistochemistry plays only a small role in subtyping this group of tumor. Immunohistochemistry may be useful to confirm ductal (luminal) differentiation by CEA and EMA and abluminal (myoepithelial) differentiation by SMA, calponin, p63, CK14, S100, GFAP, and vimentin as it is routinely performed in salivary gland [97].

## Minimalistic Approach to Subclassify a Poorly Differentiated Non-small Cell Carcinoma in Small Specimens

Due to the increasing demand for molecular analysis, pathologists are expected to subtype the tumor and simultaneously preserve diagnostic tissue for further testing. In order to achieve this goal, a minimal panel of immunohistochemistry should be applied. Unrestrained use of immunohistochemistry should be avoided [65].

Among the readily available and well-investigated markers, a number of recent studies in the literature found efficacy in TTF-1 and Napsin A as adenomarker and p63, p40, and CK5/6 as squamous marker, based on high sensitivity in those squamous markers (particularly p63 and p40, though less so for CK5/6) and high specificity in adenomarkers [2, 4, 5, 11, 12, 26, 31, 39, 40, 46, 58, 59, 61]. The following approach may be useful to interpret the results from these immunohistochemistry stains [4, 9, 46] (Fig. 5.8):

1. Expression of TTF-1 and/or Napsin A favors adenocarcinoma differentiation, even though the expression is weak or focal.
2. Diffuse p63, p40, and/or CK5/6 expression favors squamous cell carcinoma if TTF-1 or Napsin A is negative. p63 and p40 expressions are usually uniform in squamous cell carcinoma regardless of tumor grade, while CK5/6 can be focal in poorly differentiated tumor.
3. Negative expression of p63 and CK5/6 excludes squamous cell carcinoma. Even when TTF-1 and Napsin A are negative, adenocarcinoma is favored. Tumors with this immunoprofile are often diffusely positive for CK7.

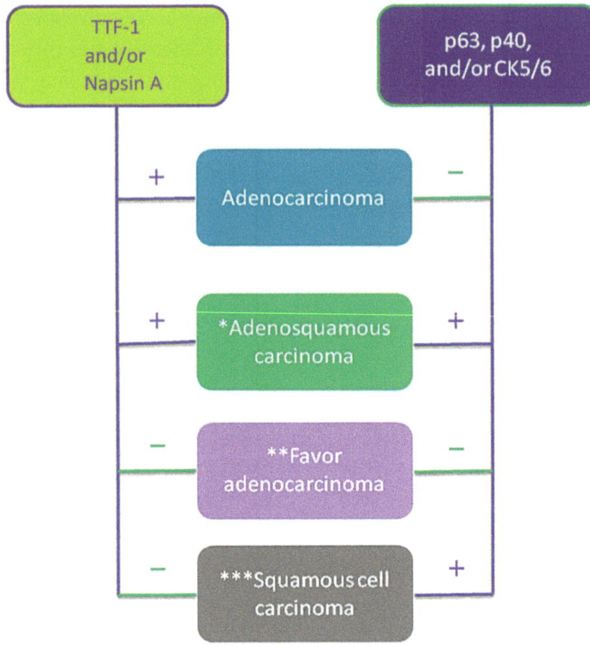


**Fig. 5.8** Minimalistic approach to subclassify a poorly differentiated non-small cell carcinoma in small specimens. (*) Positivity for both markers seen in different cell population. If the same cells express TTF-1 and p63, this is compatible with an adenocarcinoma. (**) Correlate with the clinical history to ensure that the tumor does not represent metastasis from other organs. (***) Strong and diffuse positivity for p63 or p40 is consistent with squamous cell carcinoma; focal and weak positivity for p63 and p40 is compatible with adenocarcinoma and NSCLC-NOS, respectively

4. Focal p63 expression does not necessarily exclude adenocarcinoma. When the tumor is focally p63 positive and TTF-1 (or Napsin A) negative, p40 and/or CK5/6 may correctly stratify the tumor into squamous cell carcinoma (p40/CK5/6 positive) or adenocarcinoma (p40/CK5/6 negative). If TTF-1 (or Napsin A) is also positive, the possibility of adenosquamous carcinoma should also be considered if the tumor cells staining for TTF-1 and p63 are segregated into different areas of the tissue. Expression of both markers in the same cells does not constitute evidence of adenosquamous carcinoma.

The most economical panel is a combination of TTF-1 and p40, or alternatively TTF-1 and p63, with the addition of CK5/6 in the scenario described in (4). Napsin A can be added since there are rare cases where TTF-1 is positive and Napsin A is negative, or vice versa [4, 62]. By using a panel of immunohistochemistry, discrepancies between biopsies and resections are rare [4, 5].

## References

1. Ou SH, Zell JA. Carcinoma NOS is a common histologic diagnosis and is increasing in proportion among non-small cell lung cancer histologies. J Thorac Oncol. 2009;4:1202–11.
2. Loo PS, Thomas SC, Nicolson MC, Fyfe MN, Kerr KM. Subtyping of undifferentiated non-small cell carcinomas in bronchial biopsy specimens. J Thorac Oncol. 2010;5:442–7.

3. Rossi G, Papotti M, Barbareschi M, Graziano P, Pelosi G. Morphology and a limited number of immunohistochemical markers may efficiently subtype non-small-cell lung cancer. J Clin Oncol. 2009;27:e141–2.
4. Mukhopadhyay S, Katzenstein AL. Subclassification of non-small cell lung carcinomas lacking morphologic differentiation on biopsy specimens: Utility of an immunohistochemical panel containing TTF-1, napsin A, p63, and CK5/6. Am J Surg Pathol. 2011;35:15–25.
5. Rekhtman N, Ang DC, Sima CS, Travis WD, Moreira AL. Immunohistochemical algorithm for differentiation of lung adenocarcinoma and squamous cell carcinoma based on large series of whole-tissue sections with validation in small specimens. Mod Pathol. 2011;24:1348–59.
6. Terry J, Leung S, Laskin J, Leslie KO, Gown AM, Ionescu DN. Optimal immunohistochemical markers for distinguishing lung adenocarcinomas from squamous cell carcinomas in small tumor samples. Am J Surg Pathol. 2010;34:1805–11.
7. Amatya VJ, Takeshima Y, Kohno H, et al. Caveolin-1 is a novel immunohistochemical marker to differentiate epithelioid mesothelioma from lung adenocarcinoma. Histopathology. 2009;55:10–9.
8. Au NH, Gown AM, Cheang M, et al. P63 expression in lung carcinoma: a tissue microarray study of 408 cases. Appl Immunohistochem Mol Morphol. 2004;12:240–7.
9. Bishop JA, Benjamin H, Cholakh H, Chajut A, Clark DP, Westra WH. Accurate classification of non-small cell lung carcinoma using a novel microRNA-based approach. Clin Cancer Res. 2010;16:610–9.
10. Bishop JA, Sharma R, Illei PB. Napsin A and thyroid transcription factor-1 expression in carcinomas of the lung, breast, pancreas, colon, kidney, thyroid, and malignant mesothelioma. Hum Pathol. 2010;41:20–5.
11. Brown AF, Sirohi D, Fukuoka J, et al. Tissue-preserving antibody cocktails to differentiate primary squamous cell carcinoma, adenocarcinoma, and small cell carcinoma of lung. Arch Pathol Lab Med. 2013;137:1274–81.
12. Brunnstrom H, Johansson L, Jirstrom K, Jonsson M, Jonsson P, Planck M. Immunohistochemistry in the differential diagnostics of primary lung cancer: an investigation within the Southern Swedish Lung Cancer Study. Am J Clin Pathol. 2013;140:37–46.
13. Chang YL, Lee YC, Liao WY, Wu CT. The utility and limitation of thyroid transcription factor-1 protein in primary and metastatic pulmonary neoplasms. Lung Cancer. 2004;44: 149–57.
14. Chu PG, Lyda MH, Weiss LM. Cytokeratin 14 expression in epithelial neoplasms: a survey of 435 cases with emphasis on its value in differentiating squamous cell carcinomas from other epithelial tumours. Histopathology. 2001;39:9–16.
15. Dejmek A, Naucler P, Smedjeback A, et al. Napsin A (TA02) is a useful alternative to thyroid transcription factor-1 (TTF-1) for the identification of pulmonary adenocarcinoma cells in pleural effusions. Diagn Cytopathol. 2007;35:493–7.
16. Fatima N, Cohen C, Lawson D, Siddiqui MT. TTF-1 and Napsin A double stain: a useful marker for diagnosing lung adenocarcinoma on fine-needle aspiration cell blocks. Cancer Cytopathol. 2011;119:127–33.
17. Gruver AM, Amin MB, Luthringer DJ, et al. Selective immunohistochemical markers to distinguish between metastatic high-grade urothelial carcinoma and primary poorly differentiated invasive squamous cell carcinoma of the lung. Arch Pathol Lab Med. 2012;136:1339–46.
18. Hirano T, Auer G, Maeda M, et al. Human tissue distribution of TA02, which is homologous with a new type of aspartic proteinase, napsin A. Jpn J Cancer Res. 2000;91:1015–21.
19. Hirano T, Gong Y, Yoshida K, et al. Usefulness of TA02 (napsin A) to distinguish primary lung adenocarcinoma from metastatic lung adenocarcinoma. Lung Cancer. 2003;41:155–62.
20. Inamura K, Satoh Y, Okumura S, et al. Pulmonary adenocarcinomas with enteric differentiation: histologic and immunohistochemical characteristics compared with metastatic colorectal cancers and usual pulmonary adenocarcinomas. Am J Surg Pathol. 2005;29:660–5.
21. Jain D, Mathur SR, Guleria R, Iyer VK. Utility and pattern of positivity of p40 in the diagnosis of squamous cell carcinoma of the lung by cytology: the first study on fine needle aspiration smears. Cytopathology 2014.

22. Jerome MV, Mazieres J, Groussard O, et al. Expression of TTF-1 and cytokeratins in primary and secondary epithelial lung tumours: correlation with histological type and grade. Histopathology. 2004;45:125–34.
23. Jiang B, Wu GP, Zhao YJ, Wang SC. Transcription expression and clinical significance of TTF-1 mRNA in pleural effusion of patients with lung cancer. Diagn Cytopathol. 2008;36: 849–54.
24. Johansson L. Histopathologic classification of lung cancer: Relevance of cytokeratin and TTF-1 immunophenotyping. Ann Diagn Pathol. 2004;8:259–67.
25. Kalhor N, Zander DS, Liu J. TTF-1 and p63 for distinguishing pulmonary small-cell carcinoma from poorly differentiated squamous cell carcinoma in previously pap-stained cytologic material. Mod Pathol. 2006;19:1117–23.
26. Kargi A, Gurel D, Tuna B. The diagnostic value of TTF-1, CK 5/6, and p63 immunostaining in classification of lung carcinomas. Appl Immunohistochem Mol Morphol. 2007;15:415–20.
27. Kaufmann O, Dietel M. Thyroid transcription factor-1 is the superior immunohistochemical marker for pulmonary adenocarcinomas and large cell carcinomas compared to surfactant proteins A and B. Histopathology. 2000;36:8–16.
28. Khayyata S, Yun S, Pasha T, et al. Value of P63 and CK5/6 in distinguishing squamous cell carcinoma from adenocarcinoma in lung fine-needle aspiration specimens. Diagn Cytopathol. 2009;37:178–83.
29. Khoor A, Whitsett JA, Stahlman MT, Olson SJ, Cagle PT. Utility of surfactant protein B precursor and thyroid transcription factor 1 in differentiating adenocarcinoma of the lung from malignant mesothelioma. Hum Pathol. 1999;30:695–700.
30. Kim JH, Kim YS, Choi YD, Lee JS, Park CS. Utility of napsin A and thyroid transcription factor 1 in differentiating metastatic pulmonary from non-pulmonary adenocarcinoma in pleural effusion. Acta Cytol. 2011;55:266–70.
31. Kim MJ, Shin HC, Shin KC, Ro JY. Best immunohistochemical panel in distinguishing adenocarcinoma from squamous cell carcinoma of lung: tissue microarray assay in resected lung cancer specimens. Ann Diagn Pathol. 2013;17:85–90.
32. Liu J, Farhood A. Immunostaining for thyroid transcription factor-1 on fine-needle aspiration specimens of lung tumors: a comparison of direct smears and cell block preparations. Cancer. 2004;102:109–14.
33. Maeshima AM, Omatsu M, Tsuta K, Asamura H, Matsuno Y. Immunohistochemical expression of TTF-1 in various cytological subtypes of primary lung adenocarcinoma, with special reference to intratumoral heterogeneity. Pathol Int. 2008;58:31–7.
34. Matoso A, Singh K, Jacob R, et al. Comparison of thyroid transcription factor-1 expression by 2 monoclonal antibodies in pulmonary and nonpulmonary primary tumors. Appl Immunohistochem Mol Morphol. 2010;18:142–9.
35. Monica V, Ceppi P, Righi L, et al. Desmocollin-3: a new marker of squamous differentiation in undifferentiated large-cell carcinoma of the lung. Mod Pathol. 2009;22:709–17.
36. Mukhopadhyay S, Katzenstein AL. Comparison of monoclonal napsin A, polyclonal napsin A, and TTF-1 for determining lung origin in metastatic adenocarcinomas. Am J Clin Pathol. 2012;138:703–11.
37. Myong NH. Thyroid transcription factor-1 (TTF-1) expression in human lung carcinomas: its prognostic implication and relationship with expressions of p53 and Ki-67 proteins. J Korean Med Sci. 2003;18:494–500.
38. Nakamura N, Miyagi E, Murata S, Kawaoi A, Katoh R. Expression of thyroid transcription factor-1 in normal and neoplastic lung tissues. Mod Pathol. 2002;15:1058–67.
39. Nicholson AG, Gonzalez D, Shah P, et al. Refining the diagnosis and EGFR status of non-small cell lung carcinoma in biopsy and cytologic material, using a panel of mucin staining, TTF-1, cytokeratin 5/6, and P63, and EGFR mutation analysis. J Thorac Oncol. 2010;5:436–41.
40. Noh S, Shim H. Optimal combination of immunohistochemical markers for subclassification of non-small cell lung carcinomas: A tissue microarray study of poorly differentiated areas. Lung Cancer. 2012;76:51–5.

41. Nonaka D. A study of DeltaNp63 expression in lung non-small cell carcinomas. Am J Surg Pathol. 2012;36:895–9.
42. Ocque R, Tochigi N, Ohori NP, Dacic S. Usefulness of immunohistochemical and histochemical studies in the classification of lung adenocarcinoma and squamous cell carcinoma in cytologic specimens. Am J Clin Pathol. 2011;136:81–7.
43. Ordonez NG. The diagnostic utility of immunohistochemistry in distinguishing between epithelioid mesotheliomas and squamous carcinomas of the lung: a comparative study. Mod Pathol. 2006;19:417–28.
44. Pardo J, Martinez-Penuela AM, Sola JJ, et al. Large cell carcinoma of the lung: an endangered species? Appl Immunohistochem Mol Morphol. 2009;17:383–92.
45. Pelosi G, Fraggetta F, Pasini F, et al. Immunoreactivity for thyroid transcription factor-1 in stage I non-small cell carcinomas of the lung. Am J Surg Pathol. 2001;25:363–72.
46. Pelosi G, Rossi G, Bianchi F, et al. Immunohistochemistry by means of widely agreed-upon markers (cytokeratins 5/6 and 7, p63, thyroid transcription factor-1, and vimentin) on small biopsies of non-small cell lung cancer effectively parallels the corresponding profiling and eventual diagnoses on surgical specimens. J Thorac Oncol. 2011;6:1039–49.
47. Pelosi G, Rossi G, Cavazza A, et al. DeltaNp63 (p40) distribution inside lung cancer: a driver biomarker approach to tumor characterization. Int J Surg Pathol. 2013;21:229–39.
48. Pomplun S, Wotherspoon AC, Shah G, Goldstraw P, Ladas G, Nicholson AG. Immunohistochemical markers in the differentiation of thymic and pulmonary neoplasms. Histopathology. 2002;40:152–8.
49. Righi L, Graziano P, Fornari A, et al. Immunohistochemical subtyping of nonsmall cell lung cancer not otherwise specified in fine-needle aspiration cytology: a retrospective study of 103 cases with surgical correlation. Cancer. 2011;117:3416–23.
50. Rossi G, Marchioni A, Milani M, et al. TTF-1, cytokeratin 7, 34betaE12, and CD56/NCAM immunostaining in the subclassification of large cell carcinomas of the lung. Am J Clin Pathol. 2004;122:884–93.
51. Stoll LM, Johnson MW, Gabrielson E, Askin F, Clark DP, Li QK. The utility of napsin-A in the identification of primary and metastatic lung adenocarcinoma among cytologically poorly differentiated carcinomas. Cancer Cytopathol. 2010;118:441–9.
52. Sturm N, Lantuejoul S, Laverriere MH, et al. Thyroid transcription factor 1 and cytokeratins 1, 5, 10, 14 (34betaE12) expression in basaloid and large-cell neuroendocrine carcinomas of the lung. Hum Pathol. 2001;32:918–25.
53. Suzuki A, Shijubo N, Yamada G, et al. Napsin A is useful to distinguish primary lung adenocarcinoma from adenocarcinomas of other organs. Pathol Res Pract. 2005;201:579–86.
54. Tan D, Li Q, Deeb G, et al. Thyroid transcription factor-1 expression prevalence and its clinical implications in non-small cell lung cancer: a high-throughput tissue microarray and immunohistochemistry study. Hum Pathol. 2003;34:597–604.
55. Tsuta K, Tanabe Y, Yoshida A, et al. Utility of 10 immunohistochemical markers including novel markers (desmocollin-3, glypican 3, S100A2, S100A7, and Sox-2) for differential diagnosis of squamous cell carcinoma from adenocarcinoma of the Lung. J Thorac Oncol. 2011;6:1190–9.
56. Ueno T, Linder S, Elmberger G. Aspartic proteinase napsin is a useful marker for diagnosis of primary lung adenocarcinoma. Br J Cancer. 2003;88:1229–33.
57. Wang LJ, Greaves WO, Sabo E, et al. GCDFP-15 positive and TTF-1 negative primary lung neoplasms: a tissue microarray study of 381 primary lung tumors. Appl Immunohistochem Mol Morphol. 2009;17:505–11.
58. Warth A, Muley T, Herpel E, et al. Large-scale comparative analyses of immunomarkers for diagnostic subtyping of non-small-cell lung cancer biopsies. Histopathology. 2012;61:1017–25.
59. Whithaus K, Fukuoka J, Prihoda TJ, Jagirdar J. Evaluation of napsin A, cytokeratin 5/6, p63, and thyroid transcription factor 1 in adenocarcinoma versus squamous cell carcinoma of the lung. Arch Pathol Lab Med. 2012;136:155–62.

60. Wu M, Wang B, Gil J, et al. p63 and TTF-1 immunostaining. A useful marker panel for distinguishing small cell carcinoma of lung from poorly differentiated squamous cell carcinoma of lung. Am J Clin Pathol. 2003;119:696–702.
61. Yanagita E, Imagawa N, Ohbayashi C, Itoh T. Rapid multiplex immunohistochemistry using the 4-antibody cocktail YANA-4 in differentiating primary adenocarcinoma from squamous cell carcinoma of the lung. Appl Immunohistochem Mol Morphol. 2011;19:509–13.
62. Yang M, Nonaka D. A study of immunohistochemical differential expression in pulmonary and mammary carcinomas. Mod Pathol. 2010;23:654–61.
63. Ye J, Findeis-Hosey JJ, Yang Q, et al. Combination of napsin A and TTF-1 immunohistochemistry helps in differentiating primary lung adenocarcinoma from metastatic carcinoma in the lung. Appl Immunohistochem Mol Morphol. 2011;19:313–7.
64. Yoshida A, Tsuta K, Watanabe S, et al. Frequent ALK rearrangement and TTF-1/p63 co-expression in lung adenocarcinoma with signet-ring cell component. Lung Cancer. 2011;72:309–15.
65. Rossi G, Tiseo M, Cavazza A, Colby TV. Is immunohistochemistry always required to diagnose lung cancer? Adv Anat Pathol. 2013;20:327–33.
66. Butnor KJ, Burchette JL. p40 (DeltaNp63) and keratin 34betaE12 provide greater diagnostic accuracy than p63 in the evaluation of small cell lung carcinoma in small biopsy samples. Hum Pathol. 2013;44:1479–86.
67. Chu PG, Weiss LM. Keratin expression in human tissues and neoplasms. Histopathology. 2002;40:403–39.
68. Ordonez NG. Value of cytokeratin 5/6 immunostaining in distinguishing epithelial mesothelioma of the pleura from lung adenocarcinoma. Am J Surg Pathol. 1998;22:1215–21.
69. Chen Y, Cui T, Yang L, et al. The diagnostic value of cytokeratin 5/6, 14, 17, and 18 expression in human non-small cell lung cancer. Oncology. 2011;80:333–40.
70. Miettinen M, Sarlomo-Rikala M. Expression of calretinin, thrombomodulin, keratin 5, and mesothelin in lung carcinomas of different types: an immunohistochemical analysis of 596 tumors in comparison with epithelioid mesotheliomas of the pleura. Am J Surg Pathol. 2003;27:150–8.
71. Sakai Y, Nakai T, Ohbayashi C, et al. Immunohistochemical profiling of ALK fusion gene-positive adenocarcinomas of the lung. Int J Surg Pathol. 2013;21:476–82.
72. Kitajima Y. New insights into desmosome regulation and pemphigus blistering as a desmosome-remodeling disease. Kaohsiung J Med Sci. 2013;29:1–13.
73. Fukuoka J, Dracheva T, Shih JH, et al. Desmoglein 3 as a prognostic factor in lung cancer. Hum Pathol. 2007;38:276–83.
74. Agackiran Y, Ozcan A, Akyurek N, Memis L, Findik G, Kaya S. Desmoglein-3 and Napsin A double stain, a useful immunohistochemical marker for differentiation of lung squamous cell carcinoma and adenocarcinoma from other subtypes. Appl Immunohistochem Mol Morphol. 2012;20:350–5.
75. Savci-Heijink CD, Kosari F, Aubry MC, et al. The role of desmoglein-3 in the diagnosis of squamous cell carcinoma of the lung. Am J Pathol. 2009;174:1629–37.
76. Candi E, Cipollone R. Rivetti d, V, Gonfloni S, Melino G, Knight R. p63 in epithelial development. Cell Mol Life Sci. 2008;65:3126–33.
77. Bishop JA, Teruya-Feldstein J, Westra WH, Pelosi G, Travis WD, Rekhtman N. p40 (DeltaNp63) is superior to p63 for the diagnosis of pulmonary squamous cell carcinoma. Mod Pathol. 2012;25:405–15.
78. Di Como CJ, Urist MJ, Babayan I, et al. p63 expression profiles in human normal and tumor tissues. Clin Cancer Res. 2002;8:494–501.
79. Ivan D, Hafeez DA, Prieto VG. Expression of p63 in primary cutaneous adnexal neoplasms and adenocarcinoma metastatic to the skin. Mod Pathol. 2005;18:137–42.
80. Pelosi G, Fabbri A, Bianchi F, et al. DeltaNp63 (p40) and thyroid transcription factor-1 immunoreactivity on small biopsies or cellblocks for typing non-small cell lung cancer: a novel two-hit, sparing-material approach. J Thorac Oncol. 2012;7:281–90.

81. Ordonez NG. Napsin A, expression in lung and kidney neoplasia: a review and update. Adv Anat Pathol. 2012;19:66–73.
82. Ordonez NG. Value of thyroid transcription factor-1 immunostaining in tumor diagnosis: a review and update. Appl Immunohistochem Mol Morphol. 2012;20:429–44.
83. Guazzi S, Price M, De Felice M, Damante G, Mattei MG, Di Lauro R. Thyroid nuclear factor 1 (TTF-1) contains a homeodomain and displays a novel DNA binding specificity. EMBO J. 1990;9:3631–9.
84. Yatabe Y, Mitsudomi T, Takahashi T. TTF-1 expression in pulmonary adenocarcinomas. Am J Surg Pathol. 2002;26:767–73.
85. Brasch F, Ochs M, Kahne T, et al. Involvement of napsin A in the C- and N-terminal processing of surfactant protein B in type-II pneumocytes of the human lung. J Biol Chem. 2003;278:49006–14.
86. Whitsett JA, Glasser SW. Regulation of surfactant protein gene transcription. Biochim Biophys Acta. 1998;1408:303–11.
87. Mizutani Y, Nakajima T, Morinaga S, et al. Immunohistochemical localization of pulmonary surfactant apoproteins in various lung tumors. Special reference to nonmucus producing lung adenocarcinomas. Cancer. 1988;61:532–7.
88. Zamecnik J, Kodet R. Value of thyroid transcription factor-1 and surfactant apoprotein A in the differential diagnosis of pulmonary carcinomas: a study of 109 cases. Virchows Arch. 2002;440:353–61.
89. Zhu LC, Yim J, Chiriboga L, Cassai ND, Sidhu GS, Moreira AL. DC-LAMP stains pulmonary adenocarcinoma with bronchiolar Clara cell differentiation. Hum Pathol. 2007;38:260–8.
90. Rekhtman N, Tafe LJ, Chaft JE, et al. Distinct profile of driver mutations and clinical features in immunomarker-defined subsets of pulmonary large-cell carcinoma. Mod Pathol. 2013;26:511–22.
91. Kerr KM. Classification of lung cancer: proposals for change? Arch Pathol Lab Med. 2012;136:1190–3.
92. Brambilla E, Moro D, Veale D, et al. Basal cell (basaloid) carcinoma of the lung: a new morphologic and phenotypic entity with separate prognostic significance. Hum Pathol. 1992;23: 993–1003.
93. Castro CY, Ostrowski ML, Barrios R, et al. Relationship between Epstein-Barr virus and lymphoepithelioma-like carcinoma of the lung: a clinicopathologic study of 6 cases and review of the literature. Hum Pathol. 2001;32:863–72.
94. Miettinen M. Keratin subsets in spindle cell sarcomas. Keratins are widespread but synovial sarcoma contains a distinctive keratin polypeptide pattern and desmoplakins. Am J Pathol. 1991;138:505–13.
95. Rossi G, Cavazza A, Sturm N, et al. Pulmonary carcinomas with pleomorphic, sarcomatoid, or sarcomatous elements: a clinicopathologic and immunohistochemical study of 75 cases. Am J Surg Pathol. 2003;27:311–24.
96. Takeshima Y, Amatya VJ, Kushitani K, Kaneko M, Inai K. Value of immunohistochemistry in the differential diagnosis of pleural sarcomatoid mesothelioma from lung sarcomatoid carcinoma. Histopathology. 2009;54:667–76.
97. Nagao T, Sato E, Inoue R, et al. Immunohistochemical analysis of salivary gland tumors: application for surgical pathology practice. Acta Histochem Cytochem. 2012;45:269–82.

# Chapter 6
# Adequacy and Utilization of Small Biopsy Material for Molecular Diagnosis

**Gilda da Cunha Santos**

## Clinical Application

Recent increase in the number of companion diagnostic assays for identification of individuals eligible for target therapies has expanded the use of small biopsies and cytological samples for molecular analysis.

The use of small samples, especially cytology material, for molecular tests for the diagnostic of several genomic abnormalities at the chromosomal and gene level such as specific translocations, gene rearrangements, and mutations in solid tumors has been well documented and reviewed recently in a number of publications [1–4]. Although the technical considerations and the pre-analytical variables for diagnostic and predictive assays do not differ between each other, this chapter will concentrate in assays currently in clinical practice in oncology that predict the response to approved targeted therapy to some specific biomarkers such as *EGFR* and *ALK*.

## Type of Samples and Pre-analytical Variables

The majority of non-small cell lung carcinomas (NSCLC) present with locally advanced or metastatic disease at the time of diagnosis and are not eligible for surgical resection; thus, interventional procedures required to acquire tumor tissue for diagnosis are difficult due to tumor location and patient comorbidities and most diagnostic material consists of small tissue samples, more specifically core

G. da Cunha Santos, M.D., Ph.D., FRCPC, FIAC (✉)
Department of Laboratory Medicine and Pathobiology, University of Toronto, University Health Network, 200 Elizabeth Street, 11th Floor, Eaton Wing,
Toronto, ON, Canada M5G 2C4
e-mail: gilda.santos@uhn.ca



A.L. Moreira, A. Saqi (eds.), *Diagnosing Non-small Cell Carcinoma in Small Biopsy and Cytology*, DOI 10.1007/978-1-4939-1607-8_6

needle biopsies and cytology material with minimal tumor content. Since biomarker studies have been usually structured using formalin-fixed paraffin-embedded (FFPE) tissue blocks from large surgical specimens, FFPE tissue blocks of core needle biopsies and FFPE cell blocks of fine needle aspiration (FNA) have been used more frequently in routine clinical practice for molecular assays.

More recently, studies have demonstrated optimal results using a multitude of different cytological samples for molecular tests. Good-quality DNA can be harvested from archival stained smears [5, 6]. Archival unstained cytospin preparations can also be used for molecular studies [7] as well as liquid-based preparations [3, 8]. The use of fresh cells obtained from FNA and body fluids warrants a better preservation of nucleic acids. Cryopreservation of fine-needle aspirates has been described to preserve morphology and nucleic acid integrity [9]. When using archived specimens (small biopsies or cytological samples), however, before the material can be scraped for subsequent DNA extraction, the coverslip must be removed. Recently, the "freezer method" has been described as a quick, safe, and efficient alternative to bathing slides in xylene, minimizing delays in this relatively easy, but time-consuming step [10].

One vital step, however, is the pre-analytical handling of the specimens, with attention drawn to variables affecting the collection of the sample and laboratory processing. The irreproducibility of many reported biomarkers is due at least in part to the fact that the biospecimens utilized are often procured using different collection, processing, and storage techniques. Such variability can lead to significant differences in biospecimen molecular integrity [11]. For standardized reliable assays, it has been recommended that at the time of tissue procurement, in the case of excisional/core biopsies and surgically resected specimens, the time spent between collection to fixation (cold ischemia time) should be minimized and ideally should be less than 30 min to avoid artifacts caused by degradation of nucleic acids and protein expression [12]. Overfixation should also be avoided before processing with recommended small tissue sections and fixation time of 8 h in formalin [13, 14]. Fixation times that are too short may render the tissue insufficiently protected against continuous enzymatic degradation and lead to suboptimal morphology, whereas prolonged fixation may lead to severe degradation of nucleic acids [15]. Since fixation and processing of cytological samples are steps almost always performed immediately after sample collection, it might be expected that cell blocks have better preserved material and consequently nucleic acids for obtaining consistent reliable results. In fact, FNA minimizes ischemia and produces biospecimens comprising live cells that can be quick-frozen and may provide more accurate assessments of biochemical pathway function and tumor drug sensitivity than is possible using standard FFPE tissue sections [16]. Although 10 % neutral buffered formalin has been widely used in pathology laboratories and the recommended fixative for histological and cytological samples [17, 18], its adverse effect of cross-linking of proteins and nucleic acids resulting in fragmented nucleic acids and high frequency of sequence alterations has been well documented [19, 20]. Different fixatives are routinely used for cytological specimens, especially ethanol based, and they are usually adequate for different molecular assays; however, protocols might differ from formalin-fixed material and should be adapted/validated [21, 22]. Samples fixed with acid fixatives, especially those submitted to decalcifying agents, are not recommended for molecular analysis due to degraded DNA [14]. Ethylenediaminetetraacetic acid (EDTA) is an effective decalcifying agent, has no effect on DNA quality, and should be used in samples where decalcification is required and molecular studies are anticipated [17]. For bone metastasis FNA is the procedure of choice and highly indicated since decalcification is rarely required. Cytological materials, specifically FNA samples, have some advantages over needle biopsies for molecular tests such as a naturally enriched tumor cell population with low stromal content, the possibility of sampling multiple wide areas being more representative of the target lesion, the rapid on-site evaluation (ROSE) for assessing tumor content and sample adequacy with immediate triage of material for ancillary tests including multiple molecular studies, and better DNA preservation due to immediate fixation and the use of air-dried and/or alcohol-fixed smears for long storage and future analysis.

Recent papers have highlighted that more important than the quantity of cells is the quality of the material obtained from cytological samples [23, 24]. In a large series comparing cytological and histological samples, a lack of any association between the DNA concentration and the likelihood of unsatisfactory results was identified [23]. The authors hypothesize that the lack of formalin fixation may have accounted for the complete absence of unsatisfactory test outcomes in FNA or effusions direct smears or slide preparations tested for *EGFR* mutations. The need for well-preserved tissues and cells has led to the investigation of alternative methods of preservation of specimens and standardization of protocols [21]. Novel strategies for storing fresh cells suspension have been described such as FTA cards for biobanking cytological material for future molecular analysis [25]. Residual material from the needle rinse of fine-needle aspirates stored on FTA cards yielded sufficient quantities of DNA for successful MassARRAY spectrometry [26].

## Molecular Assays

Molecular assays commonly used to detect genomic alterations are based on nucleic acid extraction and probes that target DNA or RNA. The detection technique to be employed will depend on the alteration to be detected and the type of preparation. Similarly to other laboratory tests, the pre-analytical variables such as sample collection, transportation, processing, and storage should be adequate and never overemphasized. Those variables can affect the results and standardized handling of the samples will lead to more accurate and reliable results.

The decision of which assay to use depends on the type of proposed analysis and type of specimen used.

Alterations at chromosomal and gene levels can be revealed by different techniques. An overview about the technical details and the requirements for using cytological specimens for FISH- and PCR-based analysis, as those techniques are the basis for assays used for the detection of *EGFR* mutations and *ALK* rearrangements in lung cancer, is described below.

## Fluorescence In Situ Hybridization

The technique is based on the use of nucleic acid probes labeled with fluorochromes to localize a specific target sequence in the sample tested. Probe is a sequence of nucleic acids that will hybridize to another sequence on the basis of base complementarity and allows identification and/or quantification of the target. The most commonly used probes in oncologic applications with cytological specimens are chromosome enumeration probes (CEP),. locus-specific indicator (LSI) probes, break-apart probes, and fusion probes.

A wide variety of cytological preparations have been used for FISH assays such as smears, cytospins, and FFPE cell blocks. For FFPE samples dewaxing will be the first step required. Stringent conditions might prevent nonspecific hybridization.

Factors such as reagent (including probe) concentrations and the temperature and timing of denaturation, hybridization, and slide washing contribute to the intensity of the probe signal and to the intensity of nonspecific fluorescence [27].

For FFPE samples (small biopsies and cell blocks), FISH may be performed either on 3–6 μm sections or in nuclei extracted from thick sections or cores from paraffin blocks. FISH performed on paraffin sections has the advantage of preserving specimen architecture, thus allowing the analysis to be focused on neoplastic tissue. However, sectioning causes nuclear truncation resulting in possible loss of signals in some nuclei. The technique of extraction of nuclei from thick sections yields whole nuclei, but tumor nuclei are admixed with normal nuclei from stromal and hematopoietic cells and cannot be distinguished from each other. Therefore, nuclear extraction should not be used for specimens in which tissue architecture is critical for interpretation such as *ALK* rearrangements in NSCLC. The interaction between the individuals scoring the FISH slide and a pathologist is strongly encouraged if there are any questionable findings [27].

The limitations of FISH are related to its high cost, especially at the time of the implementation of the technique, the use of specialized equipment (fluorescence microscope), and the limited number of alterations that can be detected at the same time. Alternative techniques that use bright-field microscopes are chromogenic in situ hybridization (CISH) and silver-enhanced in situ hybridization (SISH).

The application of this technique to cytological specimens has been growing and it will continue to increase due to the description of new abnormalities in solid tumors, such as the *ALK* rearrangement in lung adenocarcinomas.

## Polymerase Chain Reaction-Based Assays

Improvements and variations of the originally described protocol of polymerase chain reaction (PCR) and PCR-based assays have made this a popular, affordable, and high efficient technique. Currently, its main application is for mutation analysis in several malignant neoplasms.

The objective is to detect a specific DNA sequence (target DNA). The sequence of the target DNA should be known for designing the primers. In general, all protocols will have some adjustments for annealing temperature, cycle times, concentration of the reagents, and primer sequences in order to obtain optimal conditions for high yield and high specificity. Several strategies can confirm that the target sequence was present in the specimen by analysis of the PCR product. Subsequently, the amplicon produced by the polymerase reaction can be used for DNA sequencing and other techniques to check for the presence of any mutations.

Classic PCR followed by direct sequencing (Sanger sequencing) of areas of interest is a relatively cheap, well-established methodology, with various easily reproducible protocols published in the literature, and has been considered the "gold standard." It carries the advantage of being able to find not only the most commonly mutations present but also any additional mutation, being an exploratory technique. However, it is less sensitive and more time consuming than modern technologies, which may hamper its use in routine clinical application. Those limitations led to the investigation and development of alternative options of faster, less expensive, and high-sensitive techniques such as PCR restriction fragment length polymorphism (PCR-RFLP or fragment length analysis), locked nucleic acid PCR clamp (LNA-PCR clamp), COLD-TaqMan PCR, denaturing high-performance liquid chromatography (dHPLC), and Scorpion amplification refractory mutation system (Scorpion ARMS) that can detect common known mutations in samples with as little as 5 % of tumor cells. A list of those techniques that have been used for *EGFR* mutation testing of tumor tissue and cytological sample has been reported in detail in a recent review [28].

Pathological specimens consist of mutant and wild-type DNA from tumor cells admixed with wild-type DNA from nonneoplastic cells (normal epithelium, stromal, and hematopoietic cells). A major challenge for any molecular test is its ability to reliably detect mutations in samples consisting of a mixture of tumor cells and normal cells, especially when the tumor content is very low, such as the case for small biopsies and cytological samples [29]. The analytic sensitivity of mutation assays is defined as the allelic percentage and is a critical performance characteristic parameter to understand those assays and the minimal percentage of tumor cells necessary to accurately detect the mutation [2]. An analytic sensitivity of 5 % means that the assay can detect a mutation if it is present in at least 5 % of all alleles (normal and mutant combined). Therefore, 10 % of tumor cells would be required to be present in a sample for the detection of 5 % mutant alleles of a given gene, in case of a heterozygous mutation without amplification. In summary, for determining the minimal percentage of tumor cells required for reliable results, the analytic sensitivity of the mutation assay used should be known. However, it should be stressed that genomic abnormalities such as amplification and loss of heterozygosity might affect the percentage of the mutated allele which make impossible to calculate the percentage with certainty in all cases. The percentage of tumor cells present in biopsy specimens is usually estimated based on the fraction of surface area of the tumor tissue present in the slide. A recent article has concluded that the estimates of tumor cell percentages on H&E-stained slides are not accurate, which could result in misinterpretation of test results [29].

The authors have suggested that the estimates should be based on the number of nuclei present, which has been the method used for FFPE cell blocks by the author of this chapter, since for those cases the fraction of surface area of tumor tissue cannot be estimated. The overall cellularity (total number of normal and neoplastic nucleated cells), the tumor cellularity (total number of neoplastic cells), and the percentage of tumor present should be documented in the report. In addition, the type of fixation, the type of specimen, the type of cytological preparation, and the percentage of necrosis should also be reported. It has been also highlighted that pathologists should be cautious with the presence of lymphocytes and stromal cells (normal cells) that can dilute the tumor DNA, when selecting areas of tumor for manual or laser microdissection for DNA extraction [29]. Studies reporting *EGFR* mutation analysis using cytology have reported successful results in finding mutations in samples with as little as 1 % of tumor cells. Studies comparing the frequency of *EGFR* mutations among different types of specimens have not detected differences between biopsies and cytological samples [30, 31]. No difference was detected between FNA cell blocks and histological specimens from the same patient [32]. In the largest series consisting of histological and cytological samples, no significant differences in the failure rate, mutation rate, or mutation type were found between the two types of specimens. While tumor cellularity was significantly associated with test success or mutation rates in histology and cytology specimens, respectively, mutations could be detected in all specimen types [31]. FFPE cell blocks are as good a source of tumor cells for mutation testing as histology samples, regardless of fixative (alcohol or formalin), necrosis, or specimen type [31]. Interestingly in two large studies, pleural effusions had higher mutation rate when compared to histological specimens [30, 31]. In addition, the difference between patients with high and low abundance of EGFR mutations has been reported not significant regarding overall response rate and overall survival [33]. Therefore, it has been proposed that *EGFR* mutation testing should be attempted in any specimen. However, suboptimal samples (percentage of tumor cells below or at the same level of the test analytical sensitivity) with a negative *EGFR* mutation result should be considered for repeat testing with an alternate sample [31].

Fresh cell suspensions, smears (stained and unstained), cytospins, and FFPE cell blocks can be used to extract DNA for PCR-based assays.

## *EGFR* Mutations in Lung Cancer

In lung cancer, PCR-based assays are the methods of choice for procurement of mutations in *EGFR*. Mutations in the *EGFR* gene, such as single-nucleotide polymorphisms in exon 21 (L858R) and deletions in exon 19, constitute important biomarkers to dictate therapy against the ATP-binding site of the EGFR kinase domain, with the use of small-molecule tyrosine kinase inhibitors (TKIs), such as erlotinib and gefitinib, or monoclonal antibodies such as cetuximab. Of interest, mutations that confer resistance to these therapies, such as the T790M mutation in exon 20 of *EGFR* and mutations in *KRAS*, can also be readily recognizable by a multitude of PCR-based assays [34].

According to the recent CAP and IASLC molecular testing guideline for selection of lung cancer patients for therapy with *EGFR* and *ALK* inhibitors, laboratories may use any validated *EGFR* testing method, with the minimal number or percentage of tumor cells present in the sample being established at the discretion of each laboratory at the time of validation [18]. However, methods able to detect mutations in samples with at least 50 % of tumor cells have been recommended, with strong encouragement to use more sensitive tests, with accuracy of detecting mutations in samples with as little as 10 % of tumor cells. An example of an *EGFR*-mutated case is illustrated in Fig. 6.1. A list of recent series with more than 100 cases tested for *EGFR* mutations using cytological samples is shown in Table 6.1.

DNA can also be extracted from samples with low cellularity by the use of techniques for tumor cell enrichment such as manual microdissection and laser capture microdissection.

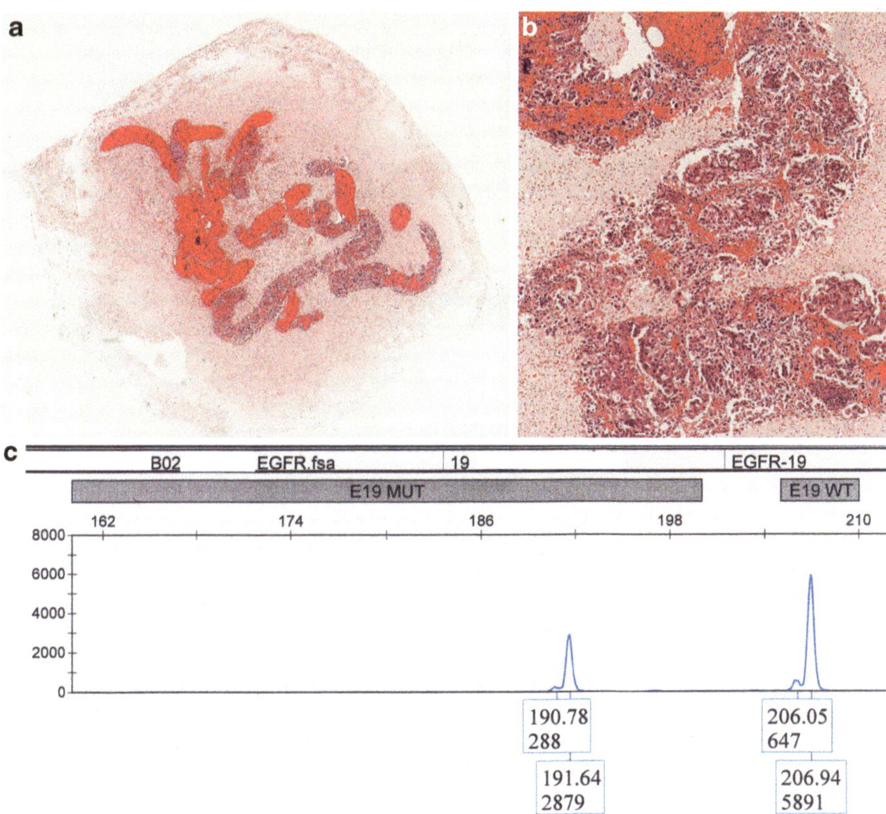


**Fig. 6.1** (**a**) Scanned cell block preparation slide of a lung fine-needle aspiration (FNA). (**b**) Formalin-fixed paraffin-embedded cell block preparation slide with high cellularity. (**c**) The inset shows *EGFR* exon 19 deletion detected by fragment analysis [(**a**) and (**b**) H&E staining. (**b**) Original magnification × 400]

**Table 6.1** Studies of *EGFR* somatic mutations using cytological specimens (publications with more than 100 cases)

| First author | Year | Patients, *n* (cytological samples) | Methods | Type of cytological samples | Type of preparations | *EGFR* mutations (%)[a] |
|---|---|---|---|---|---|---|
| Lozano | 2006 | 150 | Direct seq | FNA, PLE, PCE, BAL | AS, LBC, CB, FC | 17.3 % |
| Takano | 2007 | 117 (212[b]) | HRMA | TBNA, BB/W, PLE, PCE, FNA, Sputum | AS/CB | 41[b] |
| Molina-Vila | 2008 | 76 (268[b]) | Direct seq/Taq man assay/ length analysis | FNA, BAL, PLE, PCE | CB, FC/ LCM | 17.05[b] |
| Santis | 2011 | 126 | COLD-PCR | EBUS-TBNA | CB | 10 |
| Ma | 2012 | 269 | PCR Direct seq | Sputum BAL, BW, FNA, PLE | CB | 34.9 |
| Pang | 2012 | 140 | PCR Direct seq | FNA | AS | N/A |
| Malapelle | 2013 | 364 | Direct seq/Taq man assay/ fragment analysis | FNA | N/A | 8.8 |

[a]Considering the number of patients using cytological specimens with available material for analysis
[b]Data shown for cytology and surgical specimens together. Study did not show separate data just for the cytological samples analyzed
*PLE* pleural effusion, *HRMA* high-resolution melting analysis, *BB/W* bronchial brushing/washing, *PCE* pericardial effusion, *CB* cell blocks, *PCR* polymerase chain reaction, *FNA* fine-needle aspirates, *LCM* laser capture microdissection, *BAL* bronchoalveolar lavage

## *ALK* Rearrangements in Lung Cancer

A clinicopathologic subset of non-small cell lung carcinomas is characterized by an inversion on the short arm of chromosome 2 that juxtaposes the 5′ end of the echinoderm microtubule-associated protein-like 4 (*EML4*) gene with the 3′ end of the anaplastic lymphoma kinase (*ALK*) gene, resulting in a fusion oncogene *EML4-ALK*. Approximately 5 % of patients with NSCLC have tumors that harbor an *ALK* rearrangement [35]. Patients with lung carcinomas harboring *EML4-ALK* fusion oncogene or its variants are eligible to treatment by small-molecule inhibitors that target the ALK tyrosine kinase, specifically crizotinib. Acquired resistance has emerged as the major hurdle in the treatment of *ALK*-positive NSCLC, because patients typically relapse within 1 to 2 years of starting therapy [36]. More than 90 % of *ALK* rearrangements involve only three variants; however, up to 20 *ALK* rearrangements have been described. FISH testing using fluorescently labeled DNA probes to localize the specific genomic regions in the tumor nuclei has been developed and the *ALK* break-apart FISH set (Abbott Molecular) has received FDA approval. The commercial break-apart probe set binds to areas upstream and downstream of the common rearrangement breakpoint in exon 20 of the *ALK* gene and includes two differently colored probes: the 5′ probe labeled with green and the 3′ probe labeled in orange fluorochromes, respectively. The 3′ probe is observed as red under the microscope. In non-rearranged cells, the red and green signals are closely located or overlying resulting in a composite yellow (fused) signal. In the setting of the rearrangement, the signals (red and green) separate and splitting of the signals occur. A nucleus is considered positive when displays isolated red and green signals separated by at least 2 signal diameters. An isolated red signal without a concurrent green signal is also considered positive. A single green signal is considered negative. A sample is considered positive if ≥15 % of scored nuclei displays a positive pattern and requires counting a minimum of 50 tumor cell nuclei by a first reader. Additional 50 nuclei scored by a second reader are necessary in cases with >10 % but <50 % positive tumor cell nuclei. An example of a case with *ALK* rearrangement is illustrated in Fig. 6.2.

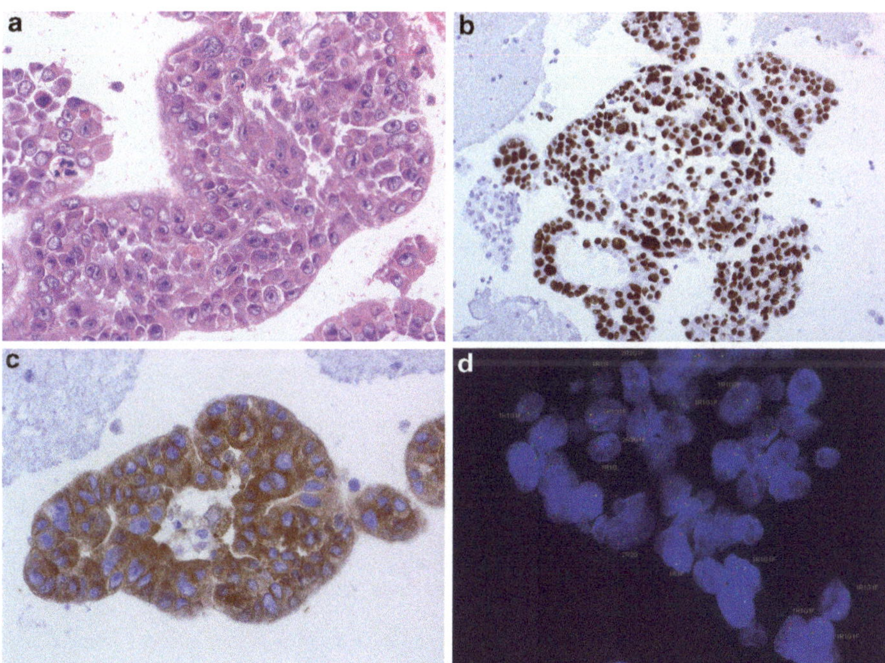

**Fig. 6.2** (**a**) Section of a formalin-fixed paraffin-embedded cell block preparation of a pleural effusion. (**b**) Immunohistochemistry for TTF-1 showing positive nuclei. (**c**) Immunohistochemistry slide positive for ALK. (**D**) Interphase fluorescence in situ hybridization (FISH) slide showing cells positive for *EML4-ALK* rearrangement using break-apart probe [(**a**) H&E staining. (**b**) Original magnification × 630. (**c**) Original magnification × 630. (**d**) Original magnification × 1,000 original magnification × 1,000]

Other methodologies can be used for the detection of *ALK* rearrangements but currently the gold standard assay for diagnosing ALK-positive tumors is FISH. Immunohistochemistry for ALK has been proposed and used in Canada and European countries as a screening test before the FISH assay or combined with FISH [37]. An extensive review about the different diagnostic tests as well as the limitations of each test has been recently published [38].

## Other Molecular Alterations

A number of other genomic alterations have been detected in NSCLC, including *Kirsten rat sarcoma viral oncogene homolog* (*KRAS*) mutation, *ROS1* rearrangement, and *c-MET* amplifications. Clinical trials have been developed for new agents targeting some of those alterations, but currently there is no need for routine clinical testing of those alterations. Although in some centers *KRAS* mutations have been routinely analyzed, a recent review about the role of *KRAS* mutation as prognostic and predictive markers in NSCLC has concluded that targeting *KRAS* remains experimental, and this oncogene cannot, at this time, be recommended routinely for the selection (or exclusion) of patients for therapy [39]. As targeted therapies become available the recommendations for testing will evolve and change over time. New technologies for high-throughput and multiplex platforms for mutational profiling of tumors including MassArray spectrometry, SNaPshot Multiplex PCR, and next generation sequencing might address the issue of the minimal volume of tissue/cells present in small biopsies and cytological samples, and the need for testing for panels of genes as markers for new-targeted therapies becomes available.

## References


1. da Cunha SG, Saieg MA, Geddie W, Leighl N. EGFR gene status in cytological samples of nonsmall cell lung carcinoma: controversies and opportunities. Cancer Cytopathol. 2011;119(2):80–91.
2. Aisner DL, Sams SB. The role of cytology specimens in molecular testing of solid tumors: techniques, limitations, and opportunities. Diagn Cytopathol. 2012;40(6):511–24.
3. Malapelle U, Bellevicine C, Zeppa P, Palombini L, Troncone G. Cytology-based gene mutation tests to predict response to anti-epidermal growth factor receptor therapy: a review. Diagn Cytopathol. 2011;39(9):703–10.
4. Savic S, Bubendorf L. Role of fluorescence in situ hybridization in lung cancer cytology. Acta Cytol. 2012;56(6):611–21.
5. Killian JK, Walker RL, Suuriniemi M, Jones L, Scurci S, Singh P, et al. Archival fine-needle aspiration cytopathology (FNAC) samples: untapped resource for clinical molecular profiling. J Mol Diagn. 2010;12(6):739–45.
6. Betz BL, Roh MH, Weigelin HC, Placido JB, Schmidt LA, Farmen S, et al. The application of molecular diagnostic studies interrogating EGFR and KRAS mutations to stained cytologic smears of lung carcinoma. Am J Clin Pathol. 2011;136(4):564–71.

7. da Cunha SG, Ko HM, Geddie WR, Boerner SL, Lai SW, Have C, et al. Targeted use of fluorescence in situ hybridization (FISH) in cytospin preparations: results of 298 fine needle aspirates of B-cell non-Hodgkin lymphoma. Cancer Cytopathol. 2010;118(5):250–8.
8. Petriella D, Galetta D, Rubini V, Savino E, Paradiso A, Simone G, et al. Molecular profiling of thin-prep FNA samples in assisting clinical management of non-small-cell lung cancer. Mol Biotechnol. 2013;54(3):913–9.
9. Ladd AC, O'Sullivan-Mejia E, Lea T, Perry J, Dumur CI, Dragoescu E, et al. Preservation of fine-needle aspiration specimens for future use in RNA-based molecular testing. Cancer Cytopathol. 2011;119(2):102–10.
10. da Cunha SG, Schroder M, Zhu JB, Saieg MA, Geddie WR, Boerner SL, et al. Minimizing delays in DNA retrieval: The "freezer method" for glass coverslip removal Letter to the editor regarding comparative study of epidermal growth factor receptor mutation analysis on cytology smears and surgical pathology specimens from primary and metastatic lung carcinomas. Cancer Cytopathol. 2013;121(9):533.
11. Moore HM, Compton CC, Alper J, Vaught JB. International approaches to advancing biospecimen science. Cancer Epidemiol Biomarkers Prev. 2011;20(5):729–32.
12. Spruessel A, Steimann G, Jung M, Lee SA, Carr T, Fentz AK, et al. Tissue ischemia time affects gene and protein expression patterns within minutes following surgical tumor excision. Biotechniques. 2004;36(6):1030–7.
13. van Maldegem F, de Wit M, Morsink F, Musler A, Weegenaar J, van Noesel CJ. Effects of processing delay, formalin fixation, and immunohistochemistry on RNA Recovery From Formalin-fixed Paraffin-embedded Tissue Sections. Diagn Mol Pathol. 2008;17(1): 51–8.
14. Babic A, Loftin IR, Stanislaw S, Wang M, Miller R, Warren SM, et al. The impact of pre-analytical processing on staining quality for H&E, dual hapten, dual color in situ hybridization and fluorescent in situ hybridization assays. Methods. 2010;52(4):287–300.
15. Groenen PJ, Blokx WA, Diepenbroek C, Burgers L, Visinoni F, Wesseling P, et al. Preparing pathology for personalized medicine: possibilities for improvement of the pre-analytical phase. Histopathology. 2011;59(1):1–7.
16. Moore HM, Compton CC, Lim MD, Vaught J, Christiansen KN, Alper J. 2009 Biospecimen research network symposium: advancing cancer research through biospecimen science. Cancer Res. 2009;69(17):6770–2.
17. Kerr KM, Bubendorf L, Edelman MJ, Marchetti A, Mok T, Novello S, et al. Panel Members. Second ESMO consensus conference on lung cancer: pathology and molecular biomarkers for non-small-cell lung cancer. Ann Oncol. 2014 Apr 8. pii: mdu145. [Epub ahead of print] Review. PubMed PMID: 24718890.
18. Lindeman NI, Cagle PT, Beasley MB, Chitale DA, Dacic S, Giaccone G, et al. Molecular testing guideline for selection of lung cancer patients for EGFR and ALK tyrosine kinase inhibitors: guideline from the College of American Pathologists, International Association for the Study of Lung Cancer, and Association for Molecular Pathology. Arch Pathol Lab Med. 2013;137(6):828–60.
19. Srinivasan M, Sedmak D, Jewell S. Effect of fixatives and tissue processing on the content and integrity of nucleic acids. Am J Pathol. 2002;161(6):1961–71.
20. Williams C, Ponten F, Moberg C, Soderkvist P, Uhlen M, Ponten J, et al. A high frequency of sequence alterations is due to formalin fixation of archival specimens. Am J Pathol. 1999;155(5):1467–71.
21. Dejmek A, Zendehrokh N, Tomaszewska M, Edsjo A. Preparation of DNA from cytological material: effects of fixation, staining, and mounting medium on DNA yield and quality. Cancer Cytopathol. 2013;121(7):344–53.
22. da Cunha SG. Standardizing preanalytical variables for molecular cytopathology. Cancer Cytopathol. 2013;121(7):341–3.
23. Pang B, Dettmer M, Ong CW, Dhewar AN, Gupta S, Lim GL, et al. The positive impact of cytological specimens for EGFR mutation testing in non-small cell lung cancer: a single South East Asian laboratory's analysis of 670 cases. Cytopathology. 2012;23(4):229–36.

24. Malapelle U, Bellevicine C, De Luca C, Salatiello M, De Stefano A, Rocco D, et al. EGFR mutations detected on cytology samples by a centralized laboratory reliably predict response to gefitinib in non-small cell lung carcinoma patients. Cancer Cytopathol. 2013;121(10):552–60.
25. da Cunha SG, Liu N, Tsao MS, Kamel-Reid S, Chin K, Geddie WR. Detection of EGFR and KRAS mutations in fine-needle aspirates stored on Whatman FTA cards: is this the tool for biobanking cytological samples in the molecular era? Cancer Cytopathol. 2010;118(6): 450–6.
26. Saieg MA, Geddie WR, Boerner SL, Liu N, Tsao M, Zhang T, et al. The use of FTA cards for preserving unfixed cytological material for high-throughput molecular analysis. Cancer Cytopathol. 2012;120(3):206–14.
27. Mascarello JT, Hirsch B, Kearney HM, Ketterling RP, Olson SB, Quigley DI, et al. Section E9 of the American College of Medical Genetics technical standards and guidelines: fluorescence in situ hybridization. Genet Med. 2011;13(7):667–75.
28. Ellison G, Zhu G, Moulis A, Dearden S, Speake G, McCormack R. EGFR mutation testing in lung cancer: a review of available methods and their use for analysis of tumour tissue and cytology samples. J Clin Pathol. 2013;66(2):79–89.
29. Smits AJ, Kummer JA, de Bruin PC, Bol M, van den Tweel JG, Seldenrijk KA, et al. The estimation of tumor cell percentage for molecular testing by pathologists is not accurate. Mod Pathol. 2014;27(2):168–74.
30. Vallee A, Sagan C, Le Loupp AG, Bach K, Dejoie T, Denis MG. Detection of EGFR gene mutations in non-small cell lung cancer: lessons from a single-institution routine analysis of 1,403 tumor samples. Int J Oncol. 2013;43(4):1045–51.
31. Shiau CJ, Babwah J, da Cunha SG, Sykes JR, Boerner SL, Geddie WR, et al. Sample features associated with success rates in population-based egfr mutation testing. J Thorac Oncol. 2014;9(7):947–56.
32. Heymann JJ, Bulman WA, Maxfield RA, Powell CA, Halmos B, Sonett J, et al. Molecular testing guidelines for lung adenocarcinoma: utility of cell blocks and concordance between fine-needle aspiration cytology and histology samples. CytoJournal. 2014;11:12.
33. Zhou Q, Zhang XC, Chen ZH, Yin XL, Yang JJ, Xu CR, et al. Relative abundance of EGFR mutations predicts benefit from gefitinib treatment for advanced non-small-cell lung cancer. J Clin Oncol. 2011;29(24):3316–21.
34. da Cunha SG, Shepherd FA, Tsao MS. EGFR mutations and lung cancer. Annu Rev Pathol. 2011;6:49–69.
35. Soda M, Choi YL, Enomoto M, Takada S, Yamashita Y, Ishikawa S, et al. Identification of the transforming EML4-ALK fusion gene in non-small-cell lung cancer. Nature. 2007;448(7153): 561–6.
36. Shaw AT, Engelman JA. ALK in lung cancer: past, present, and future. J Clin Oncol. 2013; 31(8):1105–11.
37. Sholl LM, Weremowicz S, Gray SW, Wong KK, Chirieac LR, Lindeman NI, et al. Combined use of ALK immunohistochemistry and FISH for optimal detection of ALK-rearranged lung adenocarcinomas. J Thorac Oncol. 2013;8(3):322–8.
38. Weickhardt AJ, Aisner DL, Franklin WA, Varella-Garcia M, Doebele RC, Camidge DR. Diagnostic assays for identification of anaplastic lymphoma kinase-positive non-small cell lung cancer. Cancer. 2013;119(8):1467–77.
39. Martin P, Leighl NB, Tsao MS, Shepherd FA. KRAS mutations as prognostic and predictive markers in non-small cell lung cancer. J Thorac Oncol. 2013;8(5):530–42.

# Chapter 7
# Role of Immunohistochemistry in the Detection of Targetable Mutations

**Andre Luis Moreira**

## Introduction

The discovery of targetable driver mutations in pulmonary adenocarcinomas has revolutionized the field of thoracic oncology by the introduction of oral small molecule tyrosine kinase inhibitors that target specific *EGFR* mutations and rearrangements in *ALK* gene. Testing for these is therefore now recommended for all pulmonary carcinomas diagnosed as adenocarcinoma and large cell carcinoma with adenocarcinoma immunophenotype [1] but not for squamous cell carcinoma or neuroendocrine tumors, including small cell carcinoma.

Since the majority of lung cancer patients present at an advanced stage [2], small biopsies and cytology specimens are often the only available material for diagnostic work-up and molecular characterization for predictive markers, which are essential for the selection of appropriate therapy. There has been a renewed interest in the diagnostic criteria for the subclassification of non-small cell carcinoma in biopsy specimens [3–7]. For the first time, the histological classification of lung cancer includes a diagnostic approach to small biopsy specimens [3, 8]. More importantly, small biopsy material, including cytology specimens, is now employed for molecular tests and predictive markers. Nonetheless, technical complexities during tissue acquisition and processing and relative high cost of tests have challenged the widespread use of molecular techniques in routine clinical practice. Recently, antibodies to specific molecular alterations have become available and have the potential to become instrumental in the molecular characterization of limited tumor specimens. The practical issues involving the use of immunostains for detecting mutant EGFR and ALK fusion proteins amongst others as alternatives or adjuncts to molecular testing are detailed below.

---

A.L. Moreira, M.D., Ph.D. (✉)
Department of Pathology, Memorial Sloan Kettering Cancer Center,
1275 York Ave., New York, NY 10065, USA
e-mail: moreiraa@mskcc.org

 
A.L. Moreira, A. Saqi (eds.), *Diagnosing Non-small Cell Carcinoma in Small Biopsy and Cytology*, DOI 10.1007/978-1-4939-1607-8_7

## Detection of *EGFR* Mutation in Small Biopsy Specimens

The discovery of activating mutations in tyrosine kinase domain of the *EGFR* gene and a strong association with clinical response to tyrosine kinase inhibitors gefitinib [9, 10] and erlotinib [11–14] revolutionized the field of thoracic oncology. The College of American Pathologists (CAP) in association with the International Association for the Study of Lung Cancer (IASLC) and the Association of Molecular Pathology (AMP) established guidelines for molecular testing of pulmonary carcinomas and recommended that EGFR mutation testing be performed in all adenocarcinomas and large cell carcinomas with an adenocarcinoma phenotype. In addition, they recommended that the molecular testing be able to detect all clinically relevant mutations in the *EGFR* gene [1]. Molecular testing can be performed in excised tumors and small biopsy specimens, including cytology. Though molecular profiling of adenocarcinomas has been reported in cellblock preparations [15–20] and other cytologic preparations, such as direct smears, and liquid-based cytology [21–27], the guidelines advocate the use of formalin-fixed cellblock preparations.

While molecular testing is the gold standard for mutation detection, the relatively high cost and technical complexity limit its availability outside large academic centers and referral laboratories [27]. Second, the failure rate for *EGFR* molecular testing on cytology and small biopsy samples ranges from low 2–8 % [18–29] to approximately a quarter of all cases in some studies [19, 30]. The failure rates are multifactorial and at least partly dependent upon the molecular testing technique, which may require larger amounts of tumor DNA. Currently available advanced techniques use smaller quantities of DNA for analysis with improved detection rates [21, 30–33]. In spite of efforts to obtain adequate material, it is not uncommon to have inadequate quantity or quality DNA for testing of small biopsy specimens. Therefore, many patients that could benefit from specific molecular-based therapy remain untested or undergo re-biopsy to acquire additional tissue for testing.

Immunohistochemical stains are inexpensive compared to molecular tests, widely used and available in most pathology laboratories, and most importantly, interpretable and reportable by general pathologists, who are familiar with these tests. Therefore, immunohistochemistry for mutation-specific antibodies offers an alternative and/or adjunct test to direct molecular methods. In addition, in cases with limited tumor insufficient for standard molecular tests, immunohistochemical stains for specific mutations provide a valuable tool for molecular characterization of neoplastic cells.

## EGFR Mutation-Specific Antibodies

Although there are several activating mutations in the *EGFR* gene, the two most common ones representing greater than 90 % of *EGFR* mutations are L858R point mutation in exon 21 and short 15-bp (E746-A750) in-frame deletion in exon 19 [12]. Non-15-bp deletions comprise up to 35 % of exon 19 deletions [34].

Monoclonal antibodies specific to exon 19 E746-A750 (15-bp) deletion (clone 6B6) and exon 21 L858R mutation (clone 43B2, both from Cell Signaling Technology) have been developed and are now commercially available. In the initial report describing these antibodies, the authors evaluated the performance of the pair in 340 paraffin-embedded sections of resected non-small cell lung cancer (NSCLC) specimens and showed that the antibodies had 92 % and 99 % sensitivity and specificity, respectively, when compared to direct sequencing and mass spectrometry-based DNA analysis [35]. Brevet et al., using the same pair of antibodies on surgical specimens [34], reported sensitivities of 76 % and 67 % for detecting L858R and exon 19 15-bp deletions, respectively, and positive predictive values of 100 %. The lower sensitivity for exon 19 deletions resulted from inclusion in the study of non-15-bp deletions, which the antibody Clone 6B6 does not recognize. When measuring the detection rate of only 15-bp deletions, an improved sensitivity of 80 % for the antibody has been reported [36].

Several other studies confirmed the utility of the pair of EGFR mutation-specific antibodies on tissue microarrays and whole sections of resected surgical material [37–42]. These results demonstrated the potential of these antibodies to serve as a screening tool for patients harboring *EGFR* mutations.

Different clones of mutation-specific antibodies directed against L858R (clone SP125) and exon 19 E746-A750 (15-bp) deletion (clone SP111) have been developed by Ventana Medical System also and recently reported to have sensitivities and specificities similar to the original clones [43, 44].

## Scoring of Mutation-Specific Antibodies

One of the most challenging aspects of immunohistochemistry for predictive markers is the determination of what constitutes a positive reaction. The most applied and accepted scoring method for the mutation-specific EGFR antibodies comes from Brevet et al. [34], who use a system analogous to that used for Her2/neu scoring of breast carcinomas.

The scoring is based on the evaluation of the intensity of membranous and cytoplasmic staining patterns and varies from 0 (zero) to 3+. Briefly, absence of staining of tumor cells corresponds to 0; faint cytoplasmic or incomplete membranous staining in more than 10 % tumor cells corresponds to 1+; moderate and incomplete membranous staining is 2+; and strong and complete membranous staining is regarded as 3+ (Fig. 7.1).

Jiang et al. reported that mutation detection by molecular techniques correlates with the intensity of immunohistochemical stain [45]. Accordingly, a reaction with a 1+ score is associated with false-positive results [4, 36, 45] with mutations detected by molecular techniques in only 23 % of cases [45]. Therefore, a greater number of false positives will result when a score of 1+ is interpreted as a positive reaction. Application of stringent criteria for the interpretation of a test as positive is thus important and has significant clinical implications. In fact, a large study showed that

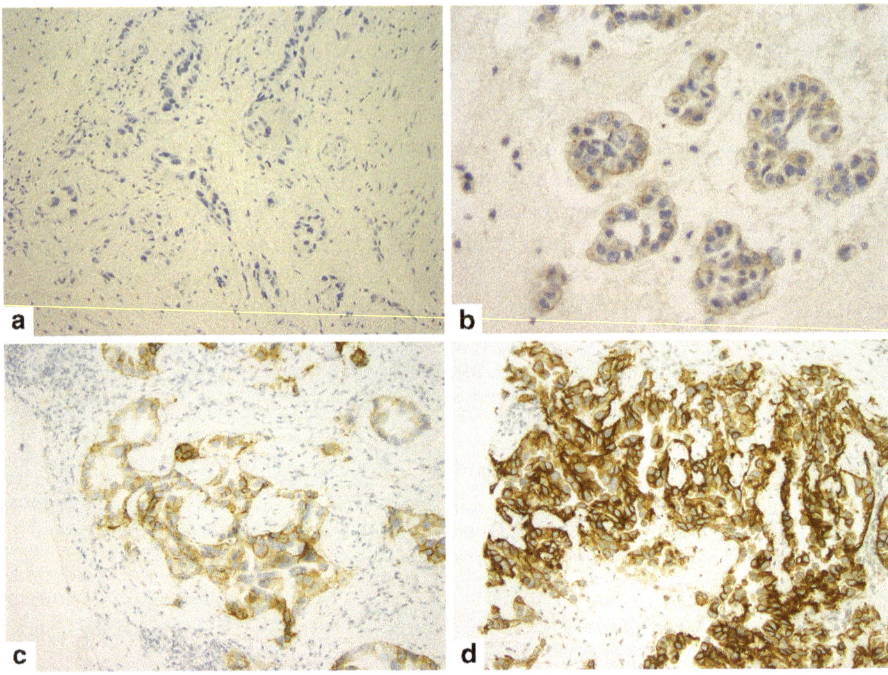


**Fig. 7.1** Scoring system for immunostaining of small biopsy specimens with mutation-specific EGFR antibodies—L858R mutation in exon 21 and 15-bp deletion in exon 19. (**a** and **b**) Negative scores. (**a**) Absence of staining, zero intensity. (**b**) Faint staining in >10 % of tumor cells, score of 1+: this pattern of immunoreactivity is associated with false-positive results. (**c**, **d**) Positive scores: a positive score corresponds to the presence of specific mutation. (**c**) Moderate but incomplete membranous staining pattern in the majority of tumor cells, scored as 2+. (**d**) Strong membranous staining pattern in the majority of tumor cells scored as 3+

administration of TKI, instead of chemotherapy, to patients without EGFR-mutated lung adenocarcinomas resulted in more harm than benefit [46].

On the contrary, scores of 2+ and 3+ with both mutation-specific EGFR antibodies [34, 36] are not associated with false-positive results, correlate with the tumor mutation profile, demonstrate high sensitivity, and have reported specificity and positive predictive values of 100 % [34, 36]. Therefore, a binary system with 2+ and 3+ regarded as positive reactions and 0 and 1+ as negative or inconclusive should be implemented.

The issue remains, however, in cases with negative or inconclusive results for EGFR mutation using this pair of antibodies (scores of 0 and 1+). Jiang et al. observed that EGFR mutations are detected in 7 % of tumors with a score of 0 by immunohistochemistry [45]. The combined sensitivity of these antibodies is approximately 70 % for the specific EGFR mutation that they are designed to detect, which means that there is at least a 30 % chance of missing an activating mutation with a negative reaction by IHC. Therefore, a negative reaction (score of 0 or 1+) should not be assumed to correspond to wild-type EGFR. Cases that are scored as negative

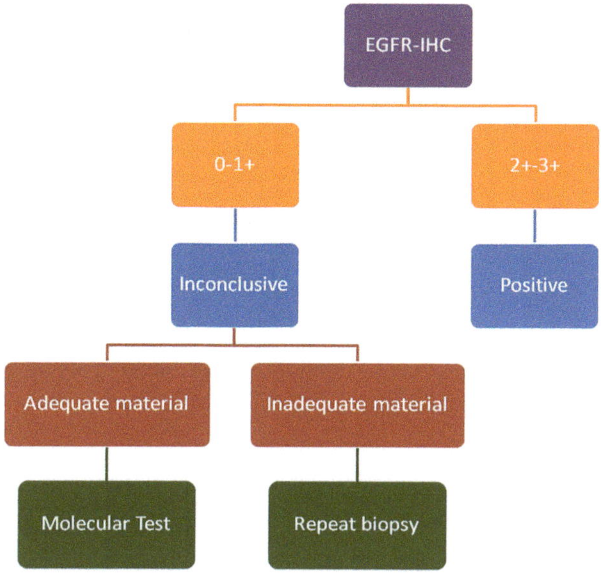


**Fig. 7.2** Algorithm for the interpretation of immunostaining with EGFR mutation-specific antibody. The pair of antibodies is designed for the detection of L858R and 15-bp deletion only. Other potential sensitizing EGFR mutations are not detected by this pair; therefore, negative or inconclusive results (score 1+) do not exclude the possibility of another mutation in the *EGFR* gene or another class of mutation such as ALK, KRAS, and others. Samples scored as negative or 1+ should be submitted to molecular tests if adequate material exists; otherwise, re-biopsy is recommended for predictive markers

for mutation-specific antibodies should still be submitted for molecular diagnostic testing that can detect other mutations in the *EGFR* gene that are unrecognized by the pair of antibodies but still confer sensitivity to tyrosine kinase inhibitors. A work flow for the use of EGFR mutation-specific antibodies is illustrated in Fig. 7.2.

## Use of Mutation-Specific Antibodies in Small Biopsy Specimen

There is a great interest in the application of these antibodies in cytology specimens, since cytologic material is the main source of tissue for patients who present with advanced stages of disease and because a small but significant proportion of cytology specimens fail molecular testing. Cytology also offers an array of specimens from aspirations of primary or metastatic sites, ultrasound-guided endobronchial biopsies (EBUS) of the lymph nodes evaluated for staging information, pleural effusions, and other exfoliative samples like bronchial lavages, brushes, washes, and sputum.

A study evaluating the application of EGFR mutant-specific antibodies to clinical specimens, including cytology samples (FNA and effusion fluid), small core

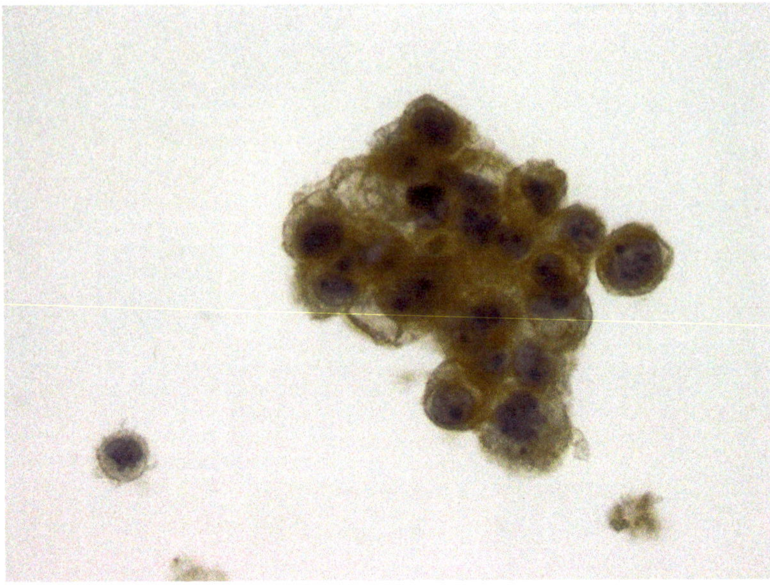

**Fig. 7.3** Microphotograph of a positive reaction with EGFR mutation-specific antibody on a liquid-based preparation (ThinPrep® slide). This positive result correlated with the detection of 15 bp deletion in exon 19 in another sample of the same tumor

biopsies, and bone biopsies showed that the pair of antibodies performs well in cytology (cellblock and ThinPrep) and small biopsy material with comparable sensitivity and specificity as that reported to excisional material [33] (Fig. 7.3). In another report, Kawahara et al. tested the performance of these two specific EGFR mutation antibodies in a relatively small sample of cytology specimens from effusions and cerebrospinal fluids and reported a sensitivity of 100 % and specificity of 92 % for both mutant-specific antibodies [47].

Moreover, Hasanovic et al. [36] showed that the mutation-specific EGFR antibodies are also useful in the assessment of mutation status in bone biopsies for stage IV patients. The decalcification process for histological evaluation of bone metastasis renders the material unsuitable for molecular testing since it affects the quality of DNA. Application of the pair of mutation-specific EGFR antibodies can provide useful information if a positive reaction is observed.

To summarize, IHC for *EGFR* mutations is useful in cytology and small biopsy specimens with scant cellularity for molecular analysis. A positive reaction by IHC in a decalcified material or small biopsy with scant cellularity can prevent the need to re-biopsy patients. Also, using a stringent cutoff of $\geq$2+ as an indicator of positivity allows for initiation of therapy with TKI in patients with advanced disease. An algorithm for the utilization of EGFR mutation-specific antibodies in small specimens that are unsuitable for molecular tests is illustrated in Fig. 7.4.

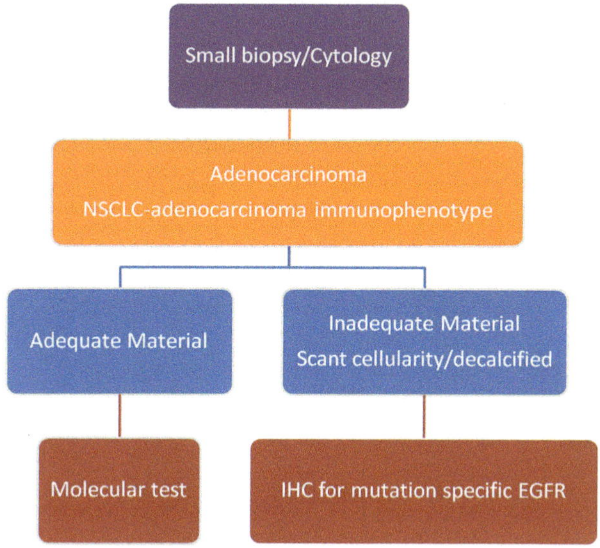


**Fig. 7.4** Algorithm for tissue utilization of small biopsy material. Samples with inadequate tumor content (scant cellularity) or processed for decalcification can be processed for EGFR mutation-specific antibody. All other biopsies that have adequate material for molecular studies should be processed as such. The CAP/IASLC/AMP recommendations suggest that priority for molecular diagnostics should be a test that can detect all mutations in the EGFR gene

## Response to TKI Therapy in EGFR Mutant Tumors Detected by Immunohistochemistry

Most reports that indicate a response to TKI in patients with EGFR mutation originate from studies that applied standard molecular techniques for the detecting mutations. As mutation-specific antibodies became available for the characterization of pulmonary adenocarcinomas, questions emerged among treating physicians as to whether mutation detection by immunohistochemistry was predictive of response to therapy with TKI.

Initial studies showed that although there was good correlation between response to therapy and mutation identified by immunohistochemistry, the best responses were noted in patients with molecular confirmation and not with mutation-specific antibody detection [40]. This discrepancy was a consequence of two factors. First discussed was the relatively low sensitivity of the antibodies; the authors compared in their analysis all EGFR mutations detectable by molecular techniques with the pair of antibodies designed to identify only two mutations (15-bp deletion in exon 19 and L858R point mutation in exon 21). Second, the criteria indicative of a positive reaction were different from those currently accepted. Inclusion of cases with weak positivity (1+) in less than 10 % of tumor cells resulted in poor correlation with mutation status and response to therapy. These conclusions do not come as a surprise given what is now known about these antibodies, including false positivity stemming from overinterpretation of faint or incomplete membranous staining in <10 % tumor cells.

In a more recent study, Kawahara A et al. [48], using the established cutoff of 2+ and 3+ as positive, demonstrated that all patients with a positive reaction for mutation-specific antibody had a significant progression-free survival compared to those with a negative reaction (0 and 1+). The authors concluded that patients with EGFR mutation detected by immunohistochemistry are good candidates for EGFR-targeted therapy.

These studies are important because they validate the correlation of immunohistochemistry detection of EGFR mutation with response to specific therapy. Considering that the results of immunohistochemistry can be available and reported within a few days, clinicians can initiate treatment of patients in need, safely, while awaiting molecular confirmation of standard molecular techniques, which may take weeks. In cases with only scant available tissue or a decalcified bone biopsy, a positive antibody reaction reduces the need to re-biopsy for further testing (Fig. 7.4).

## Specificity of EGFR Mutation-Specific Antibodies as a Marker for Lung Cancer

In the setting of disseminated metastatic disease of unknown primary, it is not uncommon to find tumors that lack expression of tissue specific markers, which makes it very difficult to pin-point the site of origin and therefore selection of appropriate therapy. Mutations in the *EGFR* gene seem to be specific to pulmonary adenocarcinomas. However, until recently, the specificity of the pair of EGFR mutation-specific antibodies in other carcinomas was unknown.

Wen et al. [49], with the working hypothesis that mutation-specific antibodies would not cross-react with overexpressed EGFR wild-type on tumors cells, evaluated the specificity of the pair of antibodies in a large series of carcinomas from non-pulmonary sites such as the breast, pancreas, colorectum, and endometrium. The authors showed that of 300 breast carcinomas, including estrogen-positive, Her2/neu-positive, and triple-negative cases, less than 1 % had a positive reaction (2+ intensity) with the anti-L858R antibody. Molecular analysis of the 2+ L858R breast carcinomas showed no mutation, indicating a false-positive result. When present, false-positive results in breast adenocarcinoma were seen only in estrogen-positive tumors and not in triple-negative carcinomas. All breast carcinomas scored 0 with the E746-A750 antibody, and all the colorectal, pancreatic carcinomas and malignant Mullerian tumors of the endometrium were negative (0 intensity) for both antibodies. These results indicate that EGFR mutation-specific antibodies can be incorporated in the diagnostic work-up of patients with disseminated metastatic diseases when pulmonary adenocarcinoma is in the differential diagnosis with a positive result to an EGFR mutation-specific antibody most likely indicating a pulmonary origin in the setting of a tumor of unknown origin. Therefore, in addition to predictive indicators for therapy with EGFR inhibitors, these antibodies are also helpful in providing a site of origin.

## ALK Rearrangement

In 2007, Soda et al. described that a subset of pulmonary adenocarcinomas showed an inversion within chromosome 2 that resulted in a transforming fusion kinase between *echinoderm microtubule-associated protein-like 4 (EML4)* in 2p21 and *anaplastic lymphoma kinase (ALK)* in 2p23.2 [50]. This fusion results in constitutive activation of ALK kinase, and transfection of this molecular alteration into cell lines was also tumorigenic [50]. *ALK* rearrangement is the second driver oncogene in pulmonary carcinoma that can be targeted by specific therapy.

Rearrangement of the *ALK* gene is present in approximately 5 % of the patients with pulmonary adenocarcinoma [50–55] and is more common in younger patients who are light or never smokers. In general, these patients present with advanced disease and are often poorly differentiated with solid or cribriform predominant histology with signet ring cell features [52–55] and psammoma bodies [56]. *ALK* rearrangement is mutually exclusive of *EGFR* or *KRAS* mutations [57] although tumors expressing double mutation with *EGFR* have been reported [58].

In 2009, crizotinib (XALKORI, Pfizer, Inc) was approved by the US Food and Drug Administration for the treatment of patients with lung adenocarcinoma harboring *ALK* rearrangement. The drug, an inhibitor of the tyrosine kinase activity of both *ALK* and the *MET* proto-oncogene, is efficacious in treating mutant *ALK* lung adenocarcinoma [59, 60].

Identification of *ALK* rearrangement in tumors is standard in the evaluation of patients with pulmonary adenocarcinoma.

## Diagnosis of *ALK* Rearrangement

The area encompassing the EML4-ALK fusion in chromosome 2 is relatively large and therefore suitable for detection by fluorescence in situ hybridization (FISH). In fact, FISH for ALK rearrangement has been licensed by the US Food and Drug Administration as a companion diagnosis for the detection of this mutation.

The Vysis ALK Dual Color, Break Apart Rearrangement Probe FISH Kit (Abbott Molecular) is the gold standard for detection of *ALK* rearrangement [59, 61, 62]. This test, however, is marred by relative high cost, limited availability, and technical complexity that require trained technicians and pathologists for its interpretation. With the added infrequency of *ALK* rearrangement in 5 % adenocarcinomas, performing FISH on all specimens is impractical and there is a great interest in developing a robust screening method for detecting this alteration. The CAP/IASLC/AMP recommendations indicate that screening of *ALK* rearrangement can be conducted with immunohistochemistry, following strict validation of the antibody in the user laboratory [1].

## Diagnosis of *ALK* Rearrangement by Immunohistochemistry

Initial analysis using the ALK-1 clone, the same antibody used to detect ALK in T-cell lymphomas, showed variable results [49, 63]. Recently, two commercially available antibodies show higher specificity and sensitivity to *ALK*-rearranged lung adenocarcinoma when compared to the ALK-1 clone. Mino-Kenudson et al. [64], using a novel antibody (clone D5F3, Cell Signaling Technology) for the detection of *ALK*-rearranged lung adenocarcinomas, showed 100 % sensitivity and 99 % specificity with excellent interobserver agreement between pathologists.

In a study by Minca EC et al. [65], D5F3 clone showed 100 % sensitivity and 100 % specificity for the detection on ALK fusion protein in paraffin-embedded tissue and cytology material, and in instances of inconclusive FISH results, negative IHC was helpful in preventing false-positive FISH. The authors concluded that the high concordance rate between FISH and IHC for ALK supports the use of IHC as a screening method for ALK status determination.

Another clone, 5A4 (Novocastra, Leica Biosystems), is commercially available for the detection of *ALK*-rearranged adenocarcinoma. Sakairi et al. correlated the results of IHC using this clone with standard FISH in 109 adenocarcinoma specimens obtained by endobronchial ultrasound-guided transbronchial needle aspiration biopsy [66]. A good correlation between the two tests was observed without any reported false-positive or false-negative cases by IHC. Savic S et al. showed that immunohistochemistry for the detection of ALK rearrangement using clone 5A4 is feasible in cytologic material with a reported sensitivity and specificity of 93.3 and 96 %, respectively [67]. The authors used cellblock material, direct smears, and liquid-based cytology in their study and reported that ALK testing with IHC is feasible on all cytology preparations.

Both antibody clones, D5F3 and 5A4, have been compared. Selinger CI [68] showed that both identified ALK rearrangement detected by FISH. IHC with D5F3 clone and 5A4 clone has been reported by several investigators as having sensitivity of 93 to 100 % and specificity of 96 to 100 %, when compared to FISH [64, 65, 67, 68].

A recent publication by the IASLC, dedicated exclusively to ALK testing in lung carcinomas, emphasized the need to validate IHC tests for ALK, since there are several available antibodies with different detection systems [69]. The report suggested the need to standardize the procedure, if results are to be comparable from different laboratories.

## Scoring of ALK Immunohistochemistry

The ALK staining pattern is predominantly cytoplasmic with a granular quality and has membranous accentuation in cases with high-intensity stain. This is in contrast to the pattern seen with EGFR mutation-specific antibodies that show predominantly membranous staining.

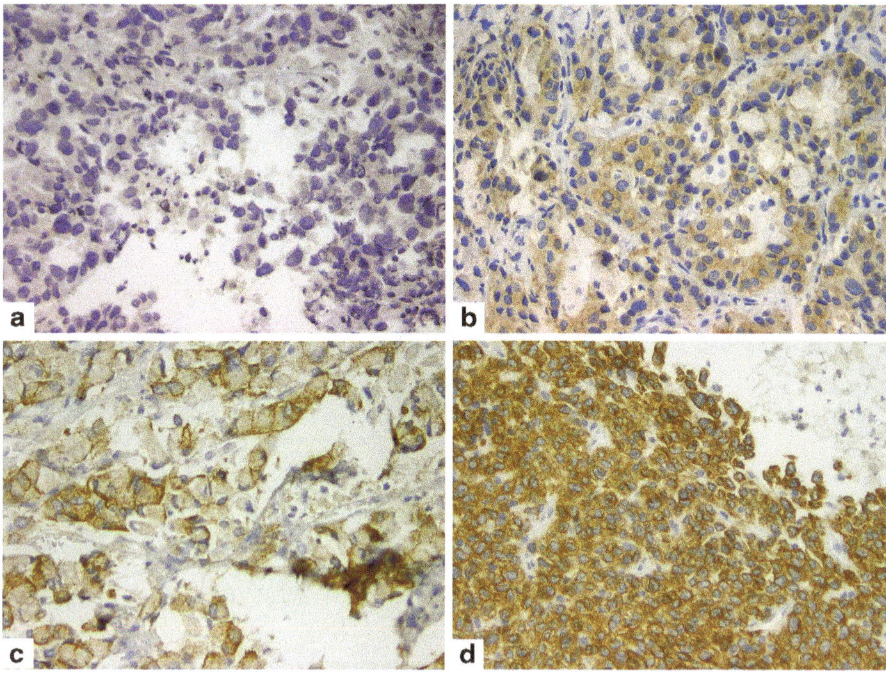


**Fig. 7.5** Scoring system for immunostaining of small biopsy specimens with antibodies that recognized rearranged ALK clone D5F3. (**a**) Absence of staining with the antibody. This has been shown to correlate lack of ALK rearrangement. (**b**) Score 1+, weak cytoplasmic staining in all tumor cells. This pattern is considered equivocal. Some authors reporting the presence of rearrangement confirmed by FISH but not others. (**c**) 2+ intensity score: this is considered a positive reaction and correlates with a positive ALK-FISH test. (**d**) 3+ intensity score: this is considered positive and correlates with a positive ALK-FISH test

In most studies, ALK staining pattern is scored from 0 (zero) to 3+: zero (no stain), 1+ (weak cytoplasmic stain, best visualized by 40× objective), 2+ (moderate cytoplasmic stain best visualized using 10× to 20× objectives), and 3+ (strong stain, seen at 2× to 4× objective) (Fig. 7.5). The definition of positivity among studies is variable, though [64–68]. Most consider 2+ and 3+ positive demonstrating good correlation with FISH tests.

As the staining intensity plays a major factor in the decision for screening algorithms, there is still considerable amount of variability when a staining pattern of 1+ is encountered, with some regarding it positive [64, 65, 68] and others considering it inconclusive with FISH follow-up [62, 69]. Some authors suggest that a diffuse reactivity in all tumor cells with an intensity of 1+ is indicative of *ALK* rearrangement [64, 65, 68], whereas others have reported that heterogeneous staining patterns is common in *ALK*-rearranged tumors [70]. The issue of a weak reactivity is more likely the result of pre-analytical problems such as fixation and antigen retrieval, as well as the clone and detection system used, rather than different levels of the fusion protein expression. Therefore, before a screening algorithm for ALK rearrangement

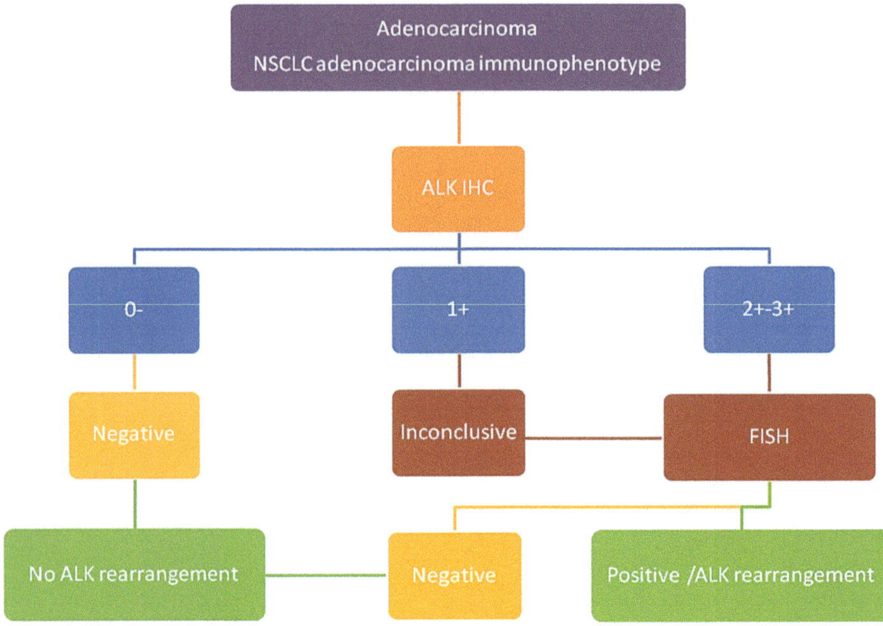


**Fig. 7.6** Algorithm for ALK screening using ALK antibody either clone D5F3 or 5A4. Since ALK FISH is the companion diagnostic test for ALK rearrangement, all positive cases should be sent for FISH test for confirmation of the arrangement. This is also true to cases scored as 1+ (equivocal). Most studies using IHC for ALK rearrangement screening suggest that a negative reaction (no staining) is indicative of native ALK. The CAP/IASLC/AMP guidelines suggest that an ALK screening algorithm using IHC should be strongly validated in each laboratory before implementation of the test. There is no agreed-upon screening algorithm for ALK rearrangement

detection can be established, a standardized procedure including pre- and post-analytical parameters needs to be outlined by competent regulatory bodies. At the time of writing this chapter, the recommendation of the CAP/IASLC/AMP is that before a screening algorithm for ALK is established, each laboratory should validate its own test with strong internal positive and negative controls.

More importantly, what appears clear from most reports on the subject is that a negative stain by IHC with either clone (D5F3 or 5A4) is indicative of negative FISH rearrangement (negative predictive value of 100 %). Therefore, in most screening algorithms that have been established outside of the United States, a negative (zero intensity) stain by IHC indicates absence of *ALK* rearrangement and no further testing is required. An example of a possible screening algorithm is illustrated in Fig. 7.6.

At least in the United States, all cases considered positive for ALK by IHC need to have confirmation of ALK rearrangement by FISH (companion diagnostic) test.

## Other Mutation-Specific Antibodies

*ROS1* is a proto-oncogene translocation identified in approximately 1–2 % of pulmonary adenocarcinomas [71] and is responsive to treatment with crizotinib, an ALK/MET inhibitor. Similar to ALK-rearranged tumors, most adenocarcinomas with this translocation are poorly differentiated and have a predominant solid, micropapillary, or cribriform growth patterns with signet ring cells and microcalcifications [72–74]. The translocation can be detected by a specific FISH probe. Due to the rarity of this mutation, most testing is conducted in tumors that are triple negative for *EGFR*, *ALK*, and *KRAS* mutations.

Recently, an antibody that detects ROS1 has become commercially available. The D4D6 clone [73, 74] has a sensitivity of 100 % and specificity of 97 % in two studies [73, 74] for the detection of ROS1 when compared to standard FISH test.

A study from Mescam-Mancini L. et al. reports good correlation between IHC and FISH test when 2+and 3+ are considered positive reaction by IHC. ROS1 antibody shows cytoplasmic staining, similar to ALK antibodies. Interestingly, the same authors reported that the antibody cross-reacts with HER/2neu mutant lung adenocarcinomas [73].

*BRAF* mutations are detected in approximately 1 to 2 % of pulmonary adenocarcinomas; the most common mutation is V600E [75]. BRAF mutations can also be targeted by specific therapy [76]. An antibody that recognizes V600E mutation is commercially available, with clone VE1 having good sensitivity and specificity for detecting mutations in pulmonary carcinomas, thyroid carcinomas, and melanoma [77–79].

## Other Uses of Mutation-Specific Antibodies

Synchronous and metachronous adenocarcinomas of the lung pose a significant challenge for diagnosis and staging of patients with lung cancer, since prognosis and clinical management are highly dependent of pathological staging.

Although pulmonary adenocarcinomas are histologically heterogeneous and therefore morphological comparison of two tumors may be sufficient for determining whether they represent metastases or separate primary tumors [80], there are still cases in which this differentiation cannot be achieved with certainty by morphology alone. At the same time, it is not uncommon to encounter a clinical situation of metachronous tumors with different histological patterns that are favored to represent separate primaries, but the clinical presentation is suggestive of metastatic disease. In these situations, most pathologists rely upon the molecular characteristics of the tumors for further differentiation.

D'Angelo SP et al. [81] evaluated 1831 resected lung adenocarcinomas from clinical stages I–III and suggested that information generated by mutational profiling following tumor excision permitted distinction between multiple primary tumors and metastases and assignment to expected directed therapy and specific clinical trials. In their evaluation of 82 multifocal adenocarcinomas of the lung, Takamochi et al. [82] showed that EGFR and KRAS mutations occurred randomly, thus suggesting that in synchronous or metachronous carcinomas, the identification of the same mutation in more than one tumor supported the concept of clonality therefore determining metastatic disease. Different mutational profiles are consistent with separate clones, therefore separate primary tumors.

Immunohistochemical stains for specific mutations can be very useful for tumor characterization in the same setting.

Knowledge of prior mutation status such as EGFR, ALK, BRAF, or ROS1 can be confirmed in most tumors if there is doubt about whether a new carcinoma is clonally related to a prior tumor. If the tumors have similar molecular profile using mutation-specific antibodies, a clonal relationship can be established. Figure 7.7 illustrates a case of a patient that presented with disease progression following tyrosine kinase inhibitor therapy. The initial diagnosis was adenocarcinoma with EGFR 15-bp deletion, and a

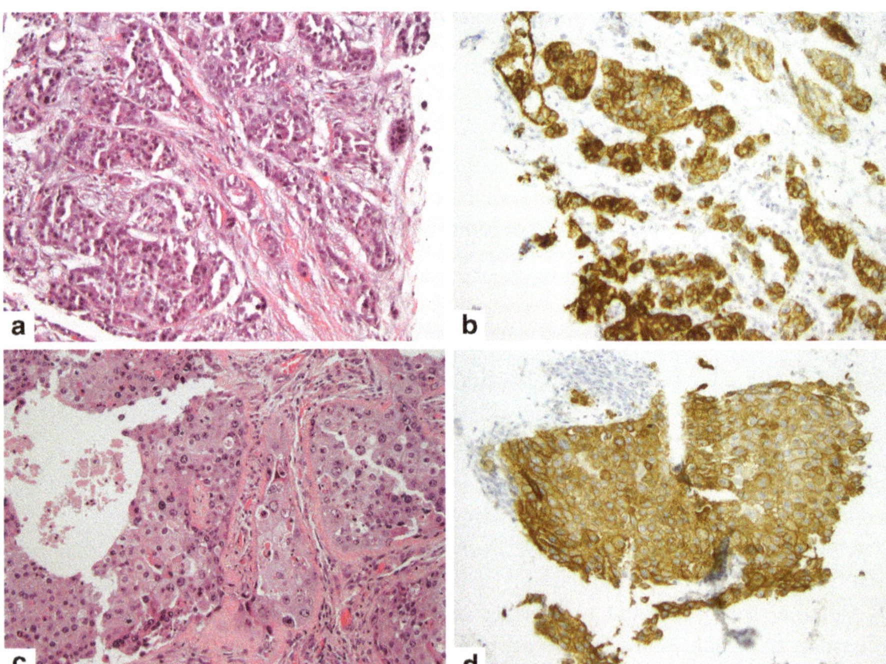


**Fig. 7.7** Example of the use of mutation-specific antibodies for the determination of clonality in metachronous tumors. In this example, the original tumor was diagnosed in a small biopsy as an adenocarcinoma (**a**) (H&E stain, ×100 original magnification). Molecular studies indicated the presence of EGFR mutation (15-bp deletion). This mutation was also detected by the EGFR mutation-specific antibody (**b**). The patient recurred under Tyrosine kinase inhibitor therapy. The new tumor had a different histology, squamous cell carcinoma (**c**) (H&E stain, original magnification ×100). The recurrent tumor was also positive for the same specific EGFR mutation antibody (**d**) thus establishing a clonal relationship. The tumor is now classified as an adenosquamous carcinoma

biopsy of the recurrent tumor showed squamous cell carcinoma histology. Immunohistochemical stain using a mutation-specific antibody confirmed that the squamous cell carcinoma carried the same mutation as the prior adenocarcinoma, thus confirming the clonality of the two tumors and establishing the diagnosis of adeno-squamous carcinoma.

## Conclusion

Although there are no established IHC screening tests, it is encouraging to see that immunohistochemical stains can be used to detect predictive markers and may have a future in the diagnostic and molecular characterization of malignant tumors. Many other predictive markers are becoming available for the characterization of specific molecular signatures in tumors. Further studies correlating their use and response to specific therapies will be determinant of their viability in the ever growing arsenal of against cancer.

## References

1. Lindeman NI, Cagle PT, Beasley MB, et al. Molecular testing guideline for selection of lung cancer patients for EGFR and ALK tyrosine kinase inhibitors: guideline from the College of American Pathologists, International Association for the Study of Lung Cancer, and Association for Molecular Pathology. J Thorac Oncol. 2013;8:823–59.
2. Molina JR, Adjei AA, Jett JR. Advances in chemotherapy of non-small cell lung cancer. Chest. 2006;130:1211–9.
3. Travis WD, Brambilla E, Noguchi M, et al. International association for the study of lung cancer/American thoracic society/European respiratory society international multidisciplinary classification of lung adenocarcinoma. J Thorac Oncol. 2011;6:244–85.
4. Edwards SL, Roberts C, McKean ME, et al. Preoperative histological classification of primary lung cancer: accuracy of diagnosis and use of the non-small cell category. J Clin Pathol. 2000;53:537–40.
5. Rekhtman N, Ang DC, Sima CS, et al. Immunohistochemical algorithm for differentiation of lung adenocarcinoma and squamous cell carcinoma based on large series of whole-tissue sections with validation in small specimens. Mod Pathol. 2011;24:1348–59.
6. Mukhopadhyay S, Katzenstein ALA. Subclassification of Non-small Cell Lung Carcinomas Lacking Morphologic Differentiation on Biopsy Specimens: Utility of an Immunohistochemical Panel Containing TTF-1, Napsin A, p63, and CK5/6. Am J Surg Pathol. 2011;35:15–25.
7. Nicholson AG, Gonzalez D, Shah P, et al. Refining the diagnosis and EGFR status of non-small cell lung carcinoma in biopsy and cytologic material, using a panel of mucin staining, TTF-1, cytokeratin 5/6, and P63, and EGFR mutation analysis. J Thorac Oncol. 2010;5:436–41.
8. Travis WD, Rekhtman N, Riley GJ, et al. Pathologic diagnosis of advanced lung cancer based on small biopsies and cytology: a paradigm shift. J Thorac Oncol. 2010;5:411–4.
9. Lynch TJ, Bell DW, Sordella R, et al. Activating mutations in the epidermal growth factor receptor underlying responsiveness of non-small-cell lung cancer to gefitinib. N Engl J Med. 2004;350:2129–39.

10. Paez JG, Janne PA, Lee JC, et al. EGFR mutations in lung cancer: correlation with clinical response to gefitinib therapy. Science. 2004;304:1497–500.
11. Pao W, Miller V, Zakowski M, et al. EGF receptor gene mutations are common in lung cancers from "never smokers" and are associated with sensitivity of tumors to gefitinib and erlotinib. Proc Natl Acad Sci USA. 2004;101:13306–11.
12. Sharma SV, Bell DW, Settleman J, et al. Epidermal growth factor receptor mutations in lung cancer. Nat Rev Cancer. 2007;7:169–81.
13. Sequist LV, Bell DW, Lynch TJ, et al. Molecular predictors of response to epidermal growth factor receptor antagonists in non-small-cell lung cancer. J Clin Oncol. 2007;25:587–95.
14. Li AR, Chitale D, Riely GJ, et al. EGFR mutations in lung adenocarcinomas: clinical testing experience and relationship to EGFR gene copy number and immunohistochemical expression. J Mol Diagn. 2008;10:242–8.
15. Rekhtman N, Brandt SM, Sigel CS, et al. Suitability of thoracic cytology for new therapeutic paradigms in non-small cell lung carcinoma: high accuracy of tumor subtyping and feasibility of EGFR and KRAS molecular testing. J Thorac Oncol. 2011;6:451–8.
16. Pan Q, Pao W, Ladanyi M. Rapid polymerase chain reaction-based detection of epidermal growth factor receptor gene mutations in lung adenocarcinomas. J Mol Diagn. 2005;7:396–403.
17. Lozano MD, Zulueta JJ, Echeveste JI, et al. Assessment of epidermal growth factor receptor and K-ras mutation status in cytological stained smears of non-small cell lung cancer patients: correlation with clinical outcomes. Oncologist. 2011;16:877–85.
18. Smouse JH, Cibas ES, Janne PA, et al. EGFR mutations are detected comparably in cytologic and surgical pathology specimens of nonsmall cell lung cancer. Cancer. 2009;117:67–72.
19. Schuurbiers OC, Looijen-Salamon MG, Ligtenberg MJ, et al. A brief retrospective report on the feasibility of epidermal growth factor receptor and KRAS mutation analysis in transesophageal ultrasound- and endobronchial ultrasound-guided fine needle cytological aspirates. J Thorac Oncol. 2010;5:1664–7.
20. Heymann J, Bulman WA, Maxfield RA, Powell CA, Halmos B, Sonett J, Beaubier NT, Crapanzano JP, Mansukhani MM, Saqi A. Molecular testing guidelines for lung adenocarcinomas: utility of cell blocks and concordance between fine needle aspiration cytology and histology samples. CytoJournal. 2014;11:12.
21. Nomoto K, Tsuta K, Takano T, et al. Detection of EGFR mutations in archived cytologic specimens of non-small cell lung cancer using high-resolution melting analysis. Am J Clin Pathol. 2006;126:608–15.
22. Boldrini L, Gisfredi S, Ursino S, et al. Mutational analysis in cytological specimens of advanced lung adenocarcinoma: a sensitive method for molecular diagnosis. J Thorac Oncol. 2007;2:1086–90.
23. Smith GD, Chadwick BE, Willmore-Payne C, et al. Detection of epidermal growth factor receptor gene mutations in cytology specimens from patients with non-small cell lung cancer utilising high-resolution melting amplicon analysis. J Clin Pathol. 2008;61:487–93.
24. Malapelle U, Bellevicine C, De Luca C, et al. EGFR mutations detected on cytology samples by a centralized laboratory reliably predict response to gefitinib in non-small cell lung carcinoma patients. Cancer Cytopathol. 2013;121:552–60.
25. Knoepp SM, Roh MH. Ancillary techniques on direct-smear aspirate slides: a significant evolution for cytopathology techniques. Cancer Cytopathol. 2013;121:120–8.
26. Khode R, Larsen DA, Culbreath BC, et al. Comparative study of epidermal growth factor receptor mutation analysis on cytology smears and surgical pathology specimens from primary and metastatic lung carcinomas. Cancer Cytopathol. 2013;121:361–9.
27. Bozzetti C, Naldi N, Nizzoli R, et al. Reliability of EGFR and KRAS mutation analysis on fine-needle aspiration washing in non-small cell lung cancer. Lung Cancer. 2013;80:35–8.
28. Ellis PM, Verma S, Sehdev S, et al. Challenges to implementation of an epidermal growth factor receptor testing strategy for non-small-cell lung cancer in a publicly funded health care system. J Thorac Oncol. 2013;8:1136–41.

29. Savic S, Tapia C, Grilli B, et al. Comprehensive epidermal growth factor receptor gene analysis from cytological specimens of non-small-cell lung cancers. Br J Cancer. 2008;98:154–60.
30. Garcia-Olive I, Monso E, Andreo F, et al. Endobronchial ultrasound-guided transbronchial needle aspiration for identifying EGFR mutations. Eur Respir J. 2010;35:391–5.
31. Akagi K, Sakai H, Sudo J, et al. Simple method to detect important epodermal growth factor receptor gene mutations with bronchoscopic specimens of lung cancer patients for gefitinib treatment. Target Oncol. 2007;2:145–51.
32. Hlinkova K, Babal P, Berzinec P, et al. Rapid and efficient detection of EGFR mutations in problematic cytologic specimens by high-resolution melting analysis. Mol Diagn Ther. 2011;15:21–9.
33. Ma ES, Ng WK, Wong CL. EGFR gene mutation study in cytology specimens. Acta Cytol. 2012;56:661–8.
34. Brevet M, Arcila M, Ladanyi M. Assessment of EGFR mutation status in lung adenocarcinoma by immunohistochemistry using antibodies specific to the two major forms of mutant EGFR. J Mol Diagn. 2010;12:169–76.
35. Yu J, Kane S, Wu J, et al. Mutation-specific antibodies for the detection of EGFR mutations in non-small-cell lung cancer. Clin Cancer Res. 2009;15:3023–8.
36. Hasanovic A, Ang D, Moreira AL, et al. Use of mutation specific antibodies to detect EGFR status in small biopsy and cytology specimens of lung adenocarcinoma. Lung Cancer. 2012;77:299–305.
37. Kawahara A, Yamamoto C, Nakashima K, et al. Molecular diagnosis of activating EGFR mutations in non-small cell lung cancer using mutation-specific antibodies for immunohistochemical analysis. Clin Cancer Res. 2010;16:3163–70.
38. Kitamura A, Hosoda W, Sasaki E, et al. Immunohistochemical detection of EGFR mutation using mutation-specific antibodies in lung cancer. Clin Cancer Res. 2010;16:3349–55.
39. Kato Y, Peled N, Wynes MW, et al. Novel epidermal growth factor receptor mutation-specific antibodies for non-small cell lung cancer: immunohistochemistry as a possible screening method for epidermal growth factor receptor mutations. J Thorac Oncol. 2010;5:1551–8.
40. Kozu Y, Tsuta K, Kohno T, et al. The usefulness of mutation-specific antibodies in detecting epidermal growth factor receptor mutations and in predicting response to tyrosine kinase inhibitor therapy in lung adenocarcinoma. Lung Cancer. 2011;73:45–50.
41. Nakamura H, Mochizuki A, Shinmyo T, et al. Immunohistochemical detection of mutated epidermal growth factor receptors in pulmonary adenocarcinoma. Anticancer Res. 2010;30: 5233–7.
42. Simonetti S, Molina MA, Queralt C, et al. Detection of EGFR mutations with mutation-specific antibodies in stage IV non-small-cell lung cancer. J Transl Med. 2010;8:135.
43. Allo G, Bandarchi B, Yanagawa N, et al. Epidermal growth factor receptor mutation-specific immunohistochemical antibodies in lung adenocarcinoma. Histopathology. 2014;64(6):826–39.
44. Seo AN, Park TI, Jin Y, et al. Novel EGFR mutation-specific antibodies for lung adenocarcinoma: Highly specific but not sensitive detection of an E746_A750 deletion in exon 19 and an L858R mutation in exon 21 by immunohistochemistry. Lung Cancer. 2014;83(3):316–23.
45. Jiang G, Fan C, Zhang X, et al. Ascertaining an appropriate diagnostic algorithm using EGFR mutation-specific antibodies to detect EGFR status in non-small-cell lung cancer. PLoS One. 2013;8:e59183.
46. Mok TS, Wu YL, Thongprasert S, et al. Gefitinib or carboplatin-paclitaxel in pulmonary adenocarcinoma. N Engl J Med. 2009;361:947–57.
47. Kawahara A, Azuma K, Sumi A, et al. Identification of non-small-cell lung cancer with activating EGFR mutations in malignant effusion and cerebrospinal fluid: rapid and sensitive detection of exon 19 deletion E746-A750 and exon 21 L858R mutation by immunocytochemistry. Lung Cancer. 2011;74:35–40.
48. Kawahara A, Taira T, Azuma K, et al. A diagnostic algorithm using EGFR mutation-specific antibodies for rapid response EGFR-TKI treatment in patients with non-small cell lung cancer. Lung Cancer. 2012;78:39–44.

49. Wen YH, Brogi E, Hasanovic A, et al. Immunohistochemical staining with EGFR mutation-specific antibodies: high specificity as a diagnostic marker for lung adenocarcinoma. Mod Pathol. 2013;26:1197–203.
50. Soda M, Choi YL, Enomoto M, et al. Identification of the transforming EML4-ALK fusion gene in non-small-cell lung cancer. Nature. 2007;448:561–6.
51. Inamura K, Takeuchi K, Togashi Y, et al. EML4-ALK lung cancers are characterized by rare other mutations, a TTF-1 cell lineage, an acinar histology, and young onset. Mod Pathol. 2009;22:508–15.
52. Inamura K, Takeuchi K, Togashi Y, et al. EML4-ALK fusion is linked to histological characteristics in a subset of lung cancers. J Thorac Oncol. 2008;3:13–7.
53. Rodig SJ, Mino-Kenudson M, Dacic S, et al. Unique clinicopathologic features characterize ALK-rearranged lung adenocarcinoma in the western population. Clin Cancer Res. 2009;15:5216–23.
54. Jokoji R, Yamasaki T, Minami S, et al. Combination of morphological feature analysis and immunohistochemistry is useful for screening of EML4-ALK-positive lung adenocarcinoma. J Clin Pathol. 2010;63:1066–70.
55. Shaw AT, Yeap BY, Mino-Kenudson M, et al. Clinical features and outcome of patients with non-small-cell lung cancer who harbor EML4-ALK. J Clin Oncol. 2009;27:4247–53.
56. Pareja FG, Mansukhani M, Bulman WA, Saqi A. ALK rearrangement: salient morphological features on cytology and surgical pathology. Abstract. J Am Soc Cytopathol. 2013;2(1 Suppl):S60.
57. Gainor JF, Varghese AM, Ou SH, et al. ALK rearrangements are mutually exclusive with mutations in EGFR or KRAS: an analysis of 1,683 patients with non-small cell lung cancer. Clin Cancer Res. 2013;19:4273–81.
58. Yang J, Zhang XC, Su J, et al. Lung cancers with concomitant EGFR mutations and ALK rearrangements: diverse responses to EGFR-TKI and crizotinib in relation to diverse receptors phosphorylation. Clin Cancer Res. 2014;20(5):1383–92.
59. Kwak EL, Bang YJ, Camidge DR, et al. Anaplastic lymphoma kinase inhibition in non-small-cell lung cancer. N Engl J Med. 2010;363:1693–703.
60. Shaw AT, Yeap BY, Solomon BJ, et al. Effect of crizotinib on overall survival in patients with advanced non-small-cell lung cancer harbouring ALK gene rearrangement: a retrospective analysis. Lancet Oncol. 2011;12:1004–12.
61. Camidge DR, Kono SA, Flacco A, et al. Optimizing the detection of lung cancer patients harboring anaplastic lymphoma kinase (ALK) gene rearrangements potentially suitable for ALK inhibitor treatment. Clin Cancer Res. 2010;16:5581–90.
62. Kim H, Yoo SB, Choe JY, et al. Detection of ALK gene rearrangement in non-small cell lung cancer: a comparison of fluorescence in situ hybridization and chromogenic in situ hybridization with correlation of ALK protein expression. J Thorac Oncol. 2011;6:1359–66.
63. Martelli MP, Sozzi G, Hernandez L, et al. EML4-ALK rearrangement in non-small cell lung cancer and non-tumor lung tissues. Am J Pathol. 2009;174:661–70.
64. Mino-Kenudson M, Chirieac LR, Law K, et al. A novel, highly sensitive antibody allows for the routine detection of ALK-rearranged lung adenocarcinomas by standard immunohistochemistry. Clin Cancer Res. 2010;16:1561–71.
65. Minca EC, Portier BP, Wang Z, et al. ALK status testing in non-small cell lung carcinoma: correlation between ultrasensitive IHC and FISH. J Mol Diagn. 2013;15:341–6.
66. Sakairi Y, Nakajima T, Yasufuku K, et al. EML4-ALK fusion gene assessment using metastatic lymph node samples obtained by endobronchial ultrasound-guided transbronchial needle aspiration. Clin Cancer Res. 2010;16:4938–45.
67. Savic S, Bode B, Diebold J, et al. Detection of ALK-positive non-small-cell lung cancers on cytological specimens: high accuracy of immunocytochemistry with the 5A4 clone. J Thorac Oncol. 2013;8:1004–11.
68. Selinger CI, Rogers TM, Russell PA, et al. Testing for ALK rearrangement in lung adenocarcinoma: a multicenter comparison of immunohistochemistry and fluorescent in situ hybridization. Mod Pathol. 2013;26:1545–53.

69. Tsao MSH, Fred R, Yatabe Y. IASLC atlas of ALK testing in lung cancer. Aurora, CO: IASLC Press; 2013.
70. Sholl LM, Weremowicz S, Gray SW, et al. Combined use of ALK immunohistochemistry and FISH for optimal detection of ALK-rearranged lung adenocarcinomas. J Thorac Oncol. 2013;8:322–8.
71. Bergethon K, Shaw AT, Ou SH, et al. ROS1 rearrangements define a unique molecular class of lung cancers. J Clin Oncol. 2012;30:863–70.
72. Go H, Kim DW, Kim D, et al. Clinicopathologic analysis of ROS1-rearranged non-small-cell lung cancer and proposal of a diagnostic algorithm. J Thorac Oncol. 2013;8:1445–50.
73. Mescam-Mancini L, Lantuejoul S, Moro-Sibilot D, et al. On the relevance of a testing algorithm for the detection of ROS1-rearranged lung adenocarcinomas. Lung Cancer. 2014;83: 168–73.
74. Sholl LM, Sun H, Butaney M, et al. ROS1 immunohistochemistry for detection of ROS1-rearranged lung adenocarcinomas. Am J Surg Pathol. 2013;37:1441–9.
75. Kinno T, Tsuta K, Shiraishi K, et al. Clinicopathological features of nonsmall cell lung carcinomas with BRAF mutations. Ann Oncol. 2014;25:138–42.
76. Liu SV, Subramaniam D, Cyriac GC, et al. Emerging protein kinase inhibitors for non-small cell lung cancer. Expert Opin Emerg Drugs. 2014;19(1):51–65.
77. Ilie M, Lassalle S, Long-Mira E, et al. Diagnostic value of immunohistochemistry for the detection of the BRAFV600E mutation in papillary thyroid carcinoma. Comparative analysis with three DNA-based assays. Thyroid. 2014;24(5):858–66.
78. Ilie M, Long E, Hofman V, et al. Diagnostic value of immunohistochemistry for the detection of the BRAFV600E mutation in primary lung adenocarcinoma Caucasian patients. Ann Oncol. 2013;24:742–8.
79. Sasaki H, Shimizu S, Tani Y, et al. Usefulness of immunohistochemistry for the detection of the BRAF V600E mutation in Japanese lung adenocarcinoma. Lung Cancer. 2013;82:51–4.
80. Girard N, Deshpande C, Lau C, et al. Comprehensive histologic assessment helps to differentiate multiple lung primary nonsmall cell carcinomas from metastases. Am J Surg Pathol. 2009;33:1752–64.
81. D'Angelo SP, Park B, Azzoli CG, et al. Reflex testing of resected stage I through III lung adenocarcinomas for EGFR and KRAS mutation: report on initial experience and clinical utility at a single center. J Thorac Cardiovasc Surg. 2011;141:476–80.
82. Takamochi K, Oh S, Matsuoka J, et al. Clonality status of multifocal lung adenocarcinomas based on the mutation patterns of EGFR and K-ras. Lung Cancer. 2012;75:313–20.

# Chapter 8
# New Discoveries for the Treatment of Lung Cancer and the Role of Small Biopsy Material

**Juliana Eng, Alexander Drilon, and Paul K. Paik**

## Adenocarcinoma of the Lung

### *EGFR-Mutant Lung Cancers*

The discovery of *EGFR* mutations in lung cancers marked the first step toward a dramatic shift in the approach to the management of patients whose tumors harbor a targetable oncogene. It was well known in the 1990s and the early 2000s that EGFR is overexpressed in a significant proportion of NSCLCs and that overexpression correlates with a poor prognosis. In the mid-1990s, the synthesis of EGFR tyrosine kinase inhibitors was first reported. Subsequent testing of these compounds (gefitinib and erlotinib) was thus undertaken in patients with advanced NSCLCs, with erlotinib receiving FDA approval after the randomized trial BR.21 revealed an overall survival advantage over placebo as a second-line therapy [1].

While the activity of these drugs was marginal across multiple studies with response rates below 10 %, a subset of patients (young, Asian, never smokers) displayed rapid, dramatic, and durable responses to therapy. Several independent groups set out to uncover a biologic substrate for these responses by sequencing tumors from responders. In 2004, three separate publications reported the landmark

J. Eng, M.D.
Department of Medicine, Thoracic Oncology Service, Memorial Sloan Kettering Cancer Center, New York, NY, USA

A. Drilon, M.D.
Department of Medicine, Thoracic Oncology Service and Developmental Therapeutics, Memorial Sloan Kettering Cancer Center, New York, NY, USA

P.K. Paik, M.D. (✉)
Department of Medicine, Thoracic Oncology Service,
Memorial Sloan Kettering Cancer Center,
300 East 66th Street, New York, NY 10065, USA
e-mail: paikp@mskcc.org



A.L. Moreira, A. Saqi (eds.), *Diagnosing Non-small Cell Carcinoma in Small Biopsy and Cytology*, DOI 10.1007/978-1-4939-1607-8_8

detection of *EGFR* mutations in lung cancers [2–4]. It is now well recognized that the presence of an activating *EGFR* mutation serves as a strong predictive factor for response to EGFR tyrosine kinase inhibitor (TKI) therapy. The prevalence of *EGFR* mutations varies between populations. In Asians, approximately 35 % of NSCLC patients have tumors that harbor an activating mutation. In contrast, these mutations are found in about 10–15 % of Caucasians [5]. Regardless of race, this incidence rises significantly in patients with a never or former light smoking history [6].

Activating *EGFR* mutations are heterozygous, somatic, and cluster around the catalytic tyrosine kinase domain. The most common of these are exon 19 deletions and exon 21 L858R point mutations which account for 85 % of all mutations. Other sensitizing mutations detected at lower frequencies include G719X, L861X, and exon 19 insertions [7]. Exon 20 insertions, on the other hand, are known to confer resistance to EGFR TKIs with rare exceptions [8]. Activating *EGFR* mutations are oncogenic and capable of transforming lung epithelial and fibroblast cells. The mutant EGFR protein remains constitutively activated and is responsible for persistent signaling through downstream growth pathways including RAF-MEK-ERK and PI3K-AKT-mTOR leading to increased cell proliferation and survival. EGFR TKIs result in the displacement of ATP in the tyrosine kinase pocket, inhibition of tyrosine kinase phosphorylation, and abrogation of downstream signaling [9].

IPASS was the first large randomized trial to demonstrate the efficacy of EGFR TKI in *EGFR*-mutant lung cancers. A clinically enriched population of East Asian never smokers with advanced lung cancers was randomized to gefitinib vs. carboplatin and paclitaxel. The use of gefitinib in patients whose tumors harbored an *EGFR* mutation resulted in dramatic and statistically significant improvements in response, quality of life, and progression-free survival over chemotherapy [10]. Multiple randomized trials have since confirmed the superiority of EGFR tyrosine kinase inhibition over chemotherapy in *EGFR*-mutant patients regardless of race or smoking history, with objective response rates (ORR) between 60 and 80 % and progression-free survival (PFS) of 8–10 months (in comparison to an ORR of 30 % and PFS of 6 months with first-line cytotoxic chemotherapy). While no difference in overall survival was noted across these trials, a finding likely secondary to crossover to EGFR TKI therapy after chemotherapy, the median OS in *EGFR*-mutant patients was 2–3 years (compared to a 1-year median OS in unselected NSCLCs) [5, 11, 12].

Unfortunately, despite the dramatic benefits offered by EGFR TKIs in *EGFR*-mutant lung cancers, the development of acquired resistance to therapy is universal. A variety of resistance mechanisms have been detected via comprehensive molecular and pathologic analysis of rebiopsy specimens at the onset of acquired resistance. Broadly, these involve the persistent reliance on EGFR signaling and abrogation of EGFR TKI activity (acquisition of an *EGFR* T790M mutation), oncogenic shift and reliance on bypass signaling pathways (*MET* amplification and *HER2* upregulation), impairment of EGFR TKI-mediated apoptosis (*BIM* deletion), and histologic transformation (epithelial-mesenchymal transition or small cell transformation) [13]. Of these, the secondary T790M mutation represents the dominant mechanism of acquired resistance and is detected in more than half of all cases [14]. The acquisition of a T790M mutation results in increased affinity of the EGFR tyrosine kinase for ATP and restored downstream signaling.

A number of strategies to target tumors with acquired resistance are currently in clinical development. While second-generation EGFR TKIs such as afatinib and dacomitinib bind irreversibly to the EGFR kinase and have activity against T790M models in silico, the clinical activity of these agents in the acquired resistance space has been minimal. However, after preclinical experiments performed by Pao and colleagues revealed the synergistic activity of afatinib and cetuximab in promoting tumor regressions in acquired resistance models, a phase II trial of the combination was launched in patients with acquired resistance to EGFR TKI therapy. The trial demonstrated an overall response rate of 30 % across patients whose tumors harbored both T790M and non-T790M-mediated resistance mechanisms [15]. Furthermore, third-generation EGFR TKIs with increased specificity for T790M and decreased activity against the wild-type EGFR kinase have resulted in response rates in the order of 60 % in T790M-mutant tumors in early reports [16]. Should these results be confirmed in larger trials, these agents are likely to be approved with an indication in EGFR TKI acquired resistance.

## *KRAS-Mutant Lung Cancers*

*KRAS* mutations were the first oncogenes to be discovered in NSCLCs and to this day remain the most prevalent driver mutations in lung adenocarcinomas. In its wild-type state, the KRAS protein serves to integrate signals from extracellular growth factors (i.e., EGF binding to EGFR resulting in receptor dimerization and activation) with downstream signaling cascades such as the RAF-MEK-ERK and PI3K-AKT-mTOR pathways. Point mutations in *KRAS* result in mutant KRAS proteins that require transforming potential secondary to impaired GTPase activity and constitutive activation. These missense mutations commonly result in the replacement of amino acids at positions 12, 13, and 61 of the protein [17].

*KRAS* mutations account for the majority of RAS mutations in human malignancies and were first described in lung cancers in 1984 by Santos and colleagues. Examination of both tumor and normal tissue from a patient with non-small cell lung cancer revealed a *KRAS* mutation only in the former, demonstrating that the aberration was somatically acquired [18]. Several investigators subsequently showed that these mutations are acquired early in oncogenesis and are important drivers of tumor growth both in vitro and in vivo.

Mutations in *KRAS* are found in approximately 25–30 % of unselected NSCLCs and tend to be mutually exclusive with other major lung cancer drivers. These are found largely in lung adenocarcinomas or adenosquamous lung carcinomas and are rarely detected in squamous cell lung carcinomas that have undergone rigorous pathologic review. Rekhtman and colleagues compared *KRAS*-mutant lung adenocarcinomas with *EGFR*-mutant and *KRAS* and *EGFR* wild-type tumors and found an overrepresentation of solid growth patterns, mucinous histology, and tumor-infiltrating lymphocytes in the former [19].

While *KRAS* mutations have been classically associated with a history of smoking, Riely and colleagues demonstrated that up to 15 % of never or light smokers harbor these driver mutations. Structurally, the type of *KRAS* mutation varies based on smoking history, with transversions (e.g., *KRAS* G12C) more commonly detected in smokers and transitions (e.g., *KRAS* G12D) in never or former light smokers [20]. As *KRAS* mutations are found in tumors from patients regardless of smoking history, testing should not discriminate based on clinical features. In general, this approach is applicable to the various other driver aberrations identified in lung cancers.

Earlier investigations into patient outcomes and a subsequent meta-analysis uncovered data supporting the role of *KRAS* mutations as negative prognostic factors for overall survival [21]; however, data across a number of subsequent studies has proved to be conflicting. One thing that is clear is that *KRAS* mutations represent a negative predictive factor for response to EGFR tyrosine kinase inhibition [22, 23]. The role of *KRAS* mutations as predictive markers of response to adjuvant cytotoxic chemotherapy remains unclear, although a recent analysis suggests that the type of mutation (i.e., those involving G12 vs. G13) may affect response [24].

Similar to *EGFR* mutations, *KRAS* mutations can be diagnosed using a variety of assays including Sanger sequencing, mass spectrometry mutational hot spot testing, and massively parallel high-throughput sequencing. The latter affords the advantage of detecting concurrent tumor suppressor gene alterations such as mutations in *TP53* and *LKB1* that are likely to play important roles in tumor biology.

Despite three decades worth of research into *KRAS*-mutant lung cancers and a variety of targeted therapeutic strategies, no approach has proven active in this population as a single agent. Recently, this landscape has begun to change with data on the combination of MEK inhibition and cytotoxic chemotherapy. Based on preclinical work establishing the activity of MEK inhibitors (i.e., selumetinib and trametinib) against *KRAS*-mutant lung cancers in vivo and in vitro and their synergy with taxanes, Janne and colleagues launched a phase II randomized study of docetaxel with or without selumetinib in patients with advanced, *KRAS*-mutant NSCLCs [25]. Statistically significant improvements in both response rate (0 % vs. 32 %, $p<0.01$) and progression-free survival (HR 0.58, CI 0.42–0.79, $p=0.01$) were noted with the addition of selumetinib. A phase III trial with a similar design is currently ongoing. In addition, Engelman and colleagues demonstrated the synergism of the combination of selumetinib and PI3K/mTOR inhibition in promoting tumor regression in a *KRAS* G12D-mutant transgenic mouse model [26]. A number of trials looking at the combination of MEK inhibition and PI3K- or mTOR-directed therapy are currently being investigated.

## *BRAF*-Mutant Lung Cancers

*BRAF* is an established proto-oncogene. The gene encodes a serine-threonine protein kinase that serves as a central mediator of MAPK signaling. Activation of upstream effectors such as KRAS results in the phosphorylation and activation of BRAF following homodimerization of BRAF monomers or heterodimerization with other RAF proteins. Activated BRAF in turn phosphorylates its primary effector MEK that activates ERK signaling and increased cell proliferation. The *BRAF* V600E activating mutation is observed in 50–70 % of cases of cutaneous melanomas and confers increased sensitivity to BRAF inhibition (vemurafenib, dabrafenib) and MEK targeting (selumetinib, trametinib). Vemurafenib, dabrafenib, and trametinib are currently FDA approved for the treatment of patients with advanced melanomas harboring these mutations based on significant improvements in survival in comparison to cytotoxic chemotherapy. Furthermore, the combination of trametinib and dabrafenib is FDA approved for the same indication after a large randomized study demonstrated improved response rates and decreased adverse effects (incidence of cutaneous squamous cell carcinomas) with the combination vs. single-agent dabrafenib [27].

Interestingly, the first report of somatic activating *BRAF* mutations in lung cancers predates the discovery of *EGFR* mutations and *ALK* rearrangements. In 2002, Davies et al. screened a panel of solid tumor cancer cell lines using direct sequencing and identified *BRAF* mutations in 3 % of lung cancer samples [28]. Various independent investigators have since confirmed the presence of these fusions in 1–4 % of unselected NSCLCs [29]. Activating missense mutations in *BRAF* are oncogenic in vitro and in vivo, confer increased kinase activity, and result in constitutive activation of BRAF-MEK-ERK signaling. *BRAF* mutations have also been confirmed to be sufficient for the initiation and maintenance of lung adenocarcinomas in transgenic mouse models [30].

Unlike in melanomas where V600E mutations comprise the majority of *BRAF* mutations (80–90 %), *BRAF* V600E is only found in about half of all lung cancer samples. The profile of the non-V600E mutants differs as well, with a higher proportion of G469A and D594G mutants in lung cancers (in contrast to V600K, V600R, or V600D mutations in melanomas). In the vast majority of cases, *BRAF* mutations do not overlap with other oncogenic mutations and are detected largely in lung adenocarcinomas. Paik and colleagues examined a series of lung adenocarcinoma patients who underwent testing for *EGFR*, *KRAS*, and *BRAF* mutations and *ALK* fusions and found a higher incidence of *BRAF* mutations in patients with a current or former smoking history [31].

A number of BRAF and MEK inhibitors are currently being investigated in *BRAF*-mutant lung cancers. A preliminary report from an ongoing phase II trial of dabrafenib for patients with advanced lung cancers with *BRAF* mutations noted a 40 % ORR and durable responses [32]. Results from an ongoing phase II study of vemurafenib in *BRAF*-mutant solid tumors including lung adenocarcinomas is likely to yield comparable results. The combination of dabrafenib and trametinib is likewise currently undergoing investigation.

It is worth pointing out that inactivating *BRAF* mutations (G466V, Y472C) have been described in a small subset of lung adenocarcinomas. As an example, the Y472C kinase domain mutation results in the development of a kinase-impaired BRAF protein that paradoxically continues to activate MEK and ERK via transactivation of CRAF. Sen and colleagues demonstrated that cell lines containing inactivating *BRAF* mutations underwent senescence and apoptosis after exposure to dasatinib. Dasatinib was found to mediate these effects via CRAF inhibition. In the same report, a patient whose tumor harbored a *BRAF* Y472C mutation developed a durable partial response to dasatinib on a phase II trial for advanced, unselected NSCLCs [33]. A phase II trial of dasatinib for patients with advanced lung cancers harboring inactivating *BRAF* mutations (and *DDR2* mutations, discussed later in this chapter) is currently ongoing.

The mechanisms of acquired resistance to BRAF inhibition in *BRAF*-mutant lung cancers are undergoing active investigation. Rudin et al. reported the development of a *KRAS* mutation in a patient with *BRAF* V600E-mutant lung cancer who developed resistance to dabrafenib after an initial durable partial response [34]. In melanomas, the acquisition of an *NRAS* mutation has been reported as a mechanism of resistance to BRAF TKIs.

## *HER2-Mutant Lung Cancers*

The *ERBB2* (*HER2*) gene encodes the membrane-bound HER2 receptor tyrosine kinase that belongs to the ERBB family. In contrast to EGFR, HER2 has no known ligand but functions to heterodimerize with other members of the ERBB family. In breast and gastric/GE junction cancers, *HER2* is an established proto-oncogene with overexpression and amplification detected in approximately 30 % and 20 % of cases, respectively. A number of HER2-directed therapies are FDA approved for the treatment of breast and/or gastric/GE junction cancers including trastuzumab, lapatinib, pertuzumab, and trastuzumab emtansine/T-DM1. These drugs are approved for use either as a single agent (T-DM1) or in combination with chemotherapy or other agents [35].

*HER2* mutations were first described in lung cancers almost concurrent with the description of *EGFR* mutations in 2004. Stephens et al. performed direct sequencing on primary lung tumors and detected intragenic *HER2* mutations [36]. Multiple investigators have since confirmed that *HER2* mutations are present in about 2–4 % of NSCLCs. Structurally, these mutations are in-frame insertions of 3–12 base pairs in exon 20 (with less common missense mutations detected in exons 19–21). Unlike in *EGFR* exon 20 mutations where significant variability exists, the majority of *HER2* exon 20 mutations involve a 12 base pair insertion causing duplication of the amino acids YVMA at codon 775. *HER2* mutations lead to increased HER2 kinase activity, enhanced downstream signaling, and increased cell survival and proliferation. These mutations are oncogenic and result in the development of non-small cell lung cancers in transgenic *HER2*-mutant mouse models. Clinically, *HER2* mutations are more frequently detected in lung adenocarcinomas from never smokers with no predilection for sex or race [37].

Irreversible tyrosine kinase inhibitors with activity against HER2 such as afatinib, dacomitinib, and neratinib have been shown to inhibit the growth of transformed *HER2*-mutant cell lines and transgenic mouse models. Responses to all three drugs have been noted in *HER2*-mutant patients on ongoing phase II trials for patients with advanced lung cancers. The combination of neratinib and temsirolimus is also currently being investigated [38] based on preclinical work performed by Perera and colleagues. This study revealed that the combination of afatinib and rapamycin was most effective (compared to single-agent afatinib, rapamycin, or trastuzumab) in causing tumor regressions in a transgenic *HER2*-mutant mouse model [39].

Unlike in breast and gastric/GE junction cancers, the value of HER2 overexpression and/or *HER2* amplification remains controversial. The prevalence of both aberrations in NSCLCs varies between series but approaches 20 % and 10 %, respectively. While responses to HER2-directed therapy (i.e., trastuzumab) have been noted in *HER2*-amplified or HER2-overexpressing lung cancers, the majority of these patients were treated with an anti-HER2 agent in combination with chemotherapy [40].

## *Lung Cancers with PI3K Pathway Activation*

Aberrations of the PI3K-AKT-mTOR pathway play important role in cancer cell cycling, metabolism, and survival. In the wild-type state, the PI3K protein serves to integrate upstream signals from growth factor receptors with downstream signaling. PI3K activation results in AKT phosphorylation and subsequent activation of mTOR (part of the mTORC1 complex), S6K1, and eI4FE. Negative regulators of this signaling cascade include PTEN and TSC [41]. While *PIK3CA*, *AKT*, and *PTEN* mutations and PTEN loss have been described in a substantial proportion of lung adenocarcinomas, the roles that these aberrations play as strong drivers of tumor growth remain in question.

The PI3K protein is a membrane-bound enzyme that is composed of a regulatory and catalytic subunit. The *PIK3CA* gene encodes a class $I_A$ catalytic isoform p110α. These somatic mutations occur with a frequency of 1–3 % in unselected NSCLCS and commonly occur within the helical (exon 9) and kinase domains (exon 20) of the gene. In a series of *PIK3CA*-mutant lung adenocarcinomas, Chaft et al. reported that 70 % of patients had tumors that harbored a second driver event including *EGFR*, *KRAS*, *BRAF*, and *MEK* mutations and *ALK* rearrangements [42]. *PIK3CA* mutations are also found in both smokers and never smokers, with a higher incidence in squamous cell lung carcinomas, as will be discussed later [43]. *PIK3CA* mutations are oncogenic in vitro and in vivo. Transgenic mice harboring the p110α H1047R transgene developed lung adenocarcinomas. Dual PI3K/mTOR inhibition (NVP-BEZ235) resulted in tumor shrinkage in this model [26]. PI3K, mTOR, and dual PI3K/mTOR inhibitors are currently in development; however, the single-agent activity of these drugs has been minimal, and development pipelines have moved toward a combinatorial therapy approach with other agents.

*PTEN* mutations are known to play important roles in a hereditary predisposition to cancer (germline mutations in Cowden syndrome). While these mutations are detected in 4 % of NSCLCs, they are largely found in squamous cell cancers [43]. *PTEN* mutations occur along the length of the gene without a predilection for specific hot spots. Inactivating and truncating mutations (e.g., R233*) are thought to result in the loss of protein function, the release of negative regulation on the PI3K-AKT axis, and the increased downstream signaling of the pathway [44]. PTEN loss can likewise be detected via IHC. Similar to *PIK3CA* mutations, *PTEN* mutations and PTEN loss are thought to potentially confer sensitivity to PI3K or mTOR inhibitors [45].

*AKT* mutations occur in approximately 1 % of unselected NSCLCs [46]. *AKT1* E17K is well described, with the mutation occurring within the pleckstrin homology domain of AKT1 [47]. AKT inhibitors are available and in clinical development.

## *ALK*-Rearranged Lung Cancers

The *ALK* gene lies on chromosome 2 and encodes the anaplastic lymphoma kinase. ALK belongs to the insulin receptor superfamily of receptor tyrosine kinases and is thought to play an important role in nervous system development. A rearrangement involving *ALK* (*NPM-ALK*) was reported in anaplastic large cell lymphomas in 1984 and has since been confirmed to be present in a substantial proportion of tumors. Missense *ALK* mutations have been identified in neuroblastomas [48].

*ALK* fusions were first reported in lung cancers in 2007. Soda et al. generated a retroviral cDNA expression library from a patient-derived lung adenocarcinoma specimen. Mouse 3T3 fibroblasts were subsequently infected with recombinant retroviruses carrying plasmid clones, and the *EML4-ALK* fusion detected in amplified cDNA recovered via PCR from transformed foci. The same group demonstrated that *EML4-ALK* was transforming in 3T3 cells and formed subcutaneous tumors in nude mice. In contrast, kinase-dead *EML4-ALK* did not lead to tumor foci or subcutaneous tumors [49]. Transgenic mice expressing *EML4-ALK* via a lung-specific promoter developed numerous lung adenocarcinomas [50].

Rearrangements involving *ALK* are structurally characterized by the presence of an intact *ALK* tyrosine kinase domain fused to several upstream partners. The latter include *EML4* (the most common, with a variety of breakpoints), *KIF5B*, *TFG*, *KLC1*, *PTPN3*, and *HIP1*. These rearrangements are formed via small chromosome 2p inversions (e.g., *EML4-ALK*) or translocations (e.g., *HIP1-ALK*). The subcellular localization of the resultant fusion proteins is thought to be dependent on the upstream partner. Rearrangements lead to constitutive activation of the ALK tyrosine kinase and signaling through the RAS-RAF-MEK and PI3K-AKT pathways [51].

*ALK* fusions are found in 3–5 % of NSCLCs [52]. They are more common in never or former light smokers from younger individuals. These rearrangements are found predominantly in lung adenocarcinomas with acinar histology or signet-ring cells [53]. *ALK* fusions can be diagnosed via a variety of tests including RT-PCR, FISH, and next-generation sequencing. The Vysis ALK Break Apart FISH Probe Kit is currently FDA approved for diagnosis. Different-colored probes flank the 5′ and 3′ regions of the highly conserved *ALK* breakpoint. In cells that do not harbor a rearrangement, fused signals represent the normal pattern. In cells with an *ALK* fusion, however, gene rearrangement results in the detection of split signals in at least 15 % of tumor cells [54].

At the time *ALK* fusions were reported in lung cancers, a phase I study of crizotinib (then positioned primarily as a MET inhibitor) was ongoing. The activity of the drug against various other kinases was subsequently evaluated using a kinase selectivity screen, with ALK and ROS1 emerging as viable targets. Shortly thereafter, patients with *ALK*-rearranged lung cancers were enrolled in a dose-escalation and a dose-expansion cohort of the trial. Responses to crizotinib in these patients were both dramatic and durable, prompting a phase II study of the drug in advanced *ALK* fusion-positive lung cancers [55]. Most recently, a positive phase III trial of crizotinib vs. chemotherapy was reported. Similar to what was previously seen in *EGFR*-mutant lung cancers treated with EGFR TKIs, crizotinib was superior to chemotherapy in *ALK*-rearranged lung cancers in terms of response rate, quality of life, and progression-free survival. Across these various studies, the use of crizotinib resulted in a 60 % ORR and 8-month PFS in *ALK* fusion-positive lung cancers [56].

Unfortunately, as with EGFR TKI therapy in *EGFR*-mutant lung cancers, the development of acquired resistance to crizotinib is universal. Mechanisms of acquired resistance include continued reliance on ALK signaling (gatekeeper and non-gatekeeper mutations, *ALK* copy number gains) and activation of bypass pathways (mutations in alternate driver oncogenes) [57]. Fortunately, the recently reported experience with second-generation ALK inhibitors (e.g., alectinib and ceritinib) has demonstrated substantial efficacy in the acquired resistance setting. Preliminary reports of the activity of these drugs note a 60–90 % response rate in patients whose tumors harbor a variety of acquired resistance mechanisms to crizotinib [56]. In addition, the use of Hsp90 inhibition is currently being investigated in this space.

## *ROS1-Rearranged Lung Cancers*

The *ROS1* gene encodes a receptor tyrosine kinase that is phylogenetically similar to ALK. While the function ROS1 in its native state is not well defined, *ROS1* rearrangements have been described in other solid tumors including glioblastomas and cholangiocarcinomas. *ROS1* fusions were first described in lung cancers in 2007 by Rikova and colleagues. A phosphoproteomic screen of NSCLC cell lines and tumors uncovered a *SLC34A2-ROS1* fusion in one cell line (HCC78) and *CD74-ROS1* in a patient-derived sample [58].

Structurally, *ROS1* fusions are characterized by the presence of an intact tyrosine kinase domain. Several upstream partners including *CD74*, *SLC34A2*, *EZR*, *CCDC6*, *TPM3*, *LRIG3*, *SDC4*, and *FIG* have been identified. Most of these fusions are formed via translocation events (with the exception of *EZR-ROS1* and *FIG-ROS1*). These rearrangement events result in ligand-independent constitutive activation of the ROS1 kinase and downstream growth factor signaling [59]. While dimerization mediated by upstream partners is responsible for ligand-independent activation in *ALK* and *RET* fusions, the exact mechanism by which this occurs in *ROS1* fusions is unclear. *ROS1* rearrangements are oncogenic in vitro and in vivo. *ROS1* fusion-expressing NIH3T3 cells form transformed foci in culture and subcutaneous tumors in nude mice [60].

ROS1 inhibition results in decreased cell proliferation and survival in a number of lung cancer models. Crizotinib resulted in dose-dependent decreases in pROS1 and cell viability in both *ROS1* fusion-transfected 3T3 and Ba/F3 cells, and a patient-derived cell line (HCC78 harboring *SLC34A2-ROS1*) [61].

Given the preclinical activity of crizotinib against *ROS1* fusion-containing lung cancer models, the same phase I trial of the drug that spurred on its eventual approval in *ALK*-rearranged lung cancers opened a dose-expansion cohort for *ROS1*-rearranged lung cancers. In a preliminary report, the overall response rate with crizotinib for advanced *ROS1*-rearranged lung cancers was approximately 60 % and comparable to the efficacy seen in *ALK* fusion-positive lung cancers. Similarly, these results were early, dramatic, and durable. Several other ROS1 inhibitors are in clinical development [62].

Investigations into the mechanisms for acquired resistance to crizotinib in *ROS1*-rearranged lung cancers are ongoing. Shaw et al. reported the acquisition of a non-gatekeeper *ROS1* G2032R in a patient with *CD74-ROS1*-rearranged lung cancer who developed resistance to crizotinib after an initial dramatic response to therapy [63].

## *RET-Rearranged Lung Cancers*

The *RET* gene is found on chromosome 10 and encodes a receptor tyrosine kinase that is involved in neural crest development. *RET* is an established proto-oncogene. Mutations and rearrangements involving *RET* are known to be integral to the pathogenesis of both benign and malignant diseases. *RET* rearrangements have been described in papillary thyroid cancers, especially those developed in the wake of previous radiation exposure [59].

In lung cancers, *RET* rearrangements were first reported by Ju and colleagues in late 2011. Whole-genome and transcriptome sequencing of tumor tissue from a young, Asian never smoker with metastatic lung adenocarcinoma revealed a *KIF5B-RET* fusion [64]. This finding was subsequently confirmed by several independent investigators using a variety of other methods including FISH and next-generation sequencing.

Similar to *ALK* and *ROS1* fusions, *RET* rearrangements are structurally characterized by the presence of an intact tyrosine kinase domain fused to a variety of upstream partners including *KIF5B*, *CCDC6*, *NCOA4*, and *TRIM33*. *RET* fusions are largely formed via paracentric inversion with the exception of *TRIM33-RET* which is formed via translocation. Upstream partners contribute coiled-coil domains that lead to ligand-independent dimerization and activation of downstream signaling including the PI3K and MAPK pathways. These fusions are oncogenic in vivo and in vitro. *RET* fusion-expressing NIH3T3 models form multiple transformed foci in culture, display anchorage-independent growth, and form subcutaneous tumors in nude mice [60, 65, 66].

While *RET* fusions are found in approximately 1–2 % of unselected lung cancers, this incidence increases to 15 % in patients with a never or former light smoking history whose tumors test negative for other known lung cancer drivers [67]. In a series of surgically resected lung cancers, Wang and colleagues demonstrated that *RET* fusion-positive lung adenocarcinomas were likely to be more poorly differentiated and found in young never smokers. Pathologic features include the presence of the solid adenocarcinoma subtype in two-thirds of patients and signet ring cells in about a third of patients. Diagnostic assays include RT-PCR, FISH, and next-generation sequencing. Unlike for *ALK* and *ROS1* fusions, IHC has not proven to be useful for the detection of *RET* rearrangements [68].

A variety of multityrosine kinase RET inhibitors have shown activity in *RET* fusion-positive lung cancer models. The proliferation of *RET* fusion-expressing Ba/F3 cells is inhibited by vandetanib, sorafenib, and sunitinib. Vandetanib treatment results in growth inhibition of a patient-derived cell line and xenograft containing *CCDC6-RET* (LC-2/ad) [69]. Clinically, durable partial responses have been reported in patients with *RET* fusion-positive lung cancers who were treated on a phase 2 trial of cabozantinib, a RET inhibitor with concomitant activity against VEGFR2 and MET [70]. Other RET inhibitors that are currently in clinical development include vandetanib, lenvatinib, ponatinib, regorafenib, and sunitinib.

## Adenosquamous Carcinomas of the Lung

Adenosquamous carcinomas of the lung are histologically mixed tumors composed of both squamous and adenocarcinoma components. These tumors represent 0.4–4 % of NSCLCs and harbor EGFR mutations and ALK rearrangements at a frequency similar to adenocarcinomas of the lung [71]. Although patients with adenosquamous carcinomas share similar clinical features as EGFR-mutant adenocarcinomas [72, 73] and respond to TKI therapy [74, 75], some studies suggest these mixed tumors portend a poor prognosis [76].

## Squamous Cell Carcinomas of the Lung

Historically, squamous cell carcinomas of the lung (SQCLCs) were the most common subtype of NSCLCs. Beginning in the 1960s and 1970s, the proportion of SQCLCs relative to lung adenocarcinomas began to decline for reasons not entirely related to smoking cessation efforts, and SQCLCs now account for 20–30 % of NSCLCs [77]. While there has been success in identifying molecularly defined subsets of patients with lung adenocarcinomas who now derive benefit from targeted therapies, the molecular landscape in SQCLCs is less defined, and research studies have only recently begun to discover potentially targetable oncogenic drivers in this disease. Below is a summary of targeted therapies currently in clinical development.

### *VEGFR*

Vascular endothelial growth factor (VEGF) is a member of the VEGF platelet-derived growth factor (PDGF) family of structurally related glycoproteins and is the key mediator of angiogenesis [78]. High tumor VEGF and VEGF receptor expression in patients with SQCLC is associated with a favorable prognosis. However, bevacizumab, a monoclonal antibody against VEGF, is not approved for the treatment of patients with SQCLCs due to safety concerns. An initial phase 2 study of chemotherapy with or without bevacizumab showed an unacceptable rate of pulmonary hemorrhage in patients with SQCLC [79]. In a subsequent small phase 2 BRIDGE study in SQCLC, bevacizumab was introduced after two cycles of cytotoxic chemotherapy and the rate of grade 3 or higher pulmonary hemorrhage was decreased at 3.2 % [80]. In a small cohort of patients with early-stage lung cancers at a high risk of bleeding (SQCLC histology, history of gross hemoptysis, or large central tumors), bevacizumab given in the adjuvant setting did not lead to hemoptysis [81]. Further exploration of the optimal use and efficacy of antiangiogenic agents in patients with SQCLC should proceed with appropriate biomarker analyses.

## *EGFR*

SQCLCs have high expression of EGFR both in frequency and intensity of staining by IHC when compared with adenocarcinomas of the lung [82]. The efficacy of cetuximab, a monoclonal antibody against EGFR, was evaluated in the FLEX trial [83], a large multinational trial that randomized patients with treatment-naïve locally advanced or metastatic NSCLCs to six cycles of cisplatin and vinorelbine with or without cetuximab. Although the group with cetuximab reached its primary endpoint of an increased OS of 1.2 months (HR 0.871, 95 % CI 0.762–0.996, $p = 0.044$), this difference was considered small, and the drug was not approved. In a prespecified secondary analysis of the FLEX data, about a third of the patients had high EGFR expression, scored by the intensity and percentage of cells positively, that was associated with an improved response rate and increased OS of 2.6 months when treated with cetuximab (HR 0.73, 95 % CI 0.58–0.93, $p = 0.011$). Importantly, a higher percentage of SQCLCs was seen in the high EGFR expression groups compared to the low EGFR expression groups. In further subset analyses comparing histologies in the high EGFR expression group, the OS benefit was seen only in patients with SQCLC (HR 0.62, 95 % CI 0.43–0.88) compared to other histologies [84]. As with the antiangiogenic agents, further biomarker studies are warranted to maximize the efficacy of cetuximab in carefully selected patients.

## *Emerging Oncogenic Targets*

As a part of The Cancer Genome Atlas project, 178 resected early-stage SQCLCs were profiled to characterize the genomic landscape and identify potential targetable aberrations (Fig. 8.1) [85]. The frequency of somatic alterations was among the highest found, with a mean of 360 exon mutations, 323 altered copy number

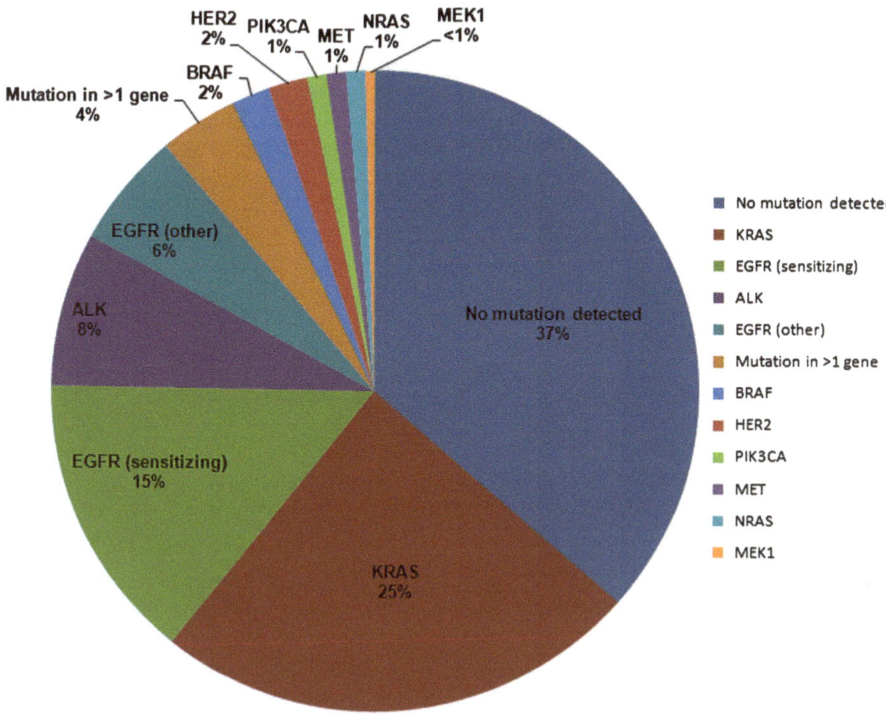


**Fig. 8.1** Frequency of oncogenic drivers in lung adenocarcinoma as part of the Lung Cancer Mutation Consortium

segments, and 165 genomic rearrangements per tumor. Statistically recurrent mutations were found in 11 genes (*TP53*, *CDKN2A*, *PTEN*, *PIK3CA*, *KEAP1*, *MLL2*, *NFE2L2*, *NOTCH1*, *RB1*, and *HLA-A*) with a mutation in *TP53* found in a large majority of the samples. Alterations impairing squamous cell differentiation were observed in 44 % of tumor samples, including overexpression and amplification of SOX2 and TP63; loss-of-function mutations in *NOTCH1*, *NOTCH2*, and *ASCL4*; and focal deletions in *FOXP1*. Alterations in oxidative stress response pathway genes were present in 34 % of cases, including mutation and copy number alterations of *NFE2L2* and *KEAP1* and/or deletions of *CUL3*. While no *EGFR* exon 19 deletions or L858R substitutions were identified, two *EGFR* L861Q substitutions were identified, and *EGFR* amplification was demonstrated in 7 % of cases. Only one sample harbored a *KRAS* codon 61 mutation.

The opportunities for potential therapeutic targets in SQCLC were supported by the observation that 96 % of tumors contained one or more mutations in tyrosine kinases, serine/threonine kinases, phosphatidylinositol-3-OH kinase (PI3K) catalytic and regulatory subunits, nuclear hormone receptors, G-protein-coupled receptors, proteases, and tyrosine phosphatases (Fig. 8.2). Targetable genetic alterations were considered present in 64 % of TCGA samples based on the availability of an

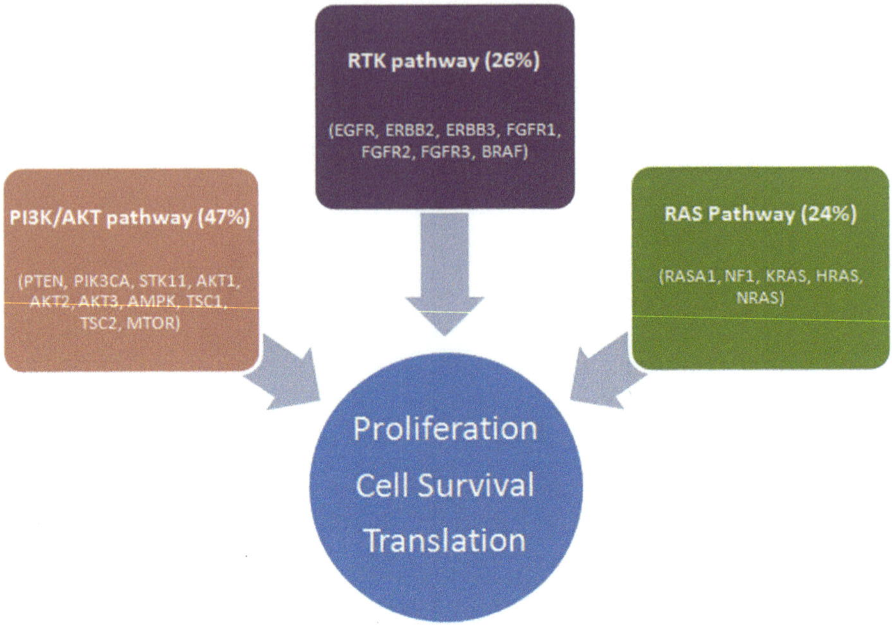


**Fig. 8.2** Alterations in targetable oncogenic pathways in SQCLCs. Sixty-nine percent of 178 SQCLCs revealed alteration in at least one of the three pathways: PI3K-AKT, RTK, and RAS. Alterations are defined by somatic mutations, homozygous deletions, and high-level, focal amplifications and, in some cases, by significant up- or downregulation of gene expression (AKT3, FGFR1, PTEN)

FDA-approved targeted therapy or one under study in clinical trials, the confirmation of the altered allele in RNA sequencing, and the mutation assessor score. Of these, mutations or amplifications were reported in three families of tyrosine kinases: the erythroblastic leukemia viral oncogene homologues (ERBBs), fibroblast growth factor receptors (FGFRs), and Janus kinases (JAKs). An alteration in at least one of the core cellular pathways known to represent potential therapeutic opportunities (PI3K-AKT, receptor tyrosine kinase (RTK), and RAS) was identified in 69 % of samples. Specifically, one of the components of the PI3K-AKT pathway was altered in 47 % of tumors, and RTK signaling was probably affected by events such as *EGFR* amplification, *BRAF* mutation, or *FGFR* amplification or mutation in 26 % of tumors. While this analysis suggests new areas for potential therapeutic development, the dependence of SQCLC on many of these alterations needs to be defined clinically.

## *FGFR*

FGFR is a transmembrane receptor tyrosine kinase that participates in the regulation of embryonal development, cell proliferation, differentiation, and angiogenesis. The FGFR family has four members, including FGFR1, FGFR2, FGFR3, and

FGFR4, and binds up to 22 FGF ligands. After binding with their FGF ligands, FGFRs undergo dimerization followed by activation of downstream signaling via PI3K-AKT and RAS-RAF-MAPK pathways central to survival in tumorigenesis.

Alterations in FGFR1–4 were seen in 27 % of tumor samples reported by TCGA, with *FGFR1* mutations or amplification in 18 % of samples [85]. In a set of 153 SQCLC tumors, Weiss and colleagues found *FGFR1* amplification in 22 % of the samples by FISH [86]. A separate study by Dutt and colleagues identified an amplification frequency of 21 % by SNP array analysis of 57 SQCLC samples [87]. In an Asian population with surgically resected SQCLC, *FGFR1* amplification was found in 13 % of 262 specimens and correlated with cigarette smoking and a shorter overall survival (51.2 vs. 115 months) [88]. A study conducted by Heist and colleagues found that *FGFR1* amplification status did not correlate with smoking history or survival in a Caucasian population [89].

In Weiss and colleagues' study, treatment with an FGFR inhibitor PD173074 resulted in tumor regression in a mouse xenograft model [87]. Malchers and colleagues found that *FGFR1*-amplified tumor cells that co-expressed MYC were more sensitive to FGFR inhibition. The authors reported two SQCLC patients with amplified *FGFR1* and high MYC expression who responded to FGFR inhibition: one responded to BGJ398, a highly specific FGFR inhibitor, and the other responded to pazopanib, a multikinase inhibitor with weak activity against FGFR [90]. FGFR inhibitors have also been found to have activity in other solid tumors such as breast cancer and gastric cancer. Several trials evaluating selective FGFR1 inhibitors are currently in early phase clinical testing [91].

## *PI3K Pathway*

The PI3K pathway is a signal transduction pathway central to cell survival, metabolism, motility, and angiogenesis. Abnormalities in this pathway including in PI3K/PTEN/AKT/mTOR are more common in SQCLC than in lung adenocarcinoma, suggesting an increased dependence on this pathway [92–94]. The TCGA analysis found 47 % of tumors to have an alteration in one of the components of the PI3K-AKT pathway [85]. The mutation rate for *PIK3CA* in SQCLC ranges from 3.6 to 6.5 % [93, 95], and *PIK3CA* amplification occurs in 42–43 % in an Asian population by FISH [94] and PCR [96], respectively. Soria and colleagues reported a loss of PTEN expression by IHC and PTEN methylation in 24 % and 35 % of NSCLC, respectively [97]. Jin and colleagues showed a *PTEN* mutation rate of 10 in SQCLC compared to 1.7 % in lung adenocarcinoma samples [44].

Spoerke and colleagues found that cell lines harboring alterations in this pathway, including *PI3K* mutation or amplification, *PTEN* loss, or receptor tyrosine kinase activation, predict for sensitivity to PI3K inhibitors [98]. There are a number of ongoing evaluations of PI3K and mTOR inhibitors in various solid tumors including in lung cancer, although no efficacy data are available to date.

## *DDR2 Mutations*

The discoidin domain receptor (DDR) is a plasma membrane receptor tyrosine kinase that regulates cell adhesion, proliferation, and extracellular remodeling upon binding to its endogenous ligand, type 1 collagen [99, 100]. Upregulation of DDR1 in NSCLC, particularly squamous tumors, has been associated with improved disease-free and overall survival [101]. Hammerman and colleagues sequenced 290 SQCLC tumors and cell lines and found 3.8 % tumors to harbor a *DDR2* mutation. These tumors showed a gain-of-function phenotype that was abrogated by treatment with dasatinib, a multikinase inhibitor with activity against both DDR1 and DDR2 [102]. Two phase II studies showed no advantage of dasatinib in unselected patients with advanced NSCLC [103, 104]. A recent case report describes a patient with chronic myelogenous leukemia (CML) and SQCLC harboring a *DDR2* mutation who was treated with dasatinib, resulting in normalization of blood counts and a near complete reduction in size of the primary lung mass [105]. A phase II trial is currently underway to investigate the efficacy of dasatinib selected in SQCLC with *DDR2* mutations.

## *IGF1R*

Insulin-like growth factor-1 receptor (IGF1R) is a cell surface receptor with tyrosine kinase activity that binds to the ligands IGF-1 or IGF-2 and activates the PI3K and RAS signaling pathways [106–108]. IGF1R protein expression is seen more commonly in SQCLC compared to other subtypes [109, 110], but thus far has not been found to be of prognostic value [111]. A phase II study with figitumumab, a monoclonal antibody against IGF1R, with paclitaxel and carboplatin showed a response rate of 78 % in patients with advanced SQCLC [112]. However, a subsequent randomized phase III trial of figitumumab with paclitaxel/carboplatin in unselected NSCLC patients was discontinued due to futility and increased toxicity [113]. Early clinical trials evaluating small molecular inhibitors of IGF1R are ongoing [114], and the utility of free IGF-1 or IGF1R protein expression as a predictive biomarker remains to be seen.

## *PDGFRA*

Platelet-derived growth factor receptor (PDGFR) tyrosine kinase, classified as PDGFRA and PDGFRB, plays a crucial role in cell proliferation and angiogenesis [115]. PDGFRA amplification occurs in 8.7 % SQCLC compared to 3.8 % of lung adenocarcinomas [116]. A randomized phase III study with the addition of sorafenib, a multi-targeted TKI that targets PDGFRA, to platinum-based chemotherapy failed to show an improved survival in patients with advanced NSCLC. A subset of

SQCLC in the study had increased mortality with the addition of sorafenib [117]. Further clinical trials are now evaluating selective anti-PDGFRA inhibitors as well as PDGFRA-targeting monoclonal antibodies [118].

## *EGFR vIII*

*EGFR* vIII is a variant of *EGFR* with deletion of exons 2–7, which was first described in human glioma [119]. A study in Japan revealed an *EGFR* vIII mutation in 8 of 252 patients, among which 7 had SQCLC [120]. Ji and colleagues examined 179 NSCLC samples and found an *EGFR* vIII mutation in 5 % SQCLC but none of the lung adenocarcinomas. The investigators also noted tumor regression in *EGFR* vIII mutant murine models treated with an irreversible EGFR inhibitor, HKI-272. Similarly cell lines that were resistant to gefitinib and erlotinib in vitro proved sensitive to HKI-272 [121]. HKI-272 is currently in the early phase of clinical development [122].

## *MET*

*MET* is a proto-oncogene located on 7q21-31 and encodes a tyrosine kinase receptor for hepatocyte growth factor. *MET* activation either by increased gene copy number or amplification leads to enhanced proliferation, motility, apoptosis resistance, and angiogenesis. *MET* amplification has been recognized as a mechanism of resistance to EGFR TKI therapy in lung adenocarcinoma [123]. MET protein expression occurs in approximately 40 % of SQCLC and associated with a poorer prognosis [124]. A phase II trial of onartuzumab, a monoclonal antibody against MET, in combination with erlotinib showed improvements in OS and PFS compared with erlotinib alone in a MET-overexpressed subgroup of advanced NSCLC, of which 30 % had SQCLC [125]. A randomized phase III study is currently evaluating onartuzumab in combination with a platinum doublet in SQCLC.

## *Small Cell Lung Cancer*

Small cell lung cancer (SCLC) is characterized by frequent inactivating mutations in the critical tumor suppressor genes *TP53* (75–90 %) [126] and *RB1* (60–90 %) [127, 128]. A mouse model with conditional inactivation of these two tumor suppressors in the lung generates lung tumors histologically and biologically similar to human SCLC [129].

Recent reports including exome, transcriptome, and limited whole-genome sequencing have provided insights into the fuller landscape of genetic alterations in SCLC [130, 131]. In addition to confirming *TP53* and *RB1* inactivation, these studies define other alterations of interest in SCLC, with potential therapeutic implications. One consistent finding from both reports was an exceptionally high degree of genomic alteration in this tumor type, including mutations, insertions, deletions, large-scale copy number alterations, and gross inter- and intra-chromosomal rearrangements. MYC family member alterations, including gene amplification of *MYC*, *MYCN*, and *MYCL1*, as well as a recurrent gene fusion involving *MYCL1*, are frequent in SCLC and may represent important drivers of SCLC oncogenesis. The tumor suppressor PTEN appears to be inactivated in approximately 10 % of SCLC, and mutations of other factors in the same signaling pathway were also identified. Other alterations implicated as potential drivers in subsets of SCLC include amplification of the tyrosine kinase FGFR1 (in a reported 6 % of cases) and of the developmental regulator and transcription factor SOX2 (in up to 27 % of cases). The therapeutic implications of the large majority of the genetic alterations documented to date in SCLC have not been defined.

Importantly, pure SCLC lacks *EGFR* mutations and *ALK* rearrangements, even in those patients with this malignancy who are never smokers [132, 133]. However, in the rare cases of SCLC transformation as a mechanism of acquired resistance to EGFR TKIs, there is persistence of the original *EGFR* mutation in the tumors confirmed on biopsy. In all cases where SCLC has been documented as a mechanism of acquired resistance to EGFR TKIs, the original tumor was a pure adenocarcinoma prior to EGFR TKI treatment, and the transformation was validated by histologic examination and confirmed by expression of neuroendocrine markers.

## *The Role of Small Biopsies in the Age of Genotype-Driven Therapy*

The majority of patients with lung cancers present with metastatic disease and are diagnosed, as a result, from small biopsy or cytology specimens alone. Bronchial biopsy samples obtained from patients with lung cancer frequently contain only limited amounts of primary carcinoma, and often one or more of the biopsy fragments will not contain tumor at all [134]. Despite these challenges, cytology can be used to distinguish histology in NSCLC with accuracy up to 96 %, and in a majority of cases, cytology is suitable for molecular analysis as well [135].

As evident in the preceding text, oncologists are increasingly faced with the challenge of obtaining sufficient tumor material to perform standard of care or exploratory molecular analyses prior to determining a patient's treatment plan, all while minimizing the need for further invasive procedures. In tertiary cancer centers, most patients present with a pathologic diagnosis, with variable amounts of diagnostic material leftover. In addition to surgical pathology, immunohistochemistry and fluorescence in situ hybridization typically require at least 4–6 five micrometer recuts,

**Table 8.1** Targeted agents for patients with genetic alterations[a]

| Genetic alteration (i.e., driver event) | Available targeted agents with activity against driver event in lung cancer |
|---|---|
| **EGFR** mutations | Erlotinib [138], gefitinib [3], afatinib [139] |
| **ALK** rearrangements | Crizotinib [140] |
| **HER2** mutations | Trastuzumab [141], afatinib [142] |
| **BRAF** mutations | Vemurafenib [143], dabrafenib [32] |
| **MET** amplification | Crizotinib [144] |
| **ROS1** rearrangements | Crizotinib [145] |
| **RET** rearrangements | Cabozantinib [70] |

[a]Adapted from NCCN guidelines

PCR-based genotyping requires approximately 10, and next-generation sequencing requires over 10. Stepwise algorithms that prioritize specific molecular studies are clearly needed.

Recognizing the need to reassess and formally address the optimal utility of small biopsy and cytology specimens to meet the modern day clinical needs, a new lung adenocarcinoma classification has recently been published under the joint sponsorship of the International Association for the Study of Lung Cancer (IASLC), the American Thoracic Society (ATS), and the European Respiratory Society (ERS) [136]. The major changes introduced include the greater use of special stains to classify difficult cases further into adenocarcinoma or SQCLC, the diagnosis using small samples, and the need to manage tissue strategically for molecular studies. In particular, for those cases where a small biopsy specimen shows NSCLC lacking either definite squamous or adenocarcinoma morphology, the immunohistochemistry workup should be as limited as possible to preserve tissue for molecular testing. A multidisciplinary and institutional approach should be implemented to incorporate clinical information in selecting the appropriate methods for obtaining tissue samples and prioritizing molecular studies including DNA sequence analysis, fluorescence in situ hybridization, and RNA-based studies. While the list of targets will continue to evolve, recommendations for testing by the National Comprehensive Cancer Network working group are driven by the availability of rationally targeted therapies which can, in practice, be given to patients (Table 8.1).

While next-generation sequencing is ideal for patients with adequate tissue samples, as it may discover potential targets for therapy and/or generate clinical trial opportunities for patients, symptomatic patients may not have the luxury of waiting, untreated, the 4–8-week turnaround time for results. In such cases, other assays that can be completed in a shorter time period, such as IHC for mutant forms of *EGFR* or *ALK*, can be prioritized to help determine treatment plans. Indeed, immunostaining to detect mutant *EGFR* correlates well with sequencing-based assays and is particularly useful for small biopsies when the material is scant or bone biopsies in which the decalcification processes often results in DNA degradation [137].

## References

1. Shepherd FA, Rodrigues Pereira J, Ciuleanu T, et al. Erlotinib in previously treated non-small-cell lung cancer. N Engl J Med. 2005;353:123–32.
2. Pao W, Miller V, Zakowski M, et al. EGF receptor gene mutations are common in lung cancers from "never smokers" and are associated with sensitivity of tumors to gefitinib and erlotinib. Proc Natl Acad Sci USA. 2004;101:13306–11.
3. Paez JG, Janne PA, Lee JC, et al. EGFR mutations in lung cancer: correlation with clinical response to gefitinib therapy. Science. 2004;304:1497–500.
4. Lynch TJ, Bell DW, Sordella R, et al. Activating mutations in the epidermal growth factor receptor underlying responsiveness of non-small-cell lung cancer to gefitinib. N Engl J Med. 2004;350:2129–39.
5. Rosell R, Carcereny E, Gervais R, et al. Erlotinib versus standard chemotherapy as first-line treatment for European patients with advanced EGFR mutation-positive non-small-cell lung cancer (EURTAC): a multicentre, open-label, randomised phase 3 trial. Lancet Oncol. 2012;13:239–46.
6. Ladanyi M, Pao W. Lung adenocarcinoma: guiding EGFR-targeted therapy and beyond. Mod Pathol. 2008;21 Suppl 2:S16–22.
7. Mitsudomi T, Yatabe Y. Epidermal growth factor receptor in relation to tumor development: EGFR gene and cancer. FEBS J. 2010;277:301–8.
8. Arcila ME, Nafa K, Chaft JE, et al. EGFR exon 20 insertion mutations in lung adenocarcinomas: prevalence, molecular heterogeneity, and clinicopathologic characteristics. Mol Cancer Ther. 2013;12:220–9.
9. Sordella R, Bell DW, Haber DA, et al. Gefitinib-sensitizing EGFR mutations in lung cancer activate anti-apoptotic pathways. Science. 2004;305:1163–7.
10. Mok TS, Wu YL, Thongprasert S, et al. Gefitinib or carboplatin-paclitaxel in pulmonary adenocarcinoma. N Engl J Med. 2009;361:947–57.
11. Mitsudomi T, Morita S, Yatabe Y, et al. Gefitinib versus cisplatin plus docetaxel in patients with non-small-cell lung cancer harbouring mutations of the epidermal growth factor receptor (WJTOG3405): an open label, randomised phase 3 trial. Lancet Oncol. 2010;11:121–8.
12. Maemondo M, Inoue A, Kobayashi K, et al. Gefitinib or chemotherapy for non-small-cell lung cancer with mutated EGFR. N Engl J Med. 2010;362:2380–8.
13. Chong CR, Janne PA. The quest to overcome resistance to EGFR-targeted therapies in cancer. Nat Med. 2013;19:1389–400.
14. Pao W, Miller VA, Politi KA, et al. Acquired resistance of lung adenocarcinomas to gefitinib or erlotinib is associated with a second mutation in the EGFR kinase domain. PLoS Med. 2005;2:e73.
15. Janjigian YY, Groen HJ, Horn L, et al. Activity and tolerability of afatinib (BIBW 2992) and cetuximab in NSCLC patients with acquired resistance to erlotinib or gefitinib. J Clin Oncol. 2011(29).
16. Sequist LV, Soria JC, Gadgeel SM, et al. First-in-human evaluation of CO-1686, an irreversible, selective, and potent tyrosine kinase inhibitor of EGFR T790M. J Clin Oncol. 2013(31).
17. Riely GJ, Marks J, Pao W. KRAS mutations in non-small cell lung cancer. Proc Am Thorac Soc. 2009;6:201–5.
18. Santos E, Martin-Zanca D, Reddy EP, et al. Malignant activation of a K-ras oncogene in lung carcinoma but not in normal tissue of the same patient. Science. 1984;223:661–4.
19. Rekhtman N, Ang DC, Riely GJ, et al. KRAS mutations are associated with solid growth pattern and tumor-infiltrating leukocytes in lung adenocarcinoma. Mod Pathol. 2013;26:1307–19.
20. Riely GJ, Kris MG, Rosenbaum D, et al. Frequency and distinctive spectrum of KRAS mutations in never smokers with lung adenocarcinoma. Clin Cancer Res. 2008;14:5731–4.
21. Mascaux C, Iannino N, Martin B, et al. The role of RAS oncogene in survival of patients with lung cancer: a systematic review of the literature with meta-analysis. Br J Cancer. 2005;92:131–9.

22. Zhu CQ, da Cunha SG, Ding K, et al. Role of KRAS and EGFR as biomarkers of response to erlotinib in National Cancer Institute of Canada Clinical Trials Group Study BR.21. J Clin Oncol. 2008;26:4268–75.
23. Mao C, Qiu LX, Liao RY, et al. KRAS mutations and resistance to EGFR-TKIs treatment in patients with non-small cell lung cancer: a meta-analysis of 22 studies. Lung Cancer. 2010;69:272–8.
24. Shepherd FA, Domerg C, Hainaut P, et al. Pooled analysis of the prognostic and predictive effects of KRAS mutation status and KRAS mutation subtype in early-stage resected non-small-cell lung cancer in four trials of adjuvant chemotherapy. J Clin Oncol. 2013;31:2173–81.
25. Janne PA, Shaw AT, Pereira JR, et al. Selumetinib plus docetaxel for KRAS-mutant advanced non-small-cell lung cancer: a randomised, multicentre, placebo-controlled, phase 2 study. Lancet Oncol. 2013;14:38–47.
26. Engelman JA, Chen L, Tan X, et al. Effective use of PI3K and MEK inhibitors to treat mutant Kras G12D and PIK3CA H1047R murine lung cancers. Nat Med. 2008;14:1351–6.
27. Eggermont AM, Spatz A, Robert C. Cutaneous melanoma. Lancet. 2014;383:816–27.
28. Brose MS, Volpe P, Feldman M, et al. BRAF and RAS mutations in human lung cancer and melanoma. Cancer Res. 2002;62:6997–7000.
29. Pratilas CA, Hanrahan AJ, Halilovic E, et al. Genetic predictors of MEK dependence in non-small cell lung cancer. Cancer Res. 2008;68:9375–83.
30. Ji H, Wang Z, Perera SA, et al. Mutations in BRAF and KRAS converge on activation of the mitogen-activated protein kinase pathway in lung cancer mouse models. Cancer Res. 2007;67:4933–9.
31. Paik PK, Arcila ME, Fara M, et al. Clinical characteristics of patients with lung adenocarcinomas harboring BRAF mutations. J Clin Oncol. 2011;29:2046–51.
32. Planchard D, Mazieres J, Riely GJ, et al. Interim results of phase II study BRF113928 of dabrafenib in BRAF V600E mutation–positive non-small cell lung cancer (NSCLC) patients. J Clin Oncol. 2013(31).
33. Sen B, Peng S, Tang X, et al. Kinase-impaired BRAF mutations in lung cancer confer sensitivity to dasatinib. Sci Transl Med 2012;4:136ra70.
34. Rudin CM, Hong K, Streit M. Molecular characterization of acquired resistance to the BRAF inhibitor dabrafenib in a patient with BRAF-mutant non-small-cell lung cancer. J Thorac Oncol. 2013;8:e41–2.
35. Arteaga CL, Sliwkowski MX, Osborne CK, et al. Treatment of HER2-positive breast cancer: current status and future perspectives. Nat Rev Clin Oncol. 2012;9:16–32.
36. Stephens P, Hunter C, Bignell G, et al. Lung cancer: intragenic ERBB2 kinase mutations in tumours. Nature. 2004;431:525–6.
37. Arcila ME, Chaft JE, Nafa K, et al. Prevalence, clinicopathologic associations, and molecular spectrum of ERBB2 (HER2) tyrosine kinase mutations in lung adenocarcinomas. Clin Cancer Res. 2012;18:4910–8.
38. Gandhi L, Bahleda R, Tolaney SM, et al. Phase I study of neratinib in combination with temsirolimus in patients with human epidermal growth factor receptor 2-dependent and other solid tumors. J Clin Oncol. 2014;32:68–75.
39. Perera SA, Li D, Shimamura T, et al. HER2YVMA drives rapid development of adenosquamous lung tumors in mice that are sensitive to BIBW2992 and rapamycin combination therapy. Proc Natl Acad Sci USA. 2009;106:474–9.
40. Landi L, Cappuzzo F. HER2 and lung cancer. Expert Rev Anticancer Ther. 2013;13:1219–28.
41. Courtney KD, Corcoran RB, Engelman JA. The PI3K pathway as drug target in human cancer. J Clin Oncol. 2010;28:1075–83.
42. Chaft JE, Arcila ME, Paik PK, et al. Coexistence of PIK3CA and other oncogene mutations in lung adenocarcinoma-rationale for comprehensive mutation profiling. Mol Cancer Ther. 2012;11:485–91.
43. Drilon A, Rekhtman N, Ladanyi M, et al. Squamous-cell carcinomas of the lung: emerging biology, controversies, and the promise of targeted therapy. Lancet Oncol. 2012;13:e418–26.

44. Jin G, Kim MJ, Jeon HS, et al. PTEN mutations and relationship to EGFR, ERBB2, KRAS, and TP53 mutations in non-small cell lung cancers. Lung Cancer. 2010;69:279–83.
45. Neshat MS, Mellinghoff IK, Tran C, et al. Enhanced sensitivity of PTEN-deficient tumors to inhibition of FRAP/mTOR. Proc Natl Acad Sci USA. 2001;98:10314–9.
46. Malanga D, Scrima M, De Marco C, et al. Activating E17K mutation in the gene encoding the protein kinase AKT1 in a subset of squamous cell carcinoma of the lung. Cell Cycle. 2008;7:665–9.
47. Carpten JD, Faber AL, Horn C, et al. A transforming mutation in the pleckstrin homology domain of AKT1 in cancer. Nature. 2007;448:439–44.
48. Hallberg B, Palmer RH. Mechanistic insight into ALK receptor tyrosine kinase in human cancer biology. Nat Rev Cancer. 2013;13:685–700.
49. Soda M, Choi YL, Enomoto M, et al. Identification of the transforming EML4-ALK fusion gene in non-small-cell lung cancer. Nature. 2007;448:561–6.
50. Soda M, Takada S, Takeuchi K, et al. A mouse model for EML4-ALK-positive lung cancer. Proc Natl Acad Sci USA. 2008;105:19893–7.
51. Shaw AT, Engelman JA. ALK in lung cancer: past, present, and future. J Clin Oncol. 2013;31:1105–11.
52. Inamura K, Takeuchi K, Togashi Y, et al. EML4-ALK lung cancers are characterized by rare other mutations, a TTF-1 cell lineage, an acinar histology, and young onset. Mod Pathol. 2009;22:508–15.
53. Wong DW, Leung EL, So KK, et al. The EML4-ALK fusion gene is involved in various histologic types of lung cancers from nonsmokers with wild-type EGFR and KRAS. Cancer. 2009;115:1723–33.
54. Shaw AT, Solomon B, Kenudson MM. Crizotinib and testing for ALK. J Natl Compr Canc Netw. 2011;9:1335–41.
55. Camidge DR, Bang YJ, Kwak EL, et al. Activity and safety of crizotinib in patients with ALK-positive non-small-cell lung cancer: updated results from a phase 1 study. Lancet Oncol. 2012;13:1011–9.
56. Shaw AT, Kim DW, Nakagawa K, et al. Crizotinib versus chemotherapy in advanced ALK-positive lung cancer. N Engl J Med. 2013;368:2385–94.
57. Doebele RC, Pilling AB, Aisner DL, et al. Mechanisms of resistance to crizotinib in patients with ALK gene rearranged non-small cell lung cancer. Clin Cancer Res. 2012;18:1472–82.
58. Rikova K, Guo A, Zeng Q, et al. Global survey of phosphotyrosine signaling identifies oncogenic kinases in lung cancer. Cell. 2007;131:1190–203.
59. Gainor JF, Shaw AT. Novel targets in non-small cell lung cancer: ROS1 and RET fusions. Oncologist. 2013;18:865–75.
60. Takeuchi K, Soda M, Togashi Y, et al. RET, ROS1 and ALK fusions in lung cancer. Nat Med. 2012;18:378–81.
61. Yasuda H, de Figueiredo-Pontes LL, Kobayashi S, et al. Preclinical rationale for use of the clinically available multitargeted tyrosine kinase inhibitor crizotinib in ROS1-translocated lung cancer. J Thorac Oncol. 2012;7:1086–90.
62. Ou SH, Bang YJ, Camidge DR, et al. Efficacy and safety of crizotinib in patients with advanced ROS1-rearranged non-small cell lung cancer (NSCLC). J Clin Oncol. 2012(31).
63. Awad MM, Engelman JA, Shaw AT. Acquired resistance to crizotinib from a mutation in CD74-ROS1. N Engl J Med. 2013;369:1173.
64. Ju YS, Lee WC, Shin JY, et al. A transforming KIF5B and RET gene fusion in lung adenocarcinoma revealed from whole-genome and transcriptome sequencing. Genome Res. 2012;22:436–45.
65. Lipson D, Capelletti M, Yelensky R, et al. Identification of new ALK and RET gene fusions from colorectal and lung cancer biopsies. Nat Med. 2012;18:382–4.
66. Kohno T, Ichikawa H, Totoki Y, et al. KIF5B-RET fusions in lung adenocarcinoma. Nat Med. 2012;18:375–7.

67. Drilon A, Wang L, Hasanovic A, et al. Screening for RET and ROS1 fusions in an enriched cohort of pan-negative never-smokers with advanced lung adenocarcinomas to identify patients for treatment in targeted therapy trials. J Clin Oncol. 2013(31).
68. Wang R, Hu H, Pan Y, et al. RET fusions define a unique molecular and clinicopathologic subtype of non-small-cell lung cancer. J Clin Oncol. 2012;30:4352–9.
69. Suzuki M, Makinoshima H, Matsumoto S, et al. Identification of a lung adenocarcinoma cell line with CCDC6-RET fusion gene and the effect of RET inhibitors in vitro and in vivo. Cancer Sci. 2013;104:896–903.
70. Drilon A, Wang L, Hasanovic A, et al. Response to Cabozantinib in patients with RET fusion-positive lung adenocarcinomas. Cancer Discov. 2013;3:630–5.
71. Ohtsuka K, Ohnishi H, Fujiwara M, et al. Abnormalities of epidermal growth factor receptor in lung squamous-cell carcinomas, adenosquamous carcinomas, and large-cell carcinomas: tyrosine kinase domain mutations are not rare in tumors with an adenocarcinoma component. Cancer. 2007;109:741–50.
72. Shiozawa T, Ishii G, Goto K, et al. Clinicopathological characteristics of EGFR mutated adenosquamous carcinoma of the lung. Pathol Int. 2013;63:77–84.
73. Wang R, Pan Y, Li C, et al. Analysis of major known driver mutations and prognosis in resected adenosquamous lung carcinomas. J Thorac Oncol. 2014;9(6):760–8.
74. Song Z, Lin B, Shao L, et al. Therapeutic efficacy of gefitinib and erlotinib in patients with advanced lung adenosquamous carcinoma. J Chin Med Assoc. 2013;76:481–5.
75. Hata A, Katakami N, Yoshioka H. How sensitive are epidermal growth factor receptor-tyrosine kinase inhibitors for squamous cell carcinoma of the lung harboring EGFR gene-sensitive mutations? J Thorac Oncol. 2014;9:e20.
76. Mordant P, Grand B, Cazes A, et al. Adenosquamous carcinoma of the lung: surgical management, pathologic characteristics, and prognostic implications. Ann Thorac Surg. 2013;95:1189–95.
77. Travis WD. Pathology of lung cancer. Clin Chest Med. 2011;32:669–92.
78. Carmeliet P. VEGF as a key mediator of angiogenesis in cancer. Oncology 2005;69(Suppl 3):4–10.
79. Johnson DH, Fehrenbacher L, Novotny WF, et al. Randomized phase II trial comparing bevacizumab plus carboplatin and paclitaxel with carboplatin and paclitaxel alone in previously untreated locally advanced or metastatic non-small-cell lung cancer. J Clin Oncol. 2004;22:2184–91.
80. Hainsworth JD, Fang L, Huang JE, et al. BRIDGE: an open-label phase II trial evaluating the safety of bevacizumab+carboplatin/paclitaxel as first-line treatment for patients with advanced, previously untreated, squamous non-small cell lung cancer. J Thorac Oncol. 2011;6:109–14.
81. Hellmann MD, Chaft JE, Rusch V, et al. Risk of hemoptysis in patients with resected squamous cell and other high-risk lung cancers treated with adjuvant bevacizumab. Cancer Chemother Pharmacol. 2013;72:453–61.
82. Hirsch FR, Varella-Garcia M, Bunn Jr PA, et al. Epidermal growth factor receptor in non-small-cell lung carcinomas: correlation between gene copy number and protein expression and impact on prognosis. J Clin Oncol. 2003;21:3798–807.
83. Pirker R, Pereira JR, Szczesna A, et al. Cetuximab plus chemotherapy in patients with advanced non-small-cell lung cancer (FLEX): an open-label randomised phase III trial. Lancet. 2009;373:1525–31.
84. Pirker R, Pereira JR, von Pawel J, et al. EGFR expression as a predictor of survival for first-line chemotherapy plus cetuximab in patients with advanced non-small-cell lung cancer: analysis of data from the phase 3 FLEX study. Lancet Oncol. 2012;13:33–42.
85. Comprehensive genomic characterization of squamous cell lung cancers. Nature. 2012;489:519–25.

86. Weiss J, Sos ML, Seidel D, et al. Frequent and focal FGFR1 amplification associates with therapeutically tractable FGFR1 dependency in squamous cell lung cancer. Sci Transl Med. 2010;2:62ra93.
87. Dutt A, Ramos AH, Hammerman PS, et al. Inhibitor-sensitive FGFR1 amplification in human non-small cell lung cancer. PLoS One. 2011;6:e20351.
88. Kim HR, Kim DJ, Kang DR, et al. Fibroblast growth factor receptor 1 gene amplification is associated with poor survival and cigarette smoking dosage in patients with resected squamous cell lung cancer. J Clin Oncol. 2013;31:731–7.
89. Heist RS, Mino-Kenudson M, Sequist LV, et al. FGFR1 amplification in squamous cell carcinoma of the lung. J Thorac Oncol. 2012;7:1775–80.
90. Malchers F, Dietlein F, Schottle J, et al. Cell-autonomous and non-cell-autonomous mechanisms of transformation by amplified FGFR1 in lung cancer. Cancer Discov. 2014;4:246–57.
91. Lim SM, Kim HR, Shim HS, et al. Role of FGF receptors as an emerging therapeutic target in lung squamous cell carcinoma. Future Oncol. 2013;9:377–86.
92. Rekhtman N, Paik PK, Arcila ME, et al. Clarifying the spectrum of driver oncogene mutations in biomarker-verified squamous carcinoma of lung: lack of EGFR/KRAS and presence of PIK3CA/AKT1 mutations. Clin Cancer Res. 2012;18:1167–76.
93. Yamamoto H, Shigematsu H, Nomura M, et al. PIK3CA mutations and copy number gains in human lung cancers. Cancer Res. 2008;68:6913–21.
94. Okudela K, Suzuki M, Kageyama S, et al. PIK3CA mutation and amplification in human lung cancer. Pathol Int. 2007;57:664–71.
95. Kawano O, Sasaki H, Endo K, et al. PIK3CA mutation status in Japanese lung cancer patients. Lung Cancer. 2006;54:209–15.
96. Ji M, Guan H, Gao C, et al. Highly frequent promoter methylation and PIK3CA amplification in non-small cell lung cancer (NSCLC). BMC Cancer. 2011;11:147.
97. Soria JC, Lee HY, Lee JI, et al. Lack of PTEN expression in non-small cell lung cancer could be related to promoter methylation. Clin Cancer Res. 2002;8:1178–84.
98. Spoerke JM, O'Brien C, Huw L, et al. Phosphoinositide 3-kinase (PI3K) pathway alterations are associated with histologic subtypes and are predictive of sensitivity to PI3K inhibitors in lung cancer preclinical models. Clin Cancer Res. 2012;18:6771–83.
99. Ikeda K, Wang LH, Torres R, et al. Discoidin domain receptor 2 interacts with Src and Shc following its activation by type I collagen. J Biol Chem. 2002;277:19206–12.
100. Olaso E, Labrador JP, Wang L, et al. Discoidin domain receptor 2 regulates fibroblast proliferation and migration through the extracellular matrix in association with transcriptional activation of matrix metalloproteinase-2. J Biol Chem. 2002;277:3606–13.
101. Ford CE, Lau SK, Zhu CQ, et al. Expression and mutation analysis of the discoidin domain receptors 1 and 2 in non-small cell lung carcinoma. Br J Cancer. 2007;96:808–14.
102. Hammerman PS, Sos ML, Ramos AH, et al. Mutations in the DDR2 kinase gene identify a novel therapeutic target in squamous cell lung cancer. Cancer Discov. 2011;1:78–89.
103. Haura EB, Tanvetyanon T, Chiappori A, et al. Phase I/II study of the Src inhibitor dasatinib in combination with erlotinib in advanced non-small-cell lung cancer. J Clin Oncol. 2010;28:1387–94.
104. Johnson FM, Bekele BN, Feng L, et al. Phase II study of dasatinib in patients with advanced non-small-cell lung cancer. J Clin Oncol. 2010;28:4609–15.
105. Pitini V, Arrigo C, Di Mirto C, et al. Response to dasatinib in a patient with SQCC of the lung harboring a discoid-receptor-2 and synchronous chronic myelogenous leukemia. Lung Cancer. 2013;82:171–2.
106. Khandwala HM, McCutcheon IE, Flyvbjerg A, et al. The effects of insulin-like growth factors on tumorigenesis and neoplastic growth. Endocr Rev. 2000;21:215–44.
107. LeRoith D, Werner H, Beitner-Johnson D, et al. Molecular and cellular aspects of the insulin-like growth factor I receptor. Endocr Rev. 1995;16:143–63.
108. Baserga R, Hongo A, Rubini M, et al. The IGF-I receptor in cell growth, transformation and apoptosis. Biochim Biophys Acta. 1997;1332:F105–26.

109. Dziadziuszko R, Merrick DT, Witta SE, et al. Insulin-like growth factor receptor 1 (IGF1R) gene copy number is associated with survival in operable non-small-cell lung cancer: a comparison between IGF1R fluorescent in situ hybridization, protein expression, and mRNA expression. J Clin Oncol. 2010;28:2174–80.
110. Gualberto A, Dolled-Filhart M, Gustavson M, et al. Molecular analysis of non-small cell lung cancer identifies subsets with different sensitivity to insulin-like growth factor I receptor inhibition. Clin Cancer Res. 2010;16:4654–65.
111. Cappuzzo F, Tallini G, Finocchiaro G, et al. Insulin-like growth factor receptor 1 (IGF1R) expression and survival in surgically resected non-small-cell lung cancer (NSCLC) patients. Ann Oncol. 2010;21:562–7.
112. Karp DD, Paz-Ares LG, Novello S, et al. Phase II study of the anti-insulin-like growth factor type 1 receptor antibody CP-751,871 in combination with paclitaxel and carboplatin in previously untreated, locally advanced, or metastatic non-small-cell lung cancer. J Clin Oncol. 2009;27:2516–22.
113. Jassem J LC, Karp DD, Mok T, Benner RJ, Green SJ, et al. Randomized, open label, phase III trial of figitumumab in combination with paclitaxel and carboplatin versus paclitaxel and carboplatin in patients with non-small cell lung cancer. J Clin Oncol. 2010;28(15 Suppl): abstract 7500.
114. Wang D, Du L, Liu Q, et al. Receptor tyrosine kinase alterations and therapeutic opportunities in squamous cell carcinoma of the lung. Cancer Chemother Pharmacol. 2013;72:725–31.
115. Ostman A. PDGF receptors-mediators of autocrine tumor growth and regulators of tumor vasculature and stroma. Cytokine Growth Factor Rev. 2004;15:275–86.
116. Ramos AH, Dutt A, Mermel C, et al. Amplification of chromosomal segment 4q12 in non-small cell lung cancer. Cancer Biol Ther. 2009;8:2042–50.
117. Scagliotti G, Novello S, von Pawel J, et al. Phase III study of carboplatin and paclitaxel alone or with sorafenib in advanced non-small-cell lung cancer. J Clin Oncol. 2010;28:1835–42.
118. Shah GD, Loizos N, Youssoufian H, et al. Rationale for the development of IMC-3G3, a fully human immunoglobulin G subclass 1 monoclonal antibody targeting the platelet-derived growth factor receptor alpha. Cancer. 2010;116:1018–26.
119. Wong AJ, Ruppert JM, Bigner SH, et al. Structural alterations of the epidermal growth factor receptor gene in human gliomas. Proc Natl Acad Sci USA. 1992;89:2965–9.
120. Sasaki H, Kawano O, Endo K, et al. EGFRvIII mutation in lung cancer correlates with increased EGFR copy number. Oncol Rep. 2007;17:319–23.
121. Ji H, Zhao X, Yuza Y, et al. Epidermal growth factor receptor variant III mutations in lung tumorigenesis and sensitivity to tyrosine kinase inhibitors. Proc Natl Acad Sci USA. 2006;103:7817–22.
122. Ito Y, Suenaga M, Hatake K, et al. Safety, efficacy and pharmacokinetics of neratinib (HKI-272) in Japanese patients with advanced solid tumors: a Phase 1 dose-escalation study. Jpn J Clin Oncol. 2012;42:278–86.
123. Engelman JA, Zejnullahu K, Mitsudomi T, et al. MET amplification leads to gefitinib resistance in lung cancer by activating ERBB3 signaling. Science. 2007;316:1039–43.
124. Go H, Jeon YK, Park HJ, et al. High MET gene copy number leads to shorter survival in patients with non-small cell lung cancer. J Thorac Oncol. 2010;5:305–13.
125. Spigel DR, Ervin TJ, Ramlau RA, et al. Randomized phase II trial of Onartuzumab in combination with erlotinib in patients with advanced non-small-cell lung cancer. J Clin Oncol. 2013;31:4105–14.
126. Wistuba II, Gazdar AF, Minna JD. Molecular genetics of small cell lung carcinoma. Semin Oncol. 2001;28:3–13.
127. Mori N, Yokota J, Akiyama T, et al. Variable mutations of the RB gene in small-cell lung carcinoma. Oncogene. 1990;5:1713–7.
128. Arriola E, Canadas I, Arumi M, et al. Genetic changes in small cell lung carcinoma. Clin Transl Oncol. 2008;10:189–97.
129. Meuwissen R, Linn SC, Linnoila RI, et al. Induction of small cell lung cancer by somatic inactivation of both Trp53 and Rb1 in a conditional mouse model. Cancer Cell. 2003;4:181–9.

130. Peifer M, Fernandez-Cuesta L, Sos ML, et al. Integrative genome analyses identify key somatic driver mutations of small-cell lung cancer. Nat Genet. 2012;44:1104–10.
131. Rudin CM, Durinck S, Stawiski EW, et al. Comprehensive genomic analysis identifies SOX2 as a frequently amplified gene in small-cell lung cancer. Nat Genet. 2012;44:1111–6.
132. Rekhtman N MA, Lau C, et al. Analysis of EGFR and KRAS mutations in small cell carcinoma and large cell neuroendocrine carcinoma. In 14th World Conference on Lung Cancer, Amsterdam, The Netherlands. 2011:16, July 2011.
133. Varghese AM, Zakowski M, Yu HA, et al. Brief Report: Small cell lung cancers in patients who never smoked cigarettes. J Thorac Oncol. 2013;9(6):892–6.
134. Coghlin CL, Smith LJ, Bakar S, et al. Quantitative analysis of tumor in bronchial biopsy specimens. J Thorac Oncol. 2010;5:448–52.
135. Rekhtman N, Brandt SM, Sigel CS, et al. Suitability of thoracic cytology for new therapeutic paradigms in non-small cell lung carcinoma: high accuracy of tumor subtyping and feasibility of EGFR and KRAS molecular testing. J Thorac Oncol. 2011;6:451–8.
136. Travis WD, Brambilla E, Noguchi M, et al. International Association for the Study of Lung Cancer/American Thoracic Society/European Respiratory Society International Multidisciplinary Classification of Lung Adenocarcinoma. J Thorac Oncol. 2011;6:244–85.
137. Hasanovic A, Ang D, Moreira AL, et al. Use of mutation specific antibodies to detect EGFR status in small biopsy and cytology specimens of lung adenocarcinoma. Lung Cancer. 2012;77:299–305.
138. Sequist LV, Joshi VA, Janne PA, et al. Response to treatment and survival of patients with non-small cell lung cancer undergoing somatic EGFR mutation testing. Oncologist. 2007;12:90–8.
139. Sequist LV, Yang JC, Yamamoto N, et al. Phase III study of afatinib or cisplatin plus pemetrexed in patients with metastatic lung adenocarcinoma with EGFR mutations. J Clin Oncol. 2013;31:3327–34.
140. Kwak EL, Bang YJ, Camidge DR, et al. Anaplastic lymphoma kinase inhibition in non-small-cell lung cancer. N Engl J Med. 2010;363:1693–703.
141. Cappuzzo F, Bemis L, Varella-Garcia M. HER2 mutation and response to trastuzumab therapy in non-small-cell lung cancer. N Engl J Med. 2006;354:2619–21.
142. Mazieres J, Peters S, Lepage B, et al. Lung cancer that harbors an HER2 mutation: epidemiologic characteristics and therapeutic perspectives. J Clin Oncol. 2013;31:1997–2003.
143. Gautschi O, Pauli C, Strobel K, et al. A patient with BRAF V600E lung adenocarcinoma responding to vemurafenib. J Thorac Oncol. 2012;7:e23–4.
144. Ou SH, Kwak EL, Siwak-Tapp C, et al. Activity of crizotinib (PF02341066), a dual mesenchymal-epithelial transition (MET) and anaplastic lymphoma kinase (ALK) inhibitor, in a non-small cell lung cancer patient with de novo MET amplification. J Thorac Oncol. 2011;6:942–6.
145. Bergethon K, Shaw AT, Ou SH, et al. ROS1 rearrangements define a unique molecular class of lung cancers. J Clin Oncol. 2012;30:863–70.

# Chapter 9
# Evaluation of Small Biopsy Material in Patients with Multiple and Secondary Tumors

**Sara E. Monaco and Sanja Dacic**

## Introduction

Small biopsies and cytological samples are frequently utilized to evaluate multiple lung nodules, particularly in patients with a known history of malignancy, in order to determine if they represent metastases, primary lung tumor(s), or nonneoplastic lesions. The ability to make a definitive diagnosis on a small sample has a significant impact on clinical management and avoids an unnecessary invasive surgical procedure, like mediastinoscopy or wedge resection, in the setting of widespread metastatic disease or a nonneoplastic process, such as granulomatous inflammation or infection.

Initial sampling of lung lesions is usually done by fine-needle aspiration (FNA) or small core biopsies utilizing bronchoscopy or radiological image guidance [1]. In addition to rendering a morphological diagnosis, procurement of sufficient material is crucial for ancillary studies, including histochemical stains, immunostains, flow cytometry, and/or particularly molecular studies in this era of personalized medicine [2, 3]. Thus, appropriate allocation of the material is necessary to provide a definitive diagnosis with complete workup in small specimens and to reduce the need for additional tissue sampling. Though these steps are critical for managing neoplastic and nonneoplastic specimens, the focus in this chapter will be on neoplastic causes.

S.E. Monaco, M.D, (✉)
Department of Pathology, University of Pittsburgh Medical Center,
5150 Centre Ave. POB2, Suite 201, Pittsburgh, PA 15232, USA
e-mail: monacose@upmc.edu

S. Dacic, M.D, Ph.D,
Department of Pathology, University of Pittsburgh Medical Center, Pittsburgh, PA, USA

 
A.L. Moreira, A. Saqi (eds.), *Diagnosing Non-small Cell Carcinoma in Small Biopsy and Cytology*, DOI 10.1007/978-1-4939-1607-8_9

## Clinical Considerations and Staging of Multiple Lung Tumors

In patients with multiple lung tumors, the main clinical considerations are whether there is a primary lung tumor with intrapulmonary metastases, synchronous primary pulmonary tumors (e.g., occurring at the same time), metachronous primary pulmonary tumors (e.g., occurring at different times), or metastatic tumors from an extrapulmonary origin. Although the reported incidence of synchronous and metachronous tumors in the lung is between 1 and 10 %, the incidence is increasing with superior imaging capabilities and greater meticulous screening of smokers and lung cancer survivors [4–7]. Also, patients with lung cancer are now surviving longer, which translates into an increasing number of patients with multiple primary malignancies. In one study from Korea, 632 patients with non-small cell lung carcinoma were reviewed to find those with additional extrapulmonary primary tumors. The incidence of additional primaries in this group was 12.8 %. The majority (40.8 %) of patients had an extrapulmonary primary ≥6 months prior to the diagnosis of lung cancer, while the remaining had a synchronous primary diagnosed within 6 months of the lung cancer diagnosis (22.2 %) or a metachronous primary diagnosed more than 6 months after the diagnosis of lung cancer (37 %) [8]. Of these additional primary tumors in lung cancer patients, the most common sites were the stomach (25 %), colorectal (19 %), and thyroid (10.7 %). Colorectal primaries were more common in patients with lung adenocarcinoma, while gastric cancer was more prevalent in patients with lung squamous cell carcinoma [9].

Given these clinical scenarios, determining the source and assigning a classification to the tumors is essential for clinical management, because staging, prognosis, and treatment differ. This is particularly important in patients with non-pulmonary metastases that may not be surgical candidates in the setting of multiple tumors involving the lung and widespread disease.

In the current seventh edition of the American Joint Committee on Cancer (AJCC) staging, primary lung tumors with additional nodules in the same lobe are considered T3 as opposed to T4 in the sixth edition of the AJCC staging; additional tumors in the ipsilateral non-primary tumor-bearing lobe are designated T4 rather than M1; tumor cells involving the pleural fluid or contralateral lung are labeled M1a; and distant metastases are assigned M1b [10]. This illustrates that determining the etiology and relationship of multiple tumors in the lung (e.g., metastasis versus synchronous primaries) impacts lung cancer staging (Table 9.1).

In some cases, morphological comparison of tumors in small biopsies with the prior primary tumor can be helpful in determining if the two have similar or divergent features (e.g., squamous cell carcinoma and adenocarcinoma). However, a morphological comparison between two adenocarcinomas can be difficult, given that the majority of primary lung adenocarcinomas have heterogeneous histology with a variety of different patterns (e.g., solid, papillary, lepidic, micropapillary, acinar) [11], and metastasis can have similar overlapping morphological features.

In morphologically ambiguous cases, immunohistochemical stains and/or molecular studies are helpful. Positivity for site-specific immunohistochemical markers is useful in establishing a pulmonary or non-pulmonary origin (Fig. 9.1).

**Table 9.1** Staging considerations in patients with multiple lung tumors

| | Criteria | AJCC staging, 7th edition |
|---|---|---|
| Primary lung tumor with intrapulmonary metastases | Similar morphology and molecular characteristics | T3: Additional nodules in the same lobe are considered T3 |
| | | T4: Additional tumors in the ipsilateral non-primary tumor-bearing lobe |
| | | M1a: Involvement of pleural fluid or contralateral lung |
| Synchronous, independent pulmonary tumors | Tumors with different morphology, immunoprofile, or molecular characteristics occurring at the same time | Stage each separately with parentheses to indicate number |
| Metachronous, independent pulmonary tumors | Tumors with different morphology, immunoprofile, or molecular characteristics occurring at a different time | Stage each separately with parentheses to indicate number |

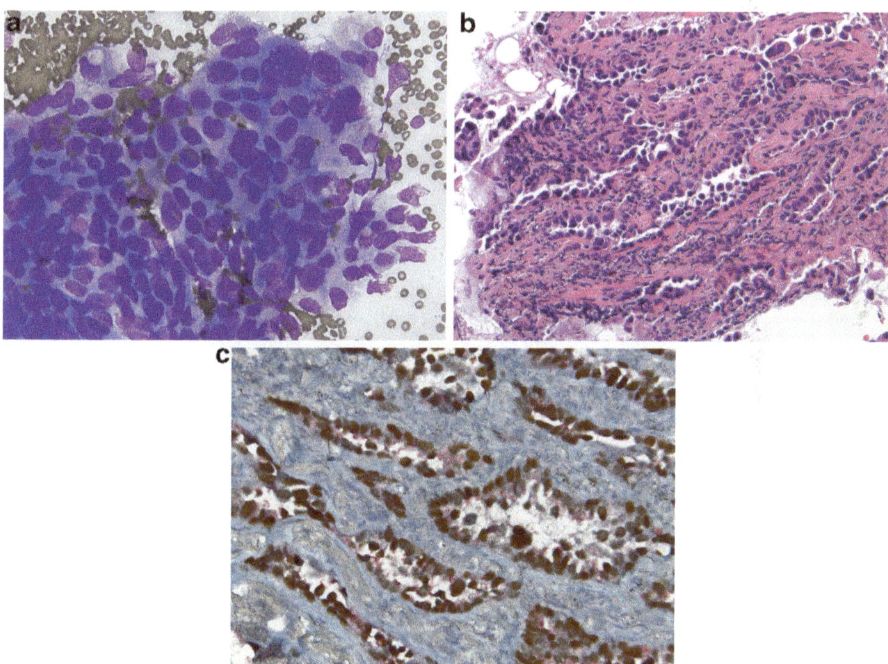


**Fig. 9.1** Adenocarcinoma of the lung with double immunostaining for TTF1 and NapsinA [(**a**) DQ stain, high power; (**b**) H&E stain, medium power; (**c**) TTF1 and NapsinA double stain]. The cytology touch preparation (**a**) shows cohesive clusters of cells with nuclear enlargement, atypia, and moderate cytoplasm, forming vague gland-like structures. The H&E stain (**b**) of the core biopsy shows an adenocarcinoma, which is *highlighted* in the image by TTF1 (*brown*, nuclear positivity) and napsinA (*red*, cytoplasmic positivity)

However, for two lung tumors that show similar morphology and immunophenotype, a comparison of molecular studies, which includes mutational profiles, loss of heterozygosity (LOH) profile, and clonality assays [12], is often the preferred approach to determine if they are synchronous, independent primaries.

The emphasis on mutational status and clonality of tumors has become prevalent since more than two-thirds of second lung cancers (synchronous or metachronous) have similar histological features as the prior lung tumor [5, 13]. In studies focusing on mutational profiles of different lung tumors with similar histology, molecular differences that are genetically unique and independent from the patient's prior tumor have been recognized [7]. However, even at the molecular level, establishing a relationship between two tumors can be difficult given that metastatic tumors may have a genetic profile that differs from the primary due to intratumoral heterogeneity or tumor progression with acquisition of additional genetic abnormalities [8, 14]. This is an important consideration particularly when molecular testing of the primary tumor is performed on cytology or small biopsy specimens, which may not be representative of the larger tumor mass.

In general, multiple tumors should be considered synchronous primaries if they have different histology or if there are morphological (e.g., associated in situ carcinoma), immunohistochemical, or molecular differences that support diagnosing two discrete primaries. In addition, if the tumors are located in different locations and temporally distinct without systemic metastases, then they may also be considered independent primary tumors. Thus, if deemed synchronous primaries based on clinical or pathological assessment, then each primary should be staged separately (Table 9.1). Intrapulmonary metastases tend to be tumors that have the same histology and occur in the same lobe without systemic metastases [5]. Given the importance of this determination for staging, meticulous description of the number of nodules, size of the nodules, and location of the nodules by the submitting clinician or radiologist that is procuring the small biopsy is crucial.

## Pathological Evaluation of Small Specimens in Patients with Multiple Lung Tumors

Small biopsies and cytology specimens obtained with minimally invasive procedures are effective at providing sufficient tissue for an accurate diagnosis and ancillary studies with little risk to the patient [15–17]. In some instances, cytological specimens have an advantage over small biopsies, given that cytological specimens utilize multiple different preparations (e.g., smears, cell blocks, ThinPrep) and stains (e.g., Diff-Quik, Papanicolaou, hematoxylin and eosin). Well-prepared cytological specimens provide better morphology without the artifactual distortion seen with formalin-fixed small biopsies and are less dependent on immunostaining for the subclassification of non-small cell carcinomas, given that keratinizing squamous cell carcinomas are easily recognized by their orangeophilia on Papanicolaou staining, which is not utilized in the analysis of small biopsies [18, 19].

In addition, endobronchial biopsies are superficial and may miss a deep tumor, which is better sampled with a transbronchial FNA or Wang needle biopsy. This is especially relevant in cases of small cell carcinomas and other tumors causing large hilar masses that compress but do not involve the superficial bronchial wall.

However, small biopsies have the advantage of potentially providing greater tumor architecture for more accurate histological subtyping. This is important because identification of adenocarcinoma subtypes may have prognostic importance. In a recent study assessing the cytological subtyping of lung adenocarcinomas using the International Association for the Study of Lung Cancer/American Thoracic Society/European Respiratory Society (IASLC/ATS/ERS) classification, it was shown that when assigning the dominant pattern subtype, there was only 40 % concordance between preoperative cytological samples and resections [20]. However, the low concordance may result from sampling. Also, formal studies comparing accuracy of dominant pattern classification based on small biopsy is lacking, and cytological patterns corresponding to known histological patterns have not been formally defined.

Reported adequacy rates of molecular studies for small specimens are variable as are preferences for cytology and/or small biopsy. For instance, one study described that approximately 15 % of tissue blocks had insufficient material for molecular studies after morphological and immunohistochemical stains are performed and an additional 15 % had insufficient or poor-quality nucleic acid for molecular studies, resulting in about 30 % of small biopsy and cytology specimens that are potentially inadequate for molecular studies [21]. Another study focused on molecular testing on cytology specimens reported that approximately 30 % of lung carcinomas with <300 tumor cells fail PCR-based studies for *EGFR* and *KRAS* mutations [22]. In contrast to these, successful molecular testing of EGFR, KRAS, or ALK was achieved in 93 % of all reflexively tested EBUS FNAs [23], and no statistically significant difference in results of ancillary studies between FNAs, core biopsies, or a combination of FNAs and core biopsies was noted on transthoracic CT-guided samples [24]. The variability among studies may be multifactorial.

The promising news is that molecular testing with whole-genome or targeted sequencing yields impressive results when detecting mutations on cytology specimens and small biopsies, which have less tissue and lower tumor cellularity than resections [15, 25]. Next-generation sequencing with targeted sequencing has enabled greater resolution, improved sensitivity, and lower cost compared to traditional sequencing methods and will likely have a significant role on small specimens in the future [26]. In addition, the combination of multiple sampling modalities, such as cytology specimens with small core biopsies, may help maximize the diagnostic yield of these procedures, and adequacy assessment during the procedure may help to ensure sufficient material. This underscores the importance of radiological-pathological correlation, immediate evaluation during the procedure (e.g., frozen section or on-site evaluation), and the use of multiple different sampling modalities in difficult or suboptimal cases.

For every case, sample management for ancillary studies is critical and begins with procuring sufficient material at the time of the procedure. Instituting an algorithm to

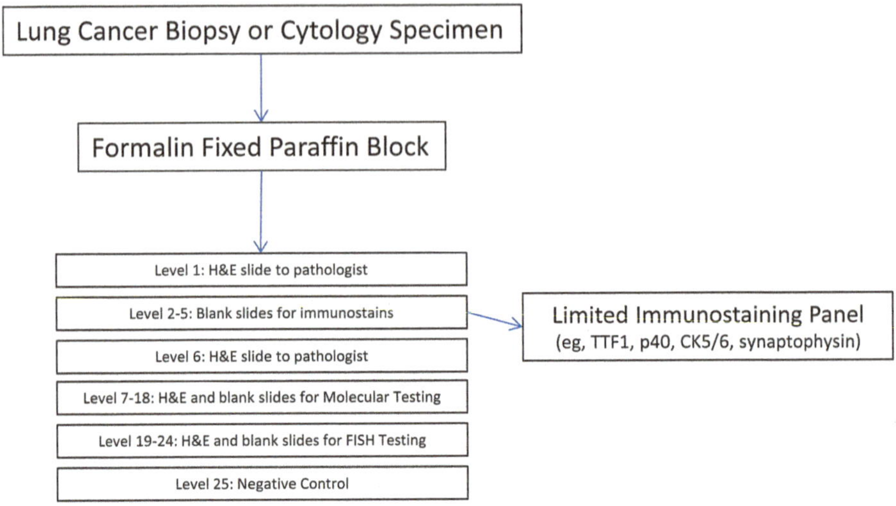


**Fig. 9.2** An example of an algorithm illustrating the triage of small biopsy and cytology materials for ancillary studies

cut blank slides upfront in the laboratory minimizes loss of tissue (Fig. 9.2). Now, to avoid the need for repeat biopsies for potential molecular studies, the trend is to conserve tissue by using focused and limited immunopanels in a staged approach guided by the clinical and radiological findings [27–29]. If there are atypical findings (e.g., TTF1 and p63 or p40 negativity), then additional immunostains are warranted to exclude a neuroendocrine tumor (e.g., synaptophysin), non-pulmonary adenocarcinoma (e.g., CDX2, PAX8, GATA3), or non-epithelial tumor.

## Adenocarcinoma

### *Clinical Presentation*

Cytology specimens and small biopsies are useful for diagnosing metastatic non-pulmonary adenocarcinomas within the lung or mediastinum, particularly when there are characteristic morphological or immunophenotypic findings. Clinically, an extrapulmonary primary should be considered in patients with a history of a prior malignancy, coincident mass lesion outside the lung, or radiological imaging showing multiple peripheral and/or bilateral lung nodules without a dominant lung mass. Nevertheless, a solitary mass can also represent a metastasis.

Some metastatic carcinomas can also present as endobronchial masses, particularly metastases from the breast, colon/rectum, kidney, and skin (e.g., melanoma) [30, 31]. By morphology, pulmonary adenocarcinomas can have morphological overlap with extrapulmonary adenocarcinomas and benign entities. Thus, a thorough clinical history is essential in distinguishing among these entities, in addition

**Table 9.2** Differential diagnosis of pulmonary adenocarcinoma in small biopsies and cytology specimens

| |
|---|
| Neoplastic |
| Poorly differentiated, nonkeratinizing squamous cell carcinoma |
| Large cell neuroendocrine carcinoma |
| Adenosquamous carcinoma |
| Salivary gland-type tumors of the bronchial glands |
| Non-epithelial tumors (e.g., sclerosing hemangioma, epithelioid sarcoma, angiosarcoma, melanoma) |
| Extrapulmonary metastatic adenocarcinomas (e.g., breast, colon) |
| Nonneoplastic |
| Benign/reactive epithelial cells (e.g., bronchial cells, squamous cells, pneumocytes) |
| Treatment-related atypia (e.g., chemotherapy, radiation) |
| Granulomatous inflammation and epithelioid histiocytes |

to performing focused immunostaining, conserving tissue in cases of atypical cytomorphological features or unexpected immunohistochemical staining results (e.g., TTF1 negative), and conducting potential molecular testing (Table 9.2).

## *Cytomorphological Features*

Primary and secondary lung adenocarcinomas have overlapping cytomorphological features, and both possibilities have to be entertained, especially in the presence of signet-ring, mucinous, or papillary features (Fig. 9.3).

## *Adenocarcinomas with Signet-Ring Cells*

Signet-ring morphology is well described in adenocarcinomas arising in the lung, stomach, and other gastrointestinal sites (Fig. 9.4). These tumors tend to be discohesive in cytological specimens and infiltrate as single cells or small nests on biopsies. With abundant cytoplasm, low nuclear-to-cytoplasmic ratios, and lack of hyperchromasia, signet-ring cells may be overlooked or dismissed as histiocytes on low magnification. Examination on high power demonstrates their subtle nuclear atypia and peripheral displacement and indentation of the nucleus by mucin, which can be highlighted by a mucicarmine stain.

Determining the site of origin in the setting of signet-ring cells requires immunohistochemical confirmation. Typically TTF1 and CK7 staining confirms a primary lung adenocarcinoma, while CK7 and CDX2 positivities are characteristic of the upper gastrointestinal tract and CK20 and CDX2 positivities of colorectal primaries (Table 9.3a). Other signet-ring mimics include plasma cell neoplasms (e.g., CD138) and malignant melanoma (e.g., S100, MelanA, HMB45).

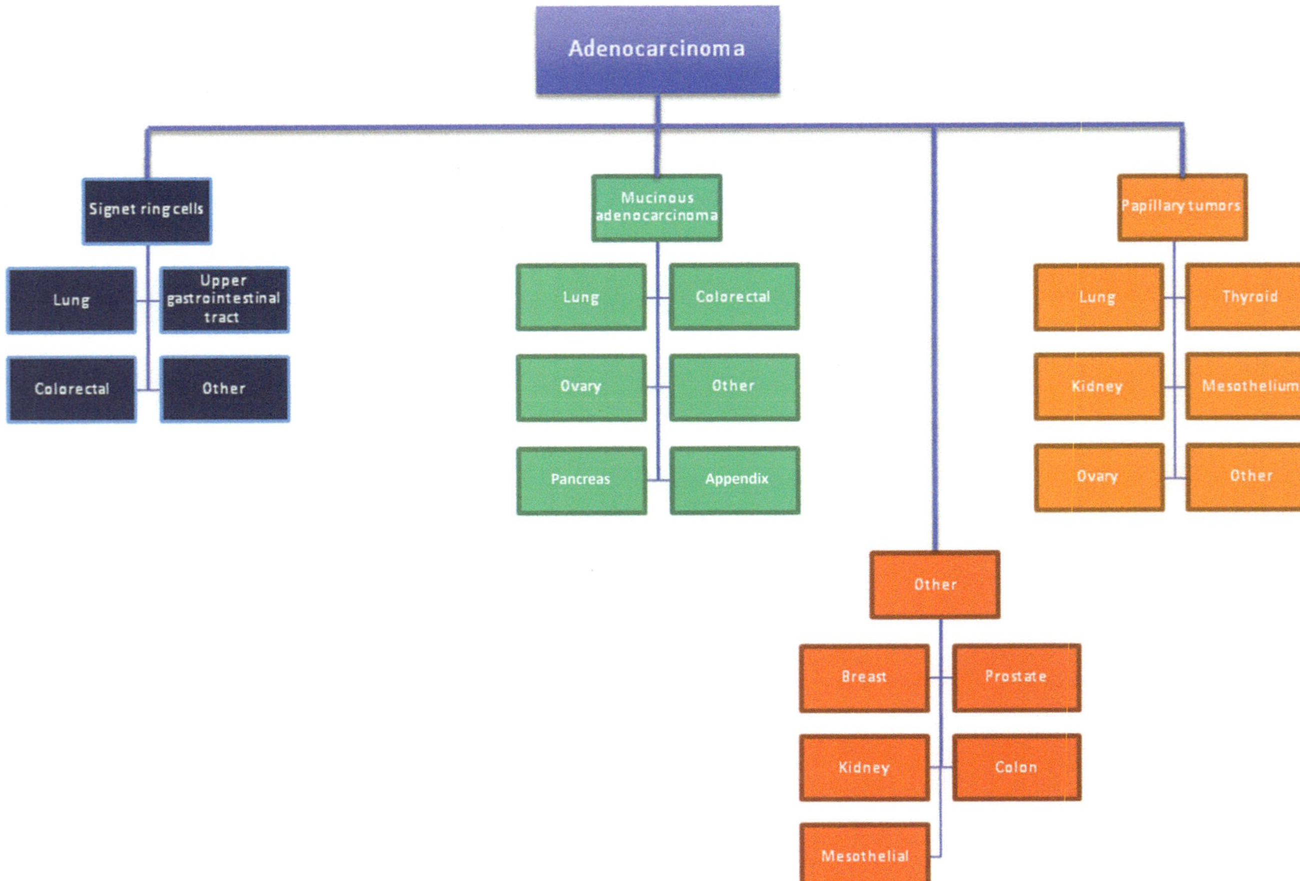


**Fig. 9.3** Differential diagnoses for adenocarcinoma involving the lung

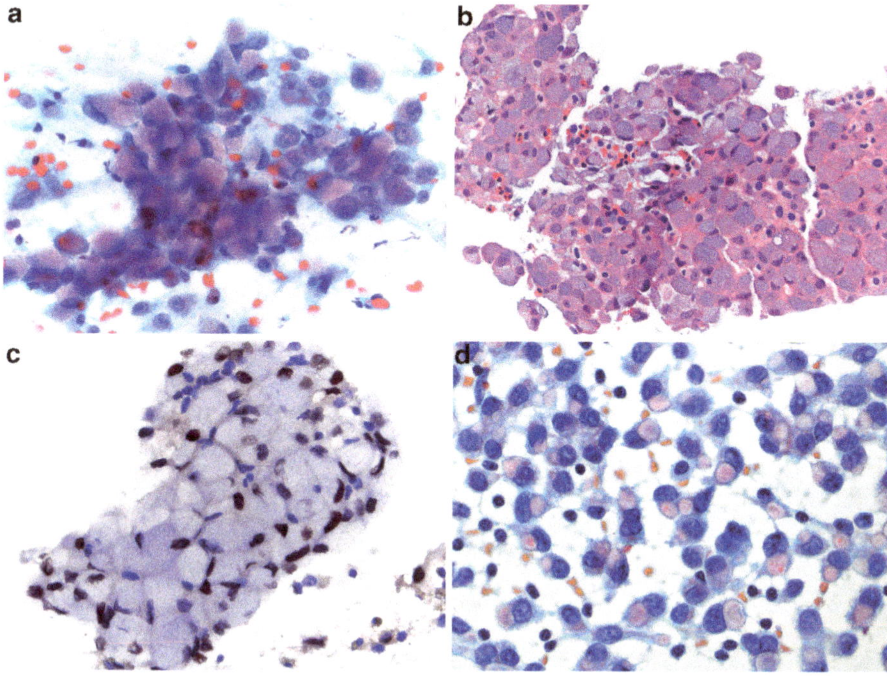

**Fig. 9.4** Signet-ring adenocarcinoma [(**a**) Pap stain, high power; (**b**) H&E stain, high power; (**c**) TTF1 stain, high power; (**d**) Pap stain, low power]. The slide (**a**) shows tumor cells with nuclear pleomorphism and eccentrically placed cytoplasm containing targetoid mucin droplets. The cell block (**b**) shows the same tumor cells with signet-ring type cells. The TTF1 stain (**c**) shows nuclear staining. Extrapulmonary sites (**d**) also have signet-ring cells [Photographs courtesy of Dr. Anjali Saqi (**a**–**c**) and Dr. John Crapanzano (**d**)]

**Table 9.3a** Immunophenotype of primary and secondary adenocarcinomas with signet-ring cells

| Primary | CK7 | CK20 | TTF1 | CDX2 |
|---|---|---|---|---|
| Lung | + | − | + | − |
| Upper GI tract | + | − | − | + |
| Colorectal | − | + | − | + |

*GI* gastrointestinal

## *Mucinous (Colloid) Adenocarcinoma*

Mucinous tumors arise in the lung, female genital tract, gastrointestinal tract, appendix, and pancreatobiliary region. Akin to signet-ring cell tumors, cells of mucinous adenocarcinomas may have low nuclear-to-cytoplasmic ratios due to their voluminous mucinous cytoplasm, but they are more cohesive and lack the indention of the

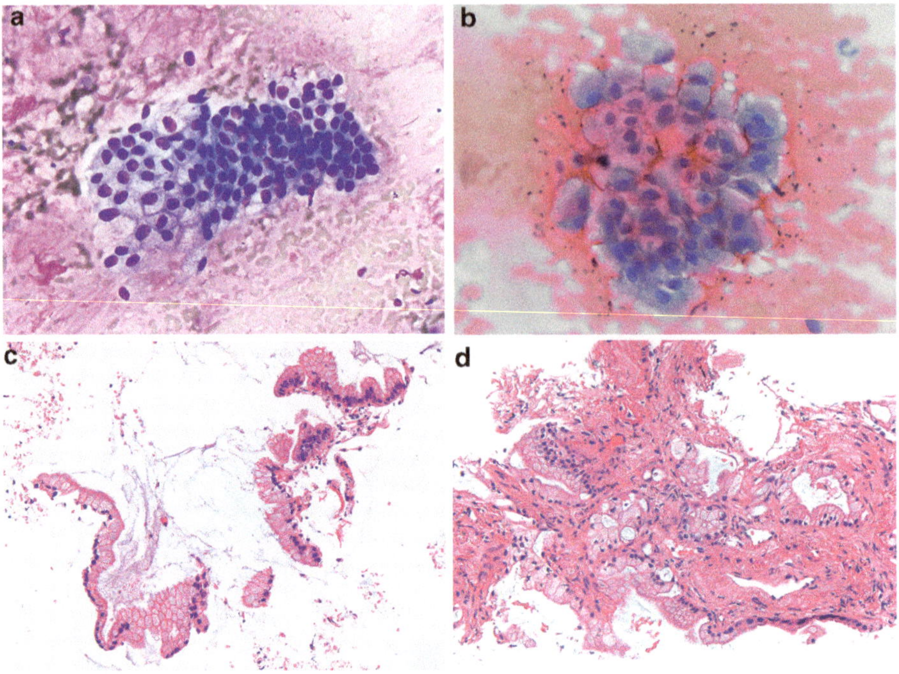

**Fig. 9.5** Mucinous adenocarcinoma of the lung [(**a**) DQ stain, high power; (**b**) Pap stain, high power; (**c**) cell block H&E stain, low power, (**d**) core biopsy, low power]. The aspirate (**a** and **b**) shows clusters of tumor cells with moderate amounts of clear, vacuolated cytoplasm and round nuclei with mild pleomorphism. The cell block (**b**) and core biopsy (**d**) show similar tumor cells with mucinous cytoplasm and basally located nuclei [Photographs courtesy of Dr. Anjali Saqi]

nucleus in signet-ring cells. In cytology specimens, there is typically thick mucinous material in the background and a "drunken honeycomb" pattern. In adenocarcinomas with mild cytological atypia, these changes can be misinterpreted as goblet cell metaplasia, which often has interspersed ciliated bronchial cells and lacks nuclear atypia, or an aggregate of histiocytes, which lacks atypia. On surgical biopsies, neoplastic cells either line alveolar walls or are suspended within mucin pools. As in cytology specimens, mucinous adenocarcinoma may go unnoticed on a small biopsy (Fig. 9.5); however, the identification of large pools of mucin should raise the possibility of the diagnosis and a search for malignant cells. Metastatic colorectal adenocarcinomas may have columnar cells and mucinous features but more commonly have oval, palisading nuclei and a background of inflammatory necrosis (Fig. 9.6).

The immunophenotype of mucinous adenocarcinomas can be ambiguous and staining has to be interpreted with caution in conjunction with the clinical history. CDX2 is a relatively specific marker generally associated with gastrointestinal or pancreatobiliary primaries. Nonetheless, primary mucinous adenocarcinomas arising in extra-gastrointestinal sites, such as the lung, ovary, and pancreas, can also express CDX2 and CK20 [32, 33]. Positivity for CK20 and negativity for TTF1 in a mucinous tumor may be seen in primary lung adenocarcinomas.

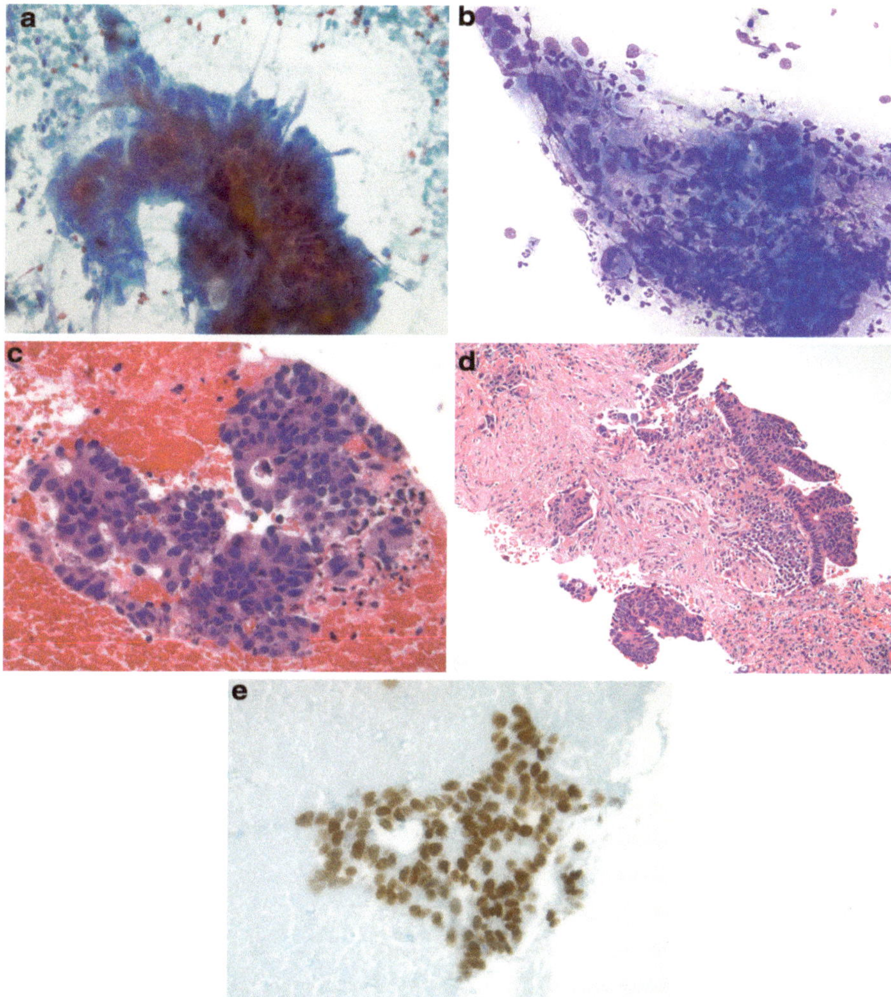


**Fig. 9.6** Metastatic colonic adenocarcinoma [(**a**) Pap stain, high power; (**b**) DQ, low power of touch imprint; (**c**) Cell block H&E stain, high power; (**d**) Core biopsy H&E stain, low power; (**e**) CDX2 immunostain]. The aspirates from adenocarcinomas of the colon typically show cohesive cells with prominent nucleoli and columnar morphology, with palisading around the edges (**a**). In addition, there is usually background necrosis (**a**) with inflammatory cells (B). The columnar morphology is usually more readily identified on the cell block sections (**c**) and core biopsy (**d**). CDX2 immunostain is useful in establishing the diagnosis (**e**) [Photographs (**b**) and (**d**) courtesy of Dr. Anjali Saqi]

However, villin and PAX8 are typically negative in these cases [34, 35]. Villin and CDX2 are typically positive in metastatic colorectal carcinomas, and PAX8 highlights ovarian mucinous tumors (Fig. 9.6). Making the distinction between synchronous and metachronous morphologically similar mucinous adenocarcinomas in the pancreas and lung may be impossible to separate either morphologically or by molecular tests as similar KRAS mutation have been described (Table 9.3b) [33].

**Table 9.3b** Immunophenotype of primary and secondary mucinous adenocarcinomas

| | CK20 | CDX2 | VILLIN | PAX8 |
|---|---|---|---|---|
| Lung | + | +/– | – | – |
| Colorectal | + | + | + | – |
| Ovary | – | + | - | + |

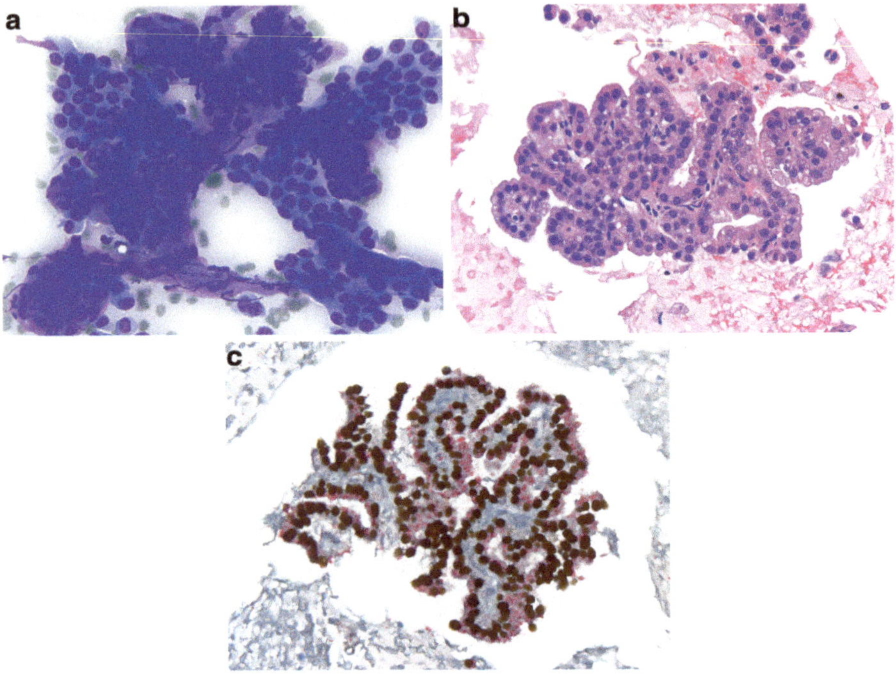

**Fig. 9.7** Papillary adenocarcinoma of the lung [(**a**) DQ stain, high power; (**b**) H&E stain, high power; (**c**) TTF1 and NapsinA double stain]. Adenocarcinomas of the lung with a papillary pattern can have transgressing vessels associated with the tumor cells on the aspirates (**a**), and show fibrovascular cores on the cell block (**b**). TTF1 and NapsinA double immunostain is helpful to conserve tissue in small specimens and shows positivity for TTF1 (*brown*, nuclear positivity) and napsinA (*red*, cytoplasmic positivity) in this lung adenocarcinoma

## *Papillary Tumors*

Papillary tumors typically arise from the lung, thyroid, kidney, mesothelium, or ovary. These tumors have fibrovascular cores and occasional psammomatous calcifications. Papillary tumors of the thyroid and lung are also associated with intranuclear inclusions, while ovarian serous papillary tumors typically have more nuclear pleomorphism (Fig. 9.7).

**Table 9.3c** Immunophenotype of primary and secondary papillary tumors in the lung

| Primary site | TTF1 | NapsinA | CK7 | Thyroglobulin | PAX8 | WT1 |
|---|---|---|---|---|---|---|
| Lung | + | + | + | – | – | –/+ |
| Thyroid | + | – | + | + | + | – |
| Ovary | – | – | + | – | + | + |
| Kidney | – | –/+ | +/– | – | + | – |
| Mesothelium | – | – | + | – | – | + |

A limited immunostain panel can resolve the differential of a papillary tumor (Table 9.3c). TTF1 is typically used to confirm lung origin but is ubiquitously expressed by papillary thyroid carcinomas. Performing additional markers, such as NapsinA for lung origin and thyroglobulin or PAX8 for thyroid origin, can discriminate between the two entities [36]. Also, in a peripheral lung mass or in a fluid cytology specimen, the possibility of a papillary epithelioid mesothelioma or papillary mesothelial hyperplasia should be considered. Given that mesothelial cells and lung adenocarcinomas both commonly express CK7 [37], TTF1 positivity can resolve the dilemma. In the absence of TTF1 staining, a panel of immunostains (e.g., for mesothelial origin: calretinin, CK5, WT1, and D2-40 and for adenocarcinoma: B72.3, BerEP4, and CEA] is recommended when lung adenocarcinoma and mesothelial origin are in consideration.

## *Additional Considerations*

Likewise, other carcinomas metastatic to the lung may not have specific features, which make their identification difficult and underscores the relevance of clinical history. This is particularly true for metastatic breast carcinomas and prostate carcinomas that can present as single or multiple lung masses and have an acinar morphology or eosinophilic granular appearance (e.g., apocrine) similar to that seen in some lung carcinomas. Clear cells suggestive of conventional (clear) cell renal carcinoma are easily identified on biopsies and cell blocks, but the recognition of cells with abundant foamy cytoplasm and discrete punched-out vacuoles associated with thin blood vessels on other cytology preparations is more subtle (Fig. 9.8).

In the absence of TTF1 staining on the initial limited panel, additional immunostains, to exclude the possibility of a poorly differentiated squamous cell carcinoma, with p40, p63, or CK5 should be performed. When reactivity with these markers is also lacking, immunostains such as CK7 and CK20 [38] and site-specific markers need to be pursued to ascertain the primary origin (Tables 9.4 and 9.5, Fig. 9.9). Also important to consider is that TTF1 can be expressed rarely by non-pulmonary and non-thyroid carcinomas, including those arising from the ovary, endometrium, and endocervix, making interpretation in conjunction with clinical history essential [41, 42].

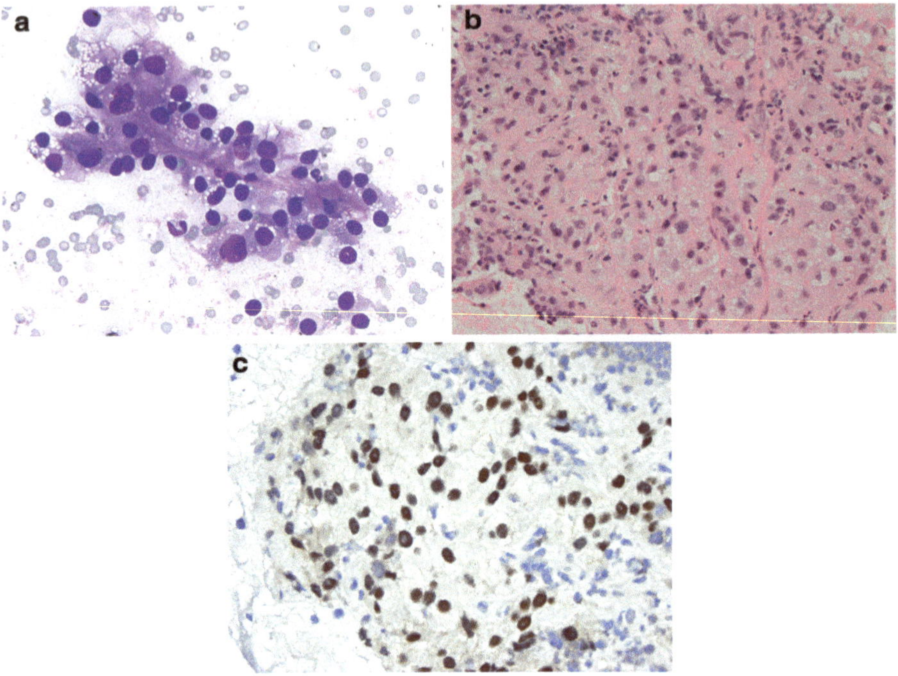


**Fig. 9.8** Metastatic renal cell carcinoma [(**a**) DQ stain, high power; (**b**) cell block H&E stain, high power; (**c**) PAX8 immunostain]. Renal cell carcinomas have tumor cells with moderate-to-abundant cytoplasm that contains discrete "punched-out" vacuoles (**a**) on the air-dried Romanowsky-stained slides. These are more obvious on cell block sections and biopsies. The morphology and immunostaining of the cell block (**b**) show strong PAX8 positivity, supporting a diagnosis of conventional (clear cell) carcinoma of the kidney [Photographs courtesy of Dr. Anjali Saqi]

## *Molecular Testing of Adenocarcinomas*

Although there are some histological associations with particular molecular abnormalities, triage based on the histological pattern of lung adenocarcinoma identified is not recommended. Thus, regardless of histological pattern, it is recommended that at a minimum all adenocarcinomas of the lung are tested for *EGFR* mutations *and ALK* rearrangements [26, 43]. Allocation of material for potential molecular studies is important, particularly on small specimens. The recommendation is to preserve tissue for the testing of *EGFR mutations and ALK* rearrangements [26, 43–45], after an extrapulmonary adenocarcinoma has been excluded, for the diagnosis of lung adenocarcinoma, adenosquamous carcinoma, and non-small cell lung carcinoma not otherwise specified, or when the possibility of an adenocarcinoma cannot entirely be excluded. In many instances, clinical management of site-specific extrapulmonary adenocarcinomas is also dependent upon ancillary testing for clinical management, such as testing for Her2/neu in gastric adenocarcinomas [46] and *BRAF and KRAS* mutations in colorectal primaries.

**Table 9.4** Summary of CK7 and CK20 profile of primary and metastatic tumors

| | | CK20 | |
|---|---|---|---|
| | | Positive | Negative |
| CK7 | Positive | GI (upper)<br>Ovary (mucinous)<br>Pancreatobiliary<br>Urothelial | Lung[a]<br>Breast<br>GI (upper)<br>Gynecological tract[b]<br>Kidney[c]<br>Pancreaticobiliary<br>Salivary gland<br>Thyroid<br>Mesothelial |
| | Negative | Colorectal<br>Merkel cell carcinoma<br>Small cell carcinoma of salivary gland | Adrenal<br>Kidney (clear cell)<br>Liver (hepatocellular carcinoma)<br>Prostate<br>Squamous cell carcinoma[d]<br>Thymic carcinoma<br>Non-epithelial tumors[e] |

*GI* gastrointestinal
[a]Small cell carcinoma can be double (CK7 and CK20) negative or CK7 positive and CK20 negative
[b]Including squamous cell carcinoma of the cervix
[c]Renal cell carcinoma (papillary and chromophobe)
[d]Squamous cell carcinoma other than that of the cervix
[e]Lymphoma, melanoma, and sarcoma

**Table 9.5** Summary of commonly used markers for carcinoma of unknown primary[a]

| Primary tumor site | Immunohistochemical stains |
|---|---|
| Breast | Hormone receptors (ER, PR, AR)<br>GATA3, mammaglobin, GCDFP15 |
| Gastrointestinal | CDX2, CK20 |
| Lung | TTF1, NapsinA |
| Ovary | PAX8, WT1 |
| Pancreatobiliary | CA19-9 |
| Prostate | NKX3.1, PSAP, PSA |
| Renal | PAX8, RCC, CD10 |
| Thyroid | PAX8, thyroglobulin, TTF1 |
| Urothelial | CK5, p63, GATA3 |

[a]Most of these stains are not entirely sensitive and specific; thus, the interpretation of the stains in the context of a panel and other features is important when making a diagnosis. For example, ER and PR may be expressed by lung adenocarcinomas and neuroendocrine tumors [39, 40]

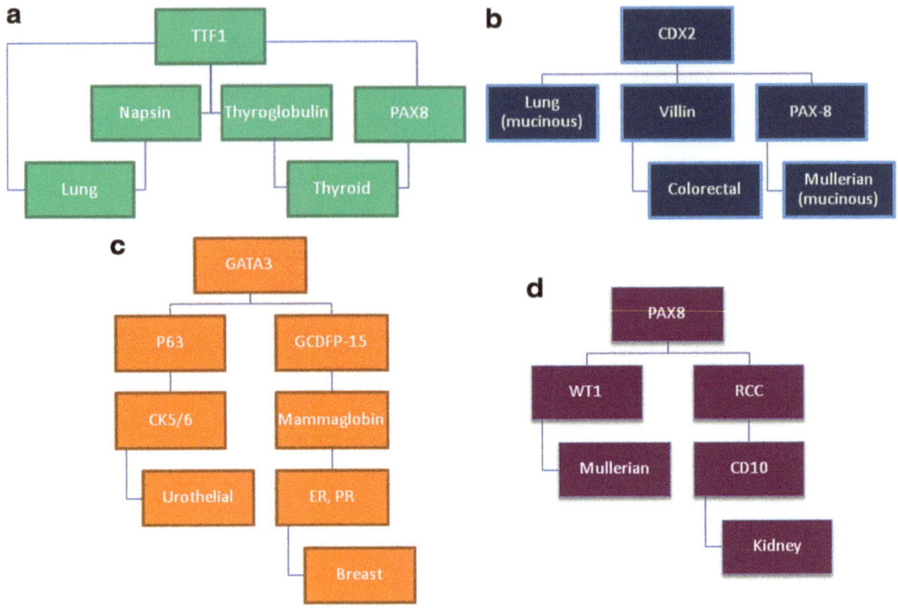


**Fig. 9.9** Differential diagnosis based on select site-specific markers. (**a**): TTF1. (**b**) CDX2. (**c**) GATA3. (**d**) PAX8

## Squamous Cell Carcinomas

Squamous cell carcinomas have different morphological subtypes, including keratinizing, nonkeratinizing, and basaloid, but the variants are not specific to a particular primary site, such that pulmonary and extrapulmonary squamous cell carcinomas can appear morphologically similar (Fig. 9.10). In addition, atypical squamous cells may represent a component of other entities, such as mucoepidermoid carcinoma or reactive processes, and resemble other neoplasms including urothelial carcinomas.

### *Well-Differentiated Squamous Cell Carcinoma*

Squamous pearls, keratinization, and intercellular bridges are the sine qua non of squamous differentiation and are readily identifiable in well-differentiated carcinomas. When present, all of these features can be seen on core biopsies. Intercellular bridges, however, are not evident on cytology smears, only on cell blocks. Meanwhile, keratinization is easily recognized as orangeophilia (i.e., orange-staining cytoplasm) on Papanicolaou-stained cytology preparations but not on hematoxylin and eosin-stained core biopsies. Additional cytomorphological features favoring squamous cell carcinoma over adenocarcinoma include greater nuclear pleomorphism, coarser chromatin with inconspicuous nucleoli, and denser cytoplasm (Fig. 9.11).

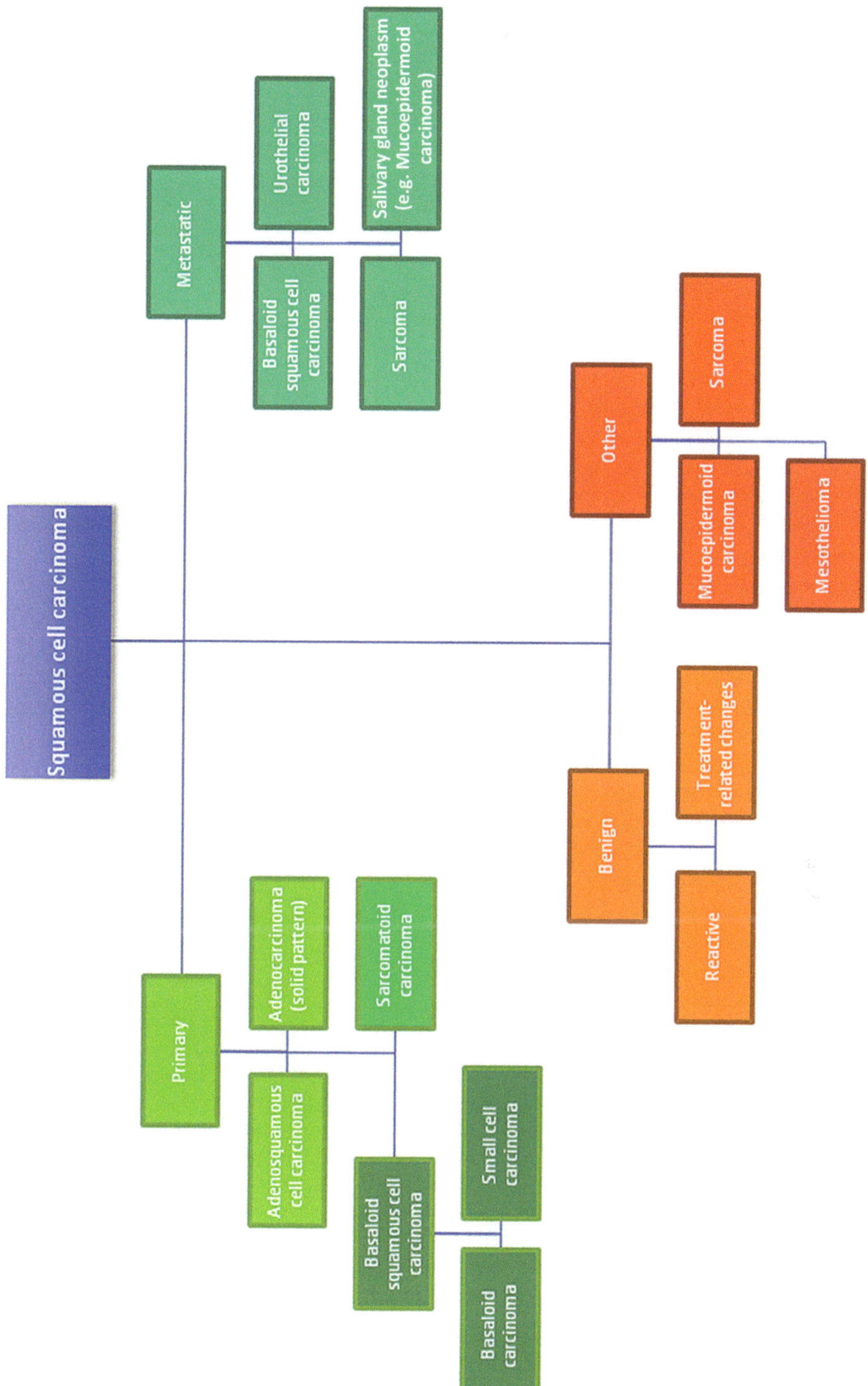


**Fig. 9.10** Differential diagnoses for squamous cell carcinoma involving the lung

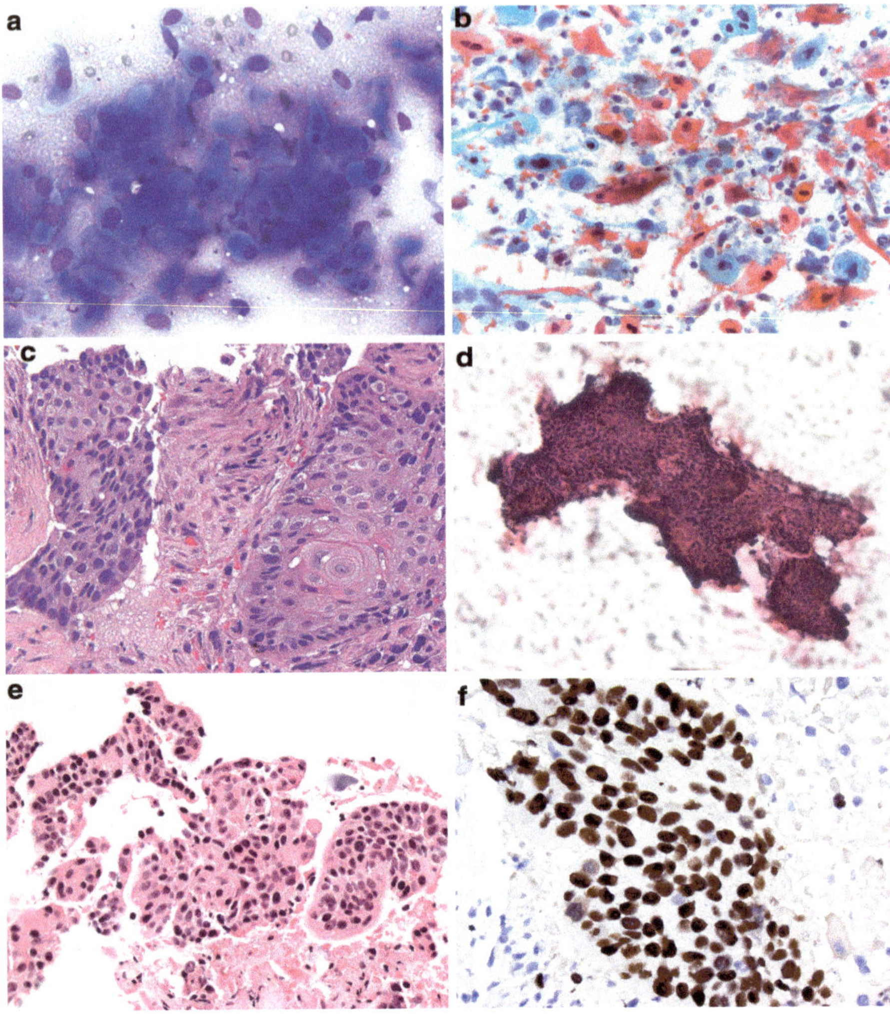


**Fig. 9.11** Squamous cell carcinoma [well-differentiated squamous cell carcinoma: (**a**) DQ stain, high power; (**b**) Pap stain, high power; (**c**) core biopsy H&E stain, high power; poorly differentiated squamous cell carcinoma: (**d**) Pap stain, high power; (**e**) cell block H&E, high power; (**f**) cell block p63, immunostain; basaloid squamous cell carcinoma: (**g**) DQ stain, high power; Pap stain, high power; (**h**) Pap stain, high power; (**i**) core biopsy H&E, high power.]. This example of well-differentiated keratinizing squamous cell carcinoma shows discohesive single cells (**a**) with dense cytoplasm showing cytoplasmic orangeophilia on the Pap-stained slide (**b**). The accompanying core biopsy shows tissue fragments with nests of an invasive squamous cell carcinoma (**c**). Poorly differentiated squamous cells arranged as a syncytial sheet (**d**) with the corresponding cell block (**e**) and p63 immunostain (**f**). Basaloid squamous cell carcinomas can mimic small cell carcinomas. The cells of basaloid squamous cell carcinomas are more cohesive and demonstrate peripheral palisading and crush artifact (**g**). The presence of occasional large cells is a clue to the diagnosis (**h**). Necrosis and apoptosis are associated with basaloid carcinomas (**i**) [Photographs courtesy of Dr. Anjali Saqi (**a**, **d**, **e**, **f**, **g**, **h** and **i**) and Dr. John Crapanzano (**b**)]

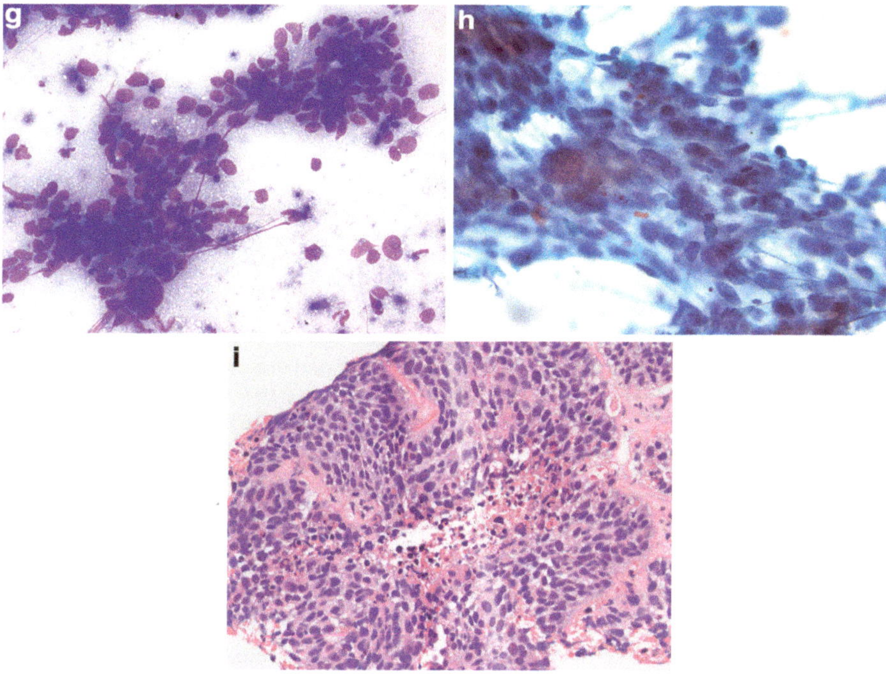


**Fig. 9.11** (continued)

## *Poorly Differentiated Squamous Cell Carcinoma*

Based on the above morphological criteria alone, nonkeratinizing, poorly differentiated squamous cell carcinomas can be difficult to differentiate from other carcinomas, including poorly differentiated adenocarcinomas and extrapulmonary metastases [47]. On FNAs, poorly differentiated adenocarcinomas and squamous cell carcinomas yield syncytial sheets or groups [48], whether they are arising from the lung or other sites, such as the head or neck (Fig. 9.11). Likewise, a core biopsy through an adenocarcinoma with a solid pattern can mimic squamous cell carcinoma.

## *Basaloid Squamous Cell Carcinoma*

Squamous cell carcinomas with basaloid features are not unique to the lung and also arise in the head and neck. Squamous cell carcinomas with basaloid features also coincide morphologically with a subtype of pulmonary large cell carcinoma, basaloid carcinoma, which is devoid of morphological squamous differentiation. Necrosis, brisk mitotic activity, apoptosis, scant cytoplasm, inconspicuous-to-pinpoint nucleoli, and nuclear molding can be seen in the basaloid variant of squamous cell carcinoma [18, 19] and pulmonary large cell basaloid carcinoma. These features can be misinterpreted as small cell carcinoma on cytology and small biopsy [49] (Fig. 9.11). Palisading of nuclei at the edge of cell clusters, the lack of prominent nuclear molding, and tightly cohesive clusters favor basaloid features over small cell carcinoma [49].

Characteristically squamous cell carcinomas are positive for p63, p40, and/or CK5/6. The sensitivity and specificity for detecting a squamous cell carcinoma is higher for p40 than for p63, which make p40 the marker of choice [50, 51]. In contrast to lung adenocarcinomas, squamous cell carcinomas do not express a site-specific marker like TTF1, which makes differentiating a primary from a metastatic squamous cell carcinomas difficult.

However, it is now well established that HPV-related squamous cell carcinomas of the head and neck, cervix, and anorectal area are positive for p16 immunostain and HPV, which can be detected by chromogenic in situ hybridization (CISH) and other methods (Fig. 9.12) [52]. Since HPV is not linked to squamous cell carcinomas of the lung, its identification supports a HPV-related metastatic squamous cell carcinoma [53]. However, some squamous cell papillomas, which are typically endobronchial and can have parenchymal involvement, are HPV(+) [54]. Positivity for p16 is defined as strong and diffuse staining of the cytoplasm and nucleus in over 70 % of the tumor cells [55]. For HPV CISH performed on formalin-fixed paraffin-embedded tissue, a dot-like pattern confers positivity but requires meticulous high-power examination to prevent a false negative interpretation [55]. The reactivity of these two markers, p16 and HPV, in a new lung squamous cell carcinoma is useful in establishing metastatic disease in the setting of a known HPV-related carcinoma or identifying an occult squamous cell carcinoma, such as a tonsillar or base of tongue primary [56]. Conversely, the absence of p16 staining and HPV identification does not exclude the possibility of a metastasis, since many squamous cell carcinomas arise secondary to non-HPV etiologies.

## *Adenosquamous Cell Carcinoma*

Metastatic squamous cell carcinomas can also be difficult to distinguish from primary lung adenosquamous carcinomas, which represent <4 % of non-small cell carcinomas and have at least 10 % of each component [57]. When two discrete components, glandular and squamous, are detected, performing TTF1 and p40 to identify adenocarcinoma and squamous carcinoma, respectively, to confirm the morphological impression is crucial (Fig. 9.13). Patients with an adenocarcinoma component may have an actionable mutation (e.g., *EGFR* mutation or ALK rearrangement) and benefit from targeted therapy [58]. Testing for *EGFR*, *KRAS*, *and ALK* is not currently recommended for patients with pure squamous cell carcinoma but should be considered on cytology and small biopsy specimens of patients with the diagnosis of squamous cell carcinoma that are never smokers; in these cases, the adenocarcinoma component as part of an adenosquamous carcinoma cannot entirely be excluded.

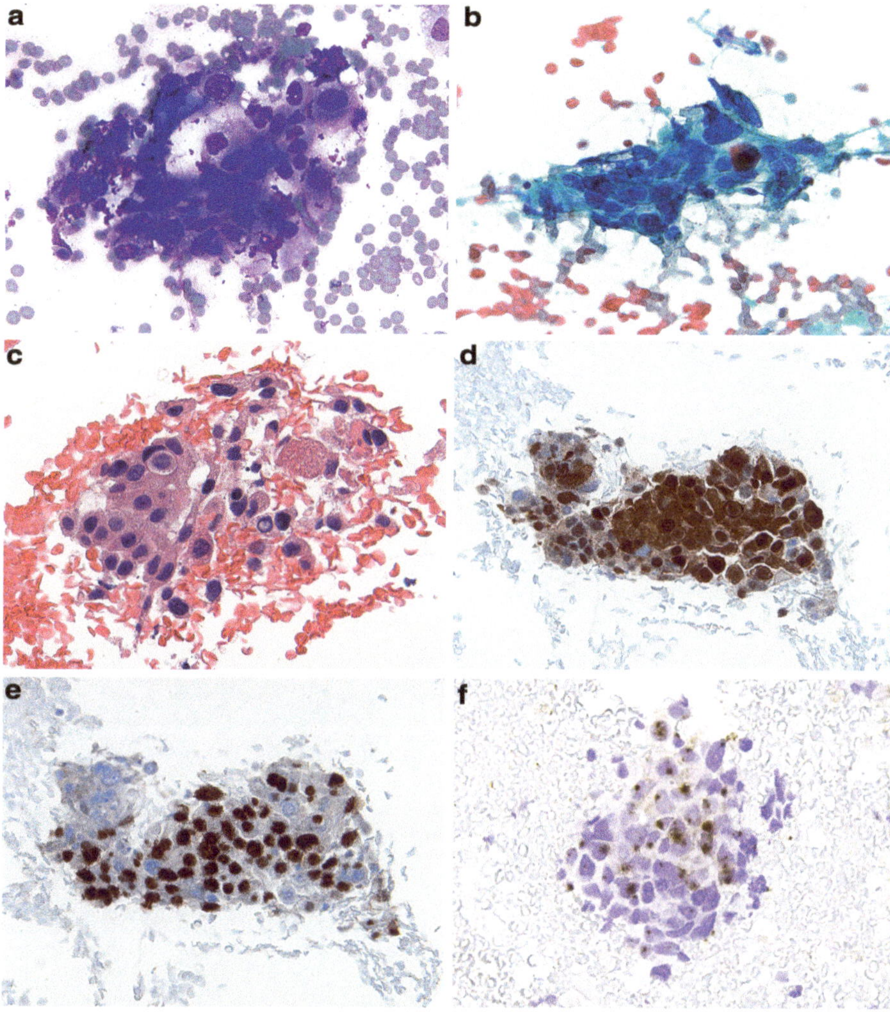


**Fig. 9.12** Metastatic HPV-positive squamous cell carcinoma [(**a**) DQ stain, high power; (**b**) Pap stain, high power; (**c**) H&E stain, high power; (**d**) p16 immunostain; (**e**) p40 immunostain; (**f**) HPV chromogenic in situ hybridization (CISH)]. The aspirates and cell block show tumor cells with nuclear pleomorphism and somewhat dense cytoplasm (**a**–**c**). The immunostains performed on the cell block reveal that the tumor cells are positive for p16 (**d**) and p40 (**e**) and positive for HPV by CISH

FISH or other studies to identify amplification or mutation in the fibroblast growth factor receptor (*FGFR*) family, as small molecule *FGFR* inhibitors, are now being investigated in patients with squamous cell carcinoma. However, this is an investigational profile, and there is no recommendation for molecular testing in these tumors [59]. Thus, accurate histological subtyping of non-small cell carcinomas influences molecular testing [12, 26, 43].

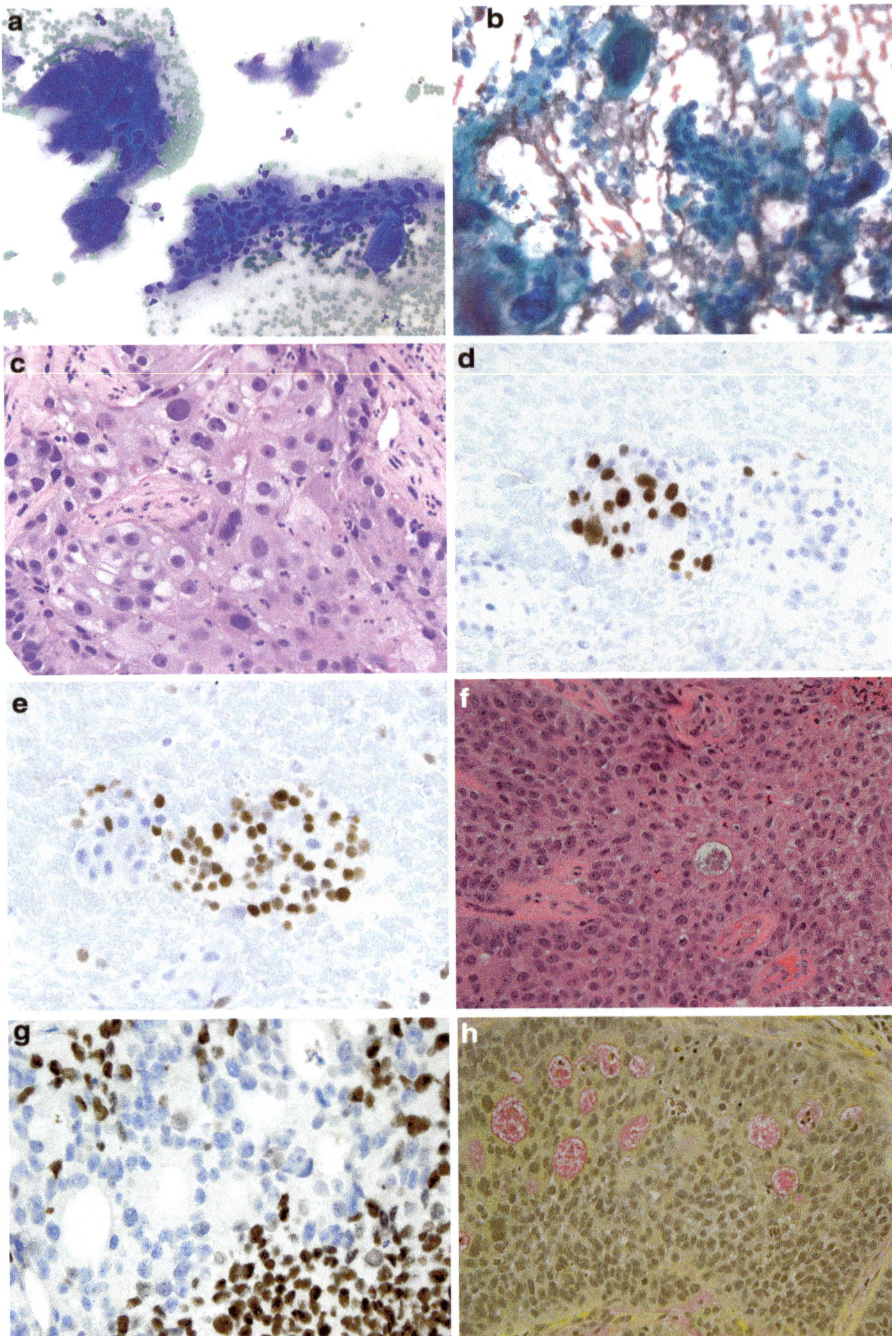


**Fig. 9.13** Adenosquamous carcinoma (**a**) DQ stain, medium power; (**b**) Pap stain, high power; (**c**) H&E stain, high power; (**d**) p40 immunostain; (**e**) TTF1 immunostain, (**f**) Histology H&E, medium power; (**g**) p63 immunostain; (**h**) mucicarmine stain, medium power). The tumor in this case shows two distinct populations, one group of tumor cells with dense cytoplasm and marked nuclear pleomorphism and a sheet of cells with round nuclei and glassy-to-vacuolated cytoplasm (**a**, **b**). Image (**c**) shows the accompanying core biopsy (**c**). The immunostains show a portion of cells staining for p40 (**d**) and another portion of tumor cells staining for TTF1 (**e**), supporting a diagnosis of adenosquamous carcinoma. Identification of gland formation can be subtle (**f**), and p63 (**g**) and mucicarmine stain (**h**) can be helpful in confirming both components [Photographs (**f**, **g**, and **h**) courtesy of Dr. Anjali Saqi]

## *Urothelial Carcinoma*

Metastatic urothelial carcinomas involving the lung can also have squamoid features. On core biopsies, the eosinophilic cytoplasm can be mistaken for squamous differentiation. Cytomorphologically, the identification of cells with blunt-ended tails, which are not orangeophilic on Papanicolaou staining (i.e., cercariform cells), and cytoplasmic eosinophilic bodies is helpful in recognizing metastatic urothelial carcinoma (Fig. 9.14).

p63 or p40 immunostaining is insufficient in differentiating squamous cell carcinoma from urothelial carcinoma, since both entities are immunoreactive for these markers [60]. GATA3, a nuclear stain, has emerged recently as helpful in distinguishing urothelial carcinoma from squamous cell carcinoma [61].

### Other Mimickers of Squamous Cell Carcinoma

Other tumors, such as sarcomas and mucoepidermoid carcinomas can mimic squamous cell carcinoma, which emphasizes the need for special stains, such as mucicarmine, and immunostains in the setting of unusual morphological findings.

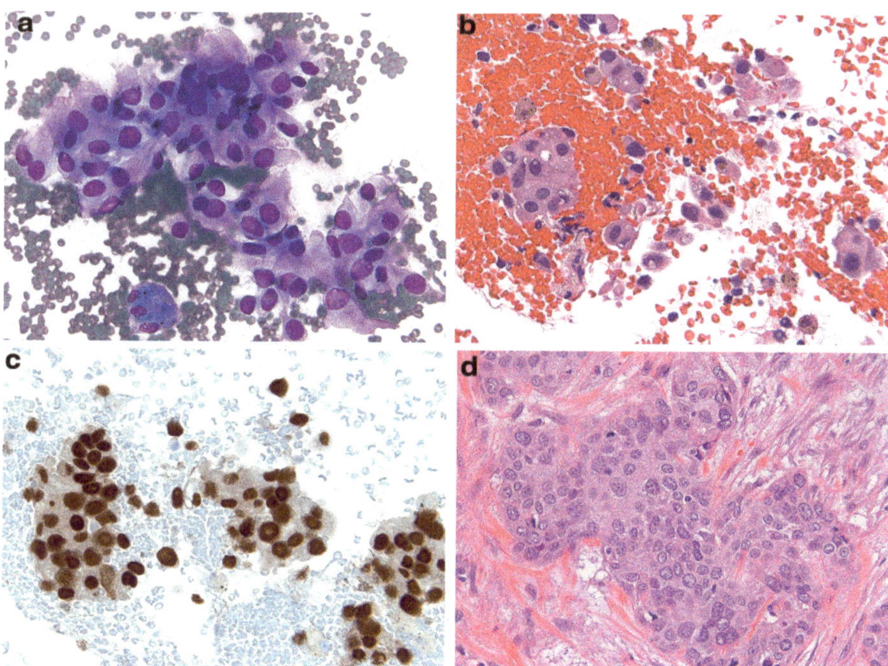


**Fig. 9.14** Metastatic urothelial carcinoma [(**a**) DQ stain, high power; (**b**) H&E stain, high power; (**c**) GATA3 immunostain; (**d**) H&E stain, high power]. The aspirates show loosely cohesive tumor cells with moderate amounts of cytoplasm, in addition to rare cells with cytoplasmic extensions imparting a tadpole-like appearance. The GATA3 immunostain shows strong nuclear positivity (**c**). The accompanying core biopsy shows infiltrative solid nests of tumor cells without prominent nucleoli

**Table 9.6** Differential diagnosis of pulmonary squamous cell carcinoma in small biopsies and cytology

| |
|---|
| Neoplastic |
| Adenocarcinoma, solid pattern |
| Adenosquamous carcinoma |
| Extrapulmonary squamous cell carcinomas (e.g., head and neck, uterine cervix, esophageal) |
| Metastatic urothelial carcinoma |
| Non-epithelial tumors (e.g., sarcoma, melanoma) |
| Salivary gland-type tumors of the bronchial glands (e.g., mucoepidermoid carcinoma) |
| Benign |
| Benign/reactive epithelial cells (e.g., squamous metaplasia, squamous atypia in the setting of fungal infection) |
| Treatment-related atypia (e.g., chemotherapy, radiation) |

**Table 9.7** Immunophenotype of primary and secondary squamous cell carcinomas in the lung

| Primary | P40 | CK5/6 | TTF1 | GATA3 | P16 | HPV CISH |
|---|---|---|---|---|---|---|
| Lung squamous cell carcinoma | + | + | – | – | – | – |
| Squamous cell carcinoma (HPV associated: anorectal, head and neck, uterine cervix) | + | + | – | – | + | + |
| Urothelial carcinoma | + | –/+ | – | + | – | – |

*ISH* in situ hybridization, *GATA3* GATA binding protein 3

Similarly, especially in small biopsies and cytology specimens of endobronchial lesions, the possibility of reactive or metaplastic squamous cells has to be entertained, particularly if there is a suspicion of infection, as fungal infections are known to be associated with squamous atypia. In these scenarios, deeper levels and special stains for organisms can be helpful to confirm the presence of infection. A summary of the differential diagnosis for a squamous cell carcinoma in the lung is seen in Table 9.6, and a list of immunohistochemical findings in the most common tumors with squamoid features is seen in Table 9.7.

## Salivary Gland-Type Tumors

Salivary gland-type tumors in the lung can represent either primaries arising from the submucosal glands of the tracheobronchial tree or metastases from the salivary glands. Primary pulmonary salivary gland-like tumors are extremely rare, accounting for <1 % of lung malignancies, with mucoepidermoid carcinomas and adenoid cystic carcinomas representing the two most common subtypes [62, 63]. Like most squamous cell carcinomas, primary pulmonary salivary gland-type tumors are morphologically and immunohistochemically indistinguishable from their metastatic counterparts, making the integration of clinical and radiological impression extremely relevant in determining the origin. Multiple pulmonary lesions presenting distant from the trachea, carina, and mainstem bronchus warrant investigation of an extrapulmonary metastasis. FISH studies are useful in recognizing salivary gland-type tumors, as novel chromosomal translocations have been identified. For example, *MECT1/MAML2* translocations are present in mucoepidermoid carcinomas, especially those that are low or intermediate grade [64], and its identification can distinguish between adenosquamous and mucoepidermoid carcinoma. In addition, adenoid cystic carcinomas are associated with MYB-NFIB chimeric fusion proteins from t(6;9) rearrangements [65].

Other helpful FISH tests for salivary gland tumors include EWSR1-ATF1 fusions in hyalinizing clear cell carcinoma of the salivary gland, ETV6-NTRK3 fusions in mammary analog secretory carcinoma of the salivary gland and breast, and Her2/neu overexpression in salivary duct carcinomas [66–68] (Table 9.8). These salivary gland tumors are exceedingly uncommon in the lung, but rare cases of metastases of the salivary gland hyalinizing clear cell carcinoma and salivary duct carcinoma to the lung have been reported [63, 69].

## Adenoid Cystic Carcinoma

Adenoid cystic carcinomas have cells with small, round nuclei and scant cytoplasm, imparting a "basaloid" appearance arranged as tubules or cribriform clusters with dense stromal globules (Fig. 9.15). The dense globules have well-defined borders and appear metachromatic on Diff-Quik stained cytology preparations, making them easily distinguishable from mucin. In small biopsies and cytology, these tumors can be difficult to differentiate from small cell carcinoma when there is a lack of the globules and a predominantly solid pattern. Adenoid cystic carcinomas, in contrast to small cell carcinomas, lack necrosis, apoptosis, positivity for neuroendocrine markers, and a high-proliferation index [63].

## Mucoepidermoid Carcinomas

Mucoepidermoid carcinomas typically have a combination of cell types, including squamoid cells, intermediate cells, and mucous cells, in varying proportions. In a tumor showing both glandular and squamous differentiation, a mucoepidermoid carcinoma should be considered, in addition to an adenosquamous and squamous cell carcinomas. When positive in the glandular component, TTF1 staining favors adenosquamous arising from the lung.

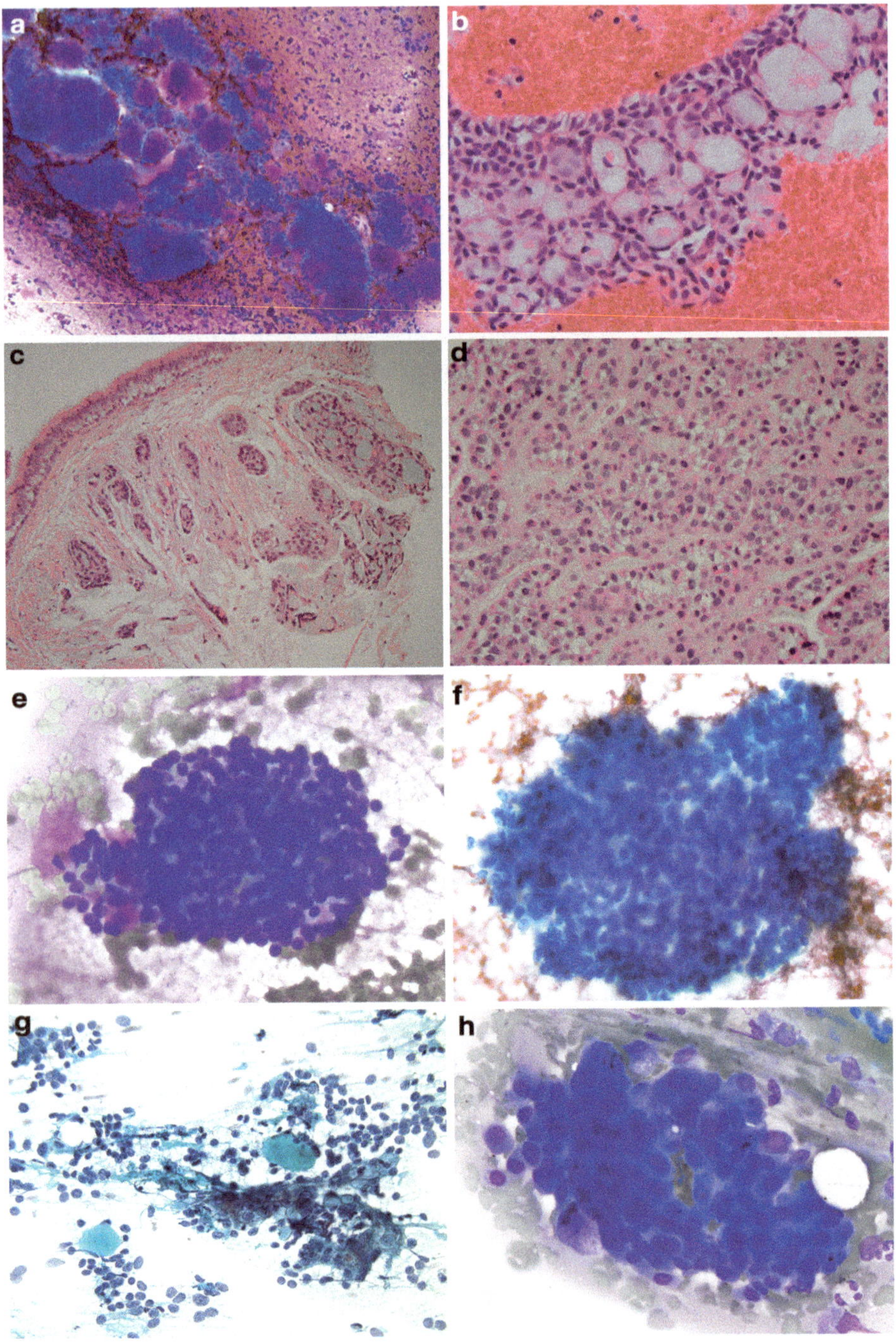


**Fig. 9.15** Primary and metastatic adenoid cystic carcinoma and mucoepidermoid carcinoma [adenoid cystic carcinoma (primary): (**a**) DQ stain, high power; (**b**) cell block H&E, high power; (**c**) core biopsy H&E, low power; (**d**) core biopsy H&E, high power;

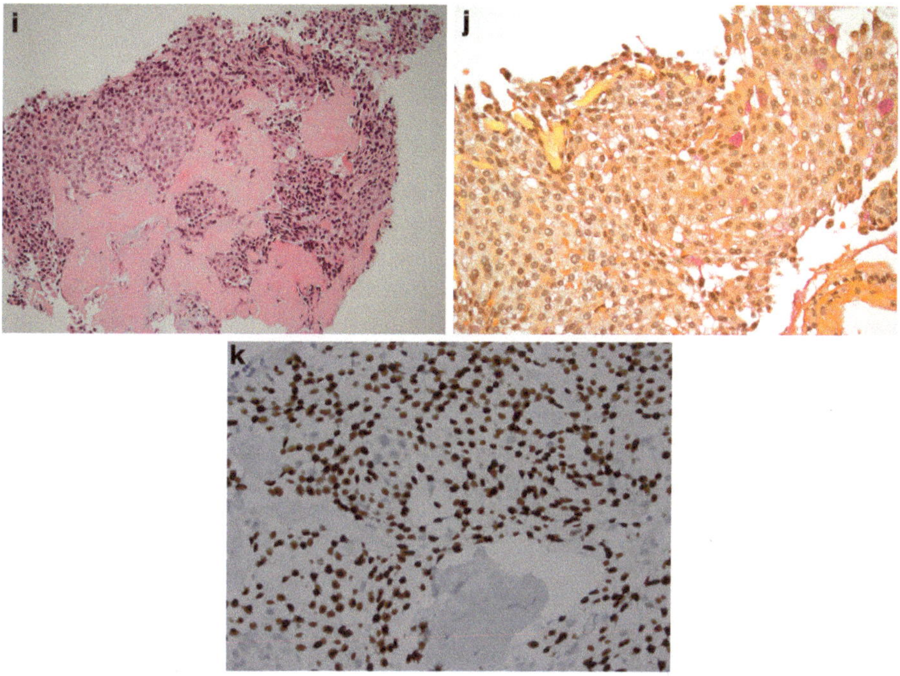

**Fig. 9.15** (continued) adenoid cystic carcinoma (metastatic): (**e**) DQ stain, high power; (**f**) Pap stain, high power; (**g**) Pap stain, medium power; and mucoepidermoid carcinoma: (**h**) DQ stain, high power; (**i**) biopsy H&E, low power; (**j**) mucicarmine stain, high power; (**k**) p63 immuno stain, low power]. The aspirates from this case show globules on the Diff-Quik stain (**a**), which appear metachromatic, and cell block (**b**). The core biopsy shows the endobronchial location (**c**). More cellular areas without discernable globules are also evident (**d**). The metastatic adenoid cystic carcinoma shows crowded clusters (**e, f**) of tumor cells with inconspicuous nucleoli and scant cytoplasm imparting a basaloid appearance. There is a conspicuous absence of background necrosis and pleomorphism. Globules can also be seen on a Pap stain (**g**). Mucoepidermoid carcinoma. Mostly epithelioid and rare mucous cells are present (**h**). The mucin-containing cells are difficult to identify on morphology (**i**) but are highlighted with mucicarmine (**j**). The remaining cells stain with p63 (**k**) [Photographs (**a–d, h–k**) courtesy of Dr. Anjali Saqi]

**Table 9.8** Chromosomal abnormalities in salivary gland-like tumors that can be detected with FISH studies in small biopsies and cytology specimens

| Salivary gland-type tumor | Gene(s) | Chromosome(s) |
|---|---|---|
| Mammary analog secretory carcinoma[a] | *ETV6-NTRK3* | t(12;15) |
| Mucoepidermoid carcinoma | *MECT1/MAML2* | t(11;19) |
| Adenoid cystic carcinoma | *MYB-NFIB* | t(6,9) |
| Salivary duct carcinoma[a] | *Her2/neu* | 17q |
| Hyalinizing clear cell carcinoma[a] | *EWSR1-ATF1* | t(12;22) |

[a]These salivary gland tumors have only rarely been reported in the lung and are seen primarily as metastases.

## Metastatic Malignant Melanoma

Malignant melanomas metastasize to many sites in the body, including the lung. On cytology, the cells tend to be discohesive. Otherwise, malignant melanomas can assume different patterns and contain cells that are enlarged, pleomorphic, monomorphic, and/or plasmacytoid. Similar variability can be seen in the nuclei, which can have binucleation, prominent nucleoli, and/or intranuclear inclusions (Fig. 9.16). When present, the identification of fine dusty, nonrefractile pigment granules is specific for distinguishing melanoma from hemosiderin and carbon [70]. But given that the vast majority of melanomas lack melanin pigment and have different morphological patterns, they can mimic large cell lymphomas, neuroendocrine tumors, and poorly differentiated non-small cell carcinomas [70].

The characteristic immunoprofile of malignant melanomas includes positivity for S100, HMB45, MelanA, MiTF, and tyrosinase. A panel of stains is typically helpful given that not all melanomas are immunoreactive for each of these markers and a subset can be S100 negative and show some cytokeratin staining [71]. Besides allocating tissue for immunohistochemical confirmation, it should also be procured

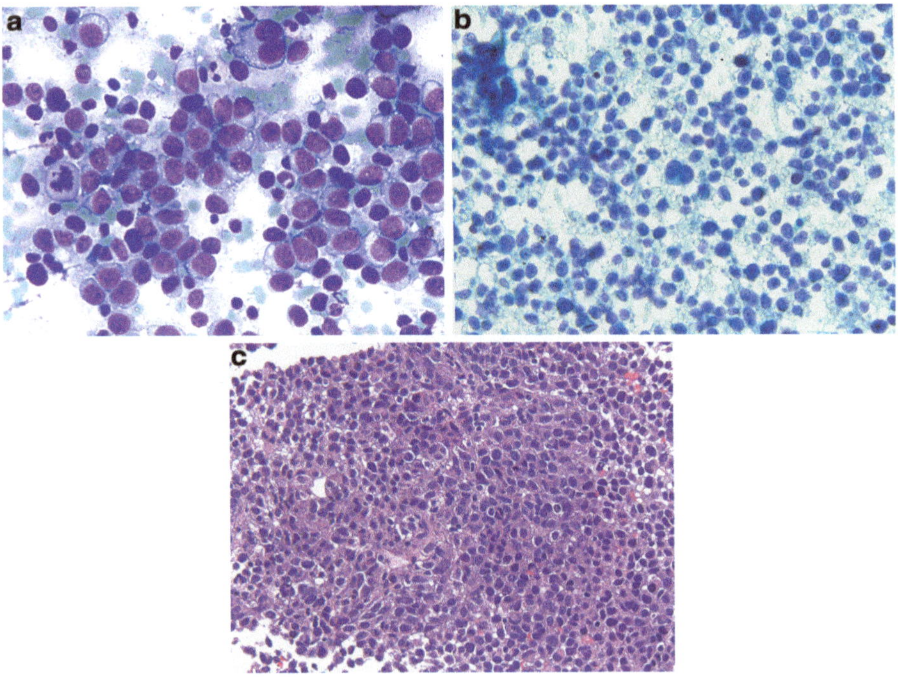


**Fig. 9.16** Metastatic malignant melanoma [(**a**) DQ stain, high power; (**b**) Pap stain, high power; (**c**) H&E stain, medium power]. Metastatic melanoma typically shows a discohesive, plasmacytoid appearance with prominent nucleoli (**a**–**c**), and in addition, binucleation is also common. These features should raise the possibility of a melanoma and prompt immunostaining for melanoma markers such as S100, HMB45, MiTF, and MelanA

for potential molecular testing. Oncologists frequently request *BRAF* and *KRAS* testing for melanomas, because there is a dramatic clinical response to targeted therapies like vemurafenib in BRAF-positive melanoma [72, 73].

## Mesenchymal Tumors

Tumors with spindle cells involving the lung are of mesenchymal or non-mesenchymal origin, present as a solitary nodule or multiple nodules, can be benign/low-malignant potential or malignant, and represent primary or metastatic disease (Fig. 9.17). In general, the differential for bland-appearing ovoid or spindle cells includes spindle cell carcinoid, solitary fibrous tumor, benign metastasizing leiomyoma, spindle cell melanoma, neurogenic tumor, Type A thymoma, and granuloma. On the opposite end of the spectrum, malignant considerations for spindle cell proliferations comprise, but are not limited to, sarcomatoid carcinoma, sarcomatoid mesothelioma, metastatic sarcoma, malignant solitary fibrous tumor, and rarely primary sarcoma arising in the lung or the vessels within the lung.

Malignant tumors with spindle cells are more likely to yield cellular diagnostic material on aspirates or touch preparations than those that are benign or low grade. Sarcomas tend to have discohesive spindle or epithelioid cells with marked nuclear atypia and a metachromatic fibrillary or chondromyxoid background on Romanowsky-based stains. Other tumors with a predominantly spindle cell component and low-grade histology are likely to yield pauci-cellular aspirates and

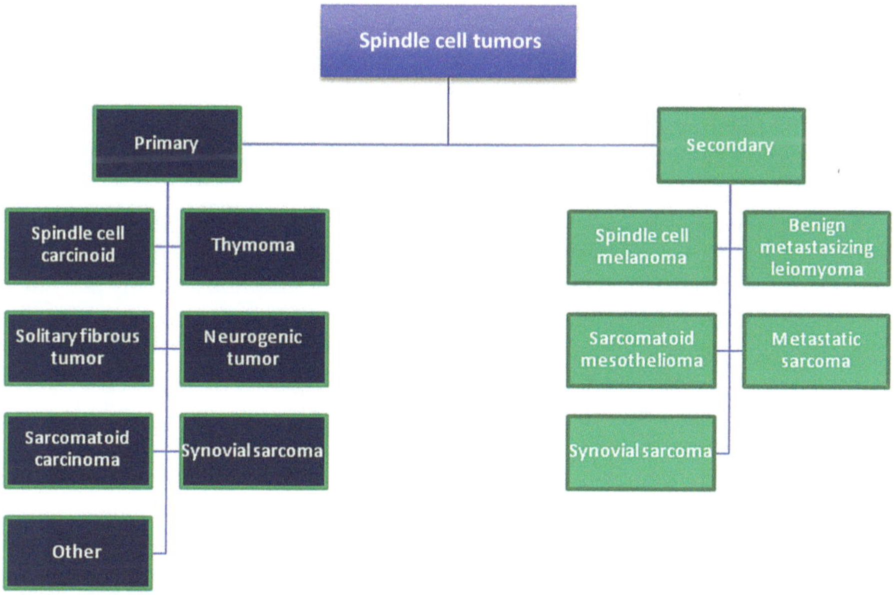


**Fig. 9.17** Differential diagnosis for spindle cell tumors involving the lung and mediastinum

**Table 9.9** Common immunophenotypes of neoplasms with spindle cells morphology

| | Keratin(s) | TTF1 | CD34 | BCL2 | Desmin | SMA | ER | PR |
|---|---|---|---|---|---|---|---|---|
| Sarcomatoid carcinoma | + | +/– | | | | | | |
| Mesothelioma | + | | | | | | | |
| Synovial sarcoma | + | | | | | | | |
| Solitary fibrous tumor | | | + | + | | | | |
| Benign metastasizing leiomyoma | | | | | + | + | + | + |
| Leiomyosarcoma | | | | | + | + | | |

*ER* estrogen receptor, *PR* progesterone receptor

touch preparations, leading to nondiagnostic or equivocal intra-procedural findings necessitating histological evaluation of the core biopsy for assessment. Even on core biopsies, a specific diagnosis may be challenging [74]. In general, hypocellularity, lack of necrosis, minimal/absent nuclear pleomorphism, and low/absent mitotic activity favor benign/low-malignant neoplasms, and those with contrasting cytomorphological features tend to be malignant.

Most spindle cell tumors are very rare in the lung. With knowledge of the clinical and imaging findings, a focused immunostain panel to differentiate among the various entities can be performed. Sarcomatoid carcinoma of the lung, which has a male predominance and arises in the lung, encompasses several subtypes (i.e., pleomorphic carcinoma, spindle cell carcinoma, giant cell carcinoma, carcinosarcoma, and pulmonary blastoma) with varying proportions of carcinoma and sarcomatoid (spindle and/or giant cell) components. Cytokeratin, considered the first-line stain in neoplasms with spindle cells suggestive of a lung primary, is helpful in identifying the epithelial component in morphologically ambiguous cases, but additional keratins (e.g., CK7, Cam5.2, CK18) may be necessary in poorly differentiated cytokeratin-negative cases (Table 9.9) [74]. A subset of sarcomatoid carcinomas stains with TTF1 and confirms a pulmonary origin [75] (Fig. 9.18). Sarcomatoid carcinomas can also express mesothelial markers and mesenchymal markers requiring cautious interpretation of the diagnosis [76].

Sarcomatoid mesotheliomas, consisting of >90 % spindle cells, classically have pleural thickening but can metastasize to the lung and distant locations. They are immunoreactive for CK and lack the diffuse staining of calretinin staining and other mesothelial markers associated with epithelioid mesothelioma [74].

Solitary fibrous tumors are associated with the pleura and can be attached to the lung by a pedicle. They are characterized by a "patternless pattern" and have malignant potential (Fig. 9.19). They typically stain with CD34, BCL2, CD99 and STAT6; few tumors are immunoreactive for desmin or actin. Spindle cell carcinoids are positive for synaptophysin and chromogranin (Fig. 9.20). Neurogenic tumors stain with S100, but this can be seen in other spindle cell tumors including spindle cell melanomas.

Benign metastasizing leiomyomas are rare tumors that present in women with a history of leiomyoma treated years earlier by a hysterectomy [77] (Fig. 9.21). They mark with desmin, smooth muscle actin, estrogen, and progesterone, and their cytological features (e.g., bland spindle cells, no mitoses or necrosis) distinguish them from leiomyosarcomas.

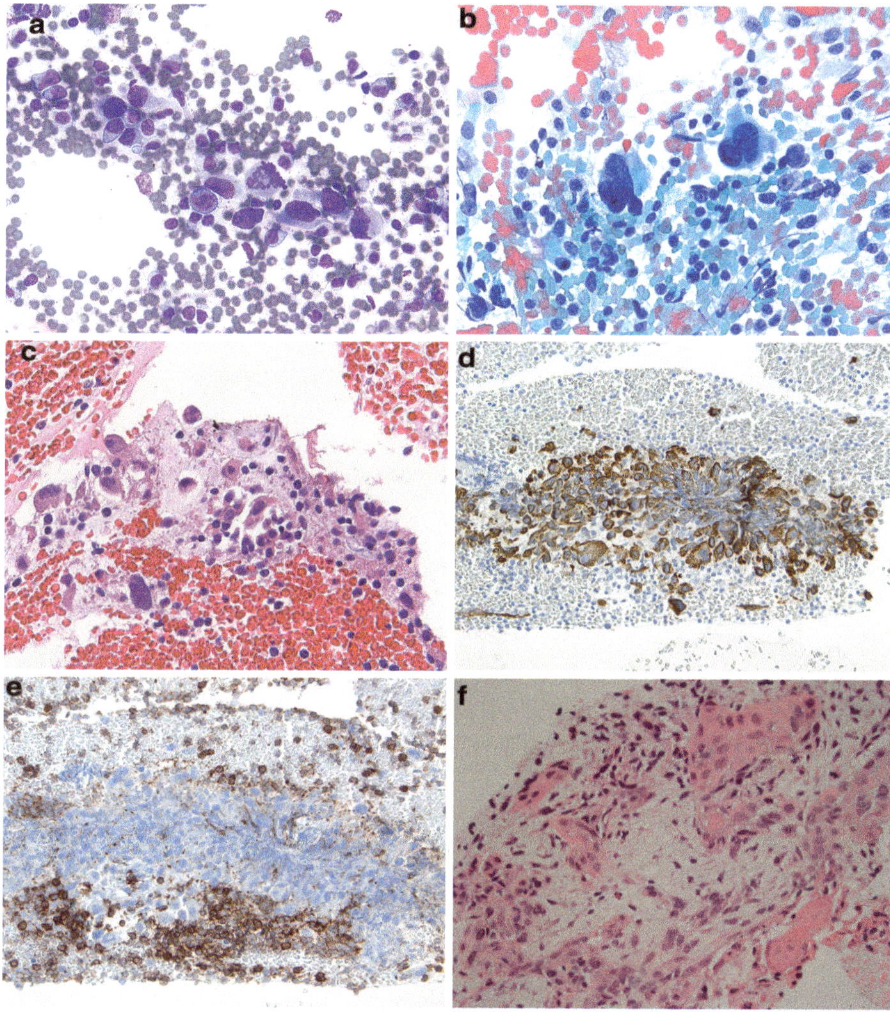


**Fig. 9.18** Sarcomatoid carcinoma of the lung [(**a**) DQ stain, high power; (**b**) Pap stain, high power; (**c**) H&E stain, medium power; (**d**) pancytokeratin immunostain, medium power; (**e**) vimentin immunostain, medium power; F. H&E, high power]. Pleomorphic spindle cells can also be seen in sarcomatoid carcinomas of the lung, and thus, cytokeratin immunoreactivity (**d**) is important to look for in a spindle cell tumor to confirm a sarcomatoid carcinoma. These tumor cells will typically be negative for vimentin (**e**), while a sarcoma would show positivity for vimentin and negativity for cytokeratin. The spindle cell component may be overlooked as a desmoplastic response (**f**) [Photograph (**f**) courtesy of Dr. Anjali Saqi]

Leiomyosarcomas and myxofibrosarcomas are the most common metastatic sarcomas in the lung, and given the proclivity for hematogenous spread, sarcomas typically will involve the lung or bone without involving the lymph nodes [78]. Primary sarcomas in the lung or thoracic cavity are rare, but vascular sarcomas and synovial sarcomas are among the most common [78]. In general, sarcomas

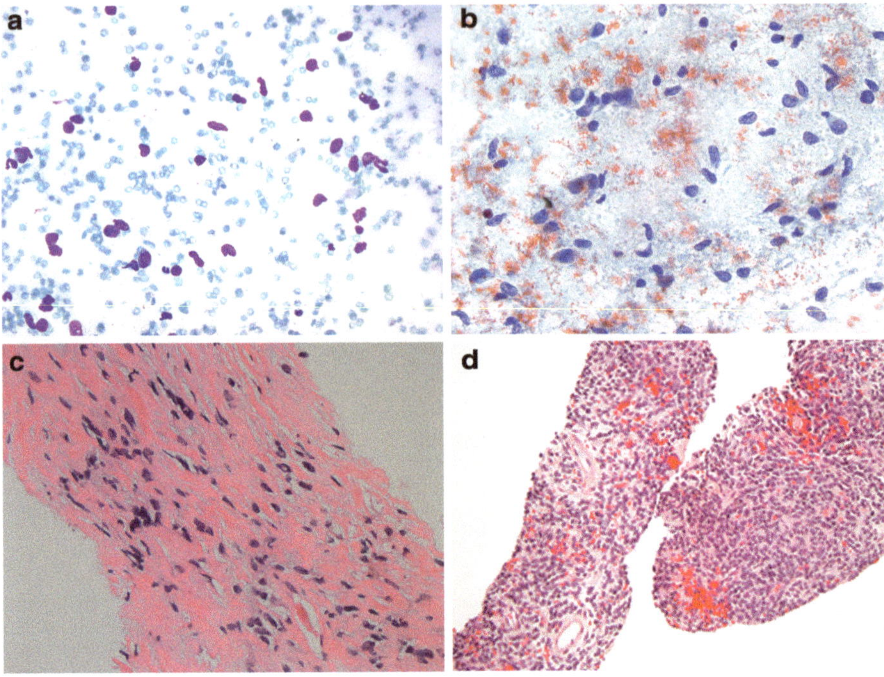


**Fig. 9.19** Solitary fibrous tumor [(**a**) DQ stain, medium power; (**b**) Pap stain, medium power; (**c**) H&E stain, high power; (**d**) H&E, medium power). Solitary fibrous tumors are spindle cell neoplasms. Cytology preparations show bland spindle cells (**a**, **b**). Similar cells, including some with atypia, are within collagenized stroma and are noted on the corresponding core biopsy (**c**). Solitary fibrous tumors can have high cellularity (**d**) as well. Malignant solitary fibrous tumors have greater cellularity, more nuclear atypia, and a high mitotic index [Photographs courtesy of Dr. Anjali Saqi (**a**–**c**) and Dr. Andre Moreira (**d**)]

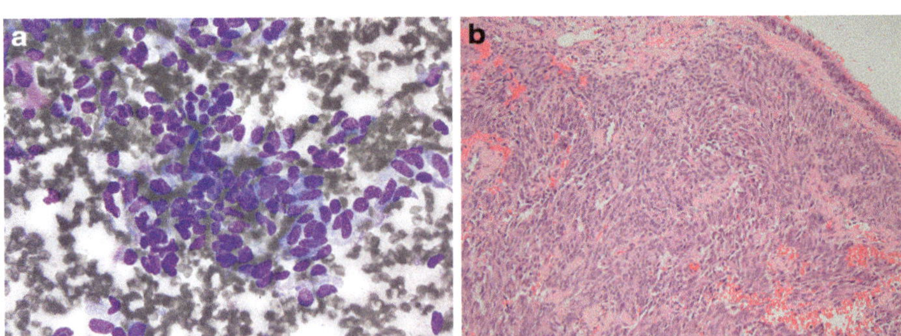


**Fig. 9.20** Spindle cell carcinoid [(**a**) DQ stain, medium power; (**b**) H&E, medium power]. The aspirate shows bland-appearing spindle cells that are loosely cohesive and singly placed (**a**). The H&E demonstrates similar cells without pleomorphism, necrosis, or mitotic activity (**b**) [Photographs courtesy of Dr. Anjali Saqi]

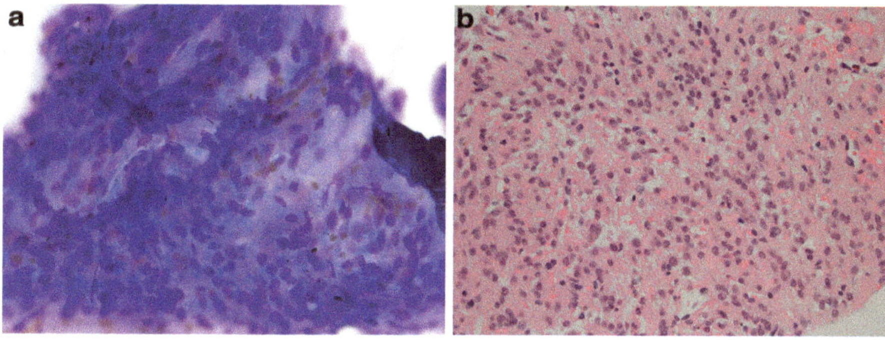

**Fig. 9.21** Benign metastasizing leiomyoma [(**a**) DQ stain, high power; (**b**) H&E, medium power]. The touch prep has a cellular spindle cells proliferation (**a**). On the H&E (**b**), no pleomorphism, necrosis, or mitotic activity is seen [Photographs courtesy of Dr. Anjali Saqi]

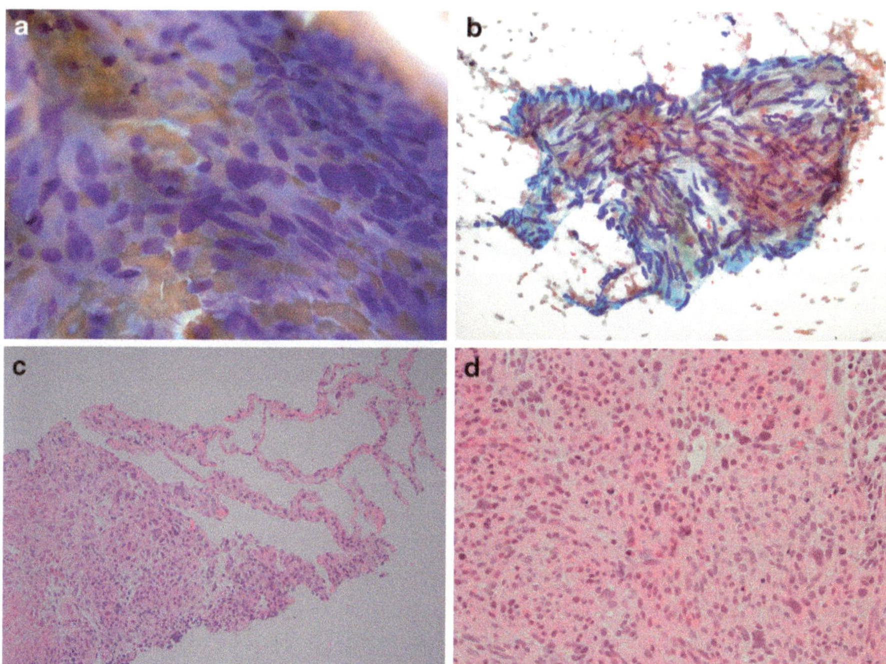

**Fig. 9.22** Metastatic leiomyosarcoma [(**a**) DQ stain, high power; (**b**) Pap stain, high power; (**c**) H&E stain, medium power; (**d**) H&E stain, high power]. Sarcomas, such as leiomyosarcomas, are typically metastatic to the lung and reveal a cellular spindle cell tumor with nuclear enlargement and pleomorphism [Photographs courtesy of Dr. Anjali Saqi (**a**, **c**, and **d**) and Dr. John Crapanzano (**b**)]

are vimentin and desmin positive and cytokeratin negative, whereas the opposite immunoprofile (cytokeratin positive, vimentin negative) is more compatible with a sarcomatoid carcinoma of the lung, provided that a synovial sarcoma has been excluded (Fig. 9.22).

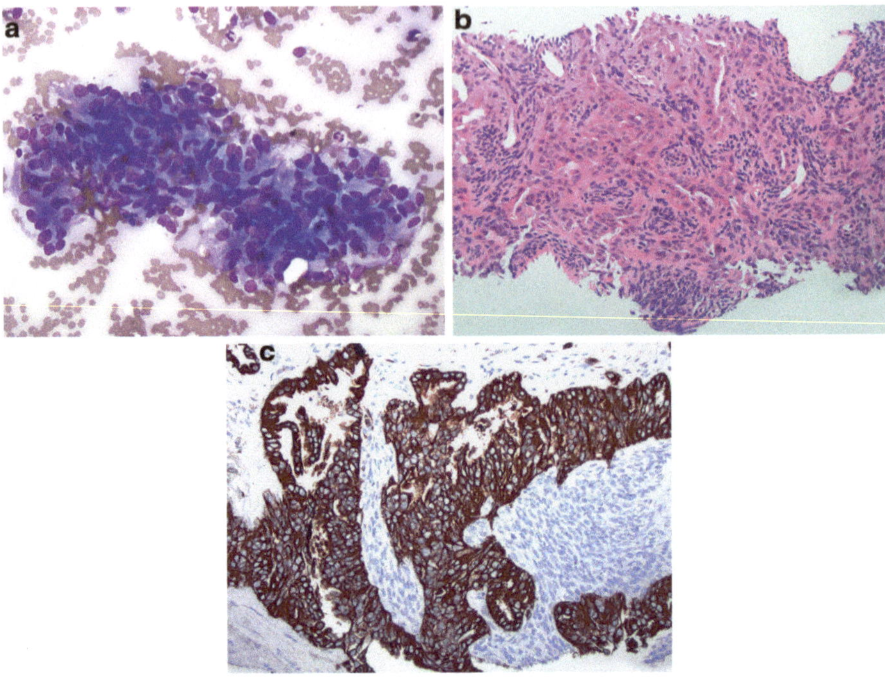

**Fig. 9.23** Synovial sarcoma [(**a**) DQ, medium power; (**b**) H&E stain, low power; (**c**) CK stain, medium power]. Synovial sarcomas can be monophasic or biphasic. The cytology shows epithelioid and ovoid cells (**a**). These are better seen on the core biopsy (**b**), and the epithelial cells are highlighted by cytokeratin immunostain (**c**) [Photographs courtesy of Dr. John Crapanzano]

Given the presence of SYT-SSX fusions in synovial sarcoma, FISH studies can confirm the diagnosis and should be considered in spindle cell tumors, including those with some staining for epithelial immunomarkers [79] (Fig. 9.23).

Malignant melanomas can also have spindle cells and mimic a spindle cell tumor. They have mild to marked nuclear atypia, and in contrast their epithelioid counterparts, they have inconspicuous nucleoli, and on cytology, the cells are more cohesive and may have intranuclear grooves [80]. They are distinguished from sarcomas by their positivity for melanoma markers, except HMB45, which is typically negative in spindle cell melanomas (Fig. 9.24).

## Malignant Lymphoma

Lymphomas can involve the lung as a primary or as secondary process. The most common lymphomas arising in the lung are extranodal marginal zone lymphomas of mucosa-associated lymphoid tissue (MALT) type; however, almost any type of lymphoma can secondarily involve the lung [81]. Clues to the diagnosis on cytology

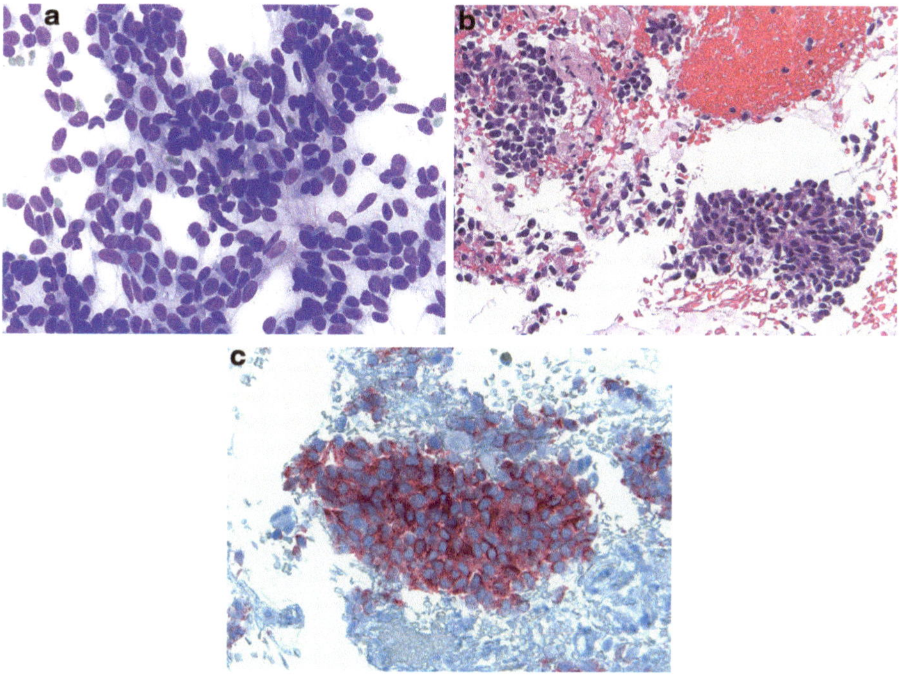

**Fig. 9.24** Metastatic spindle cell melanoma [(**a**) DQ stain, high power; (**b**) H&E stain, medium power; (**c**) MelanA immunostain, medium power]. Malignant melanoma can present with spindle cells, which have mild pleomorphism, occasional intranuclear grooves, and less prominent nucleoli than in epithelioid melanoma. This diagnosis should be considered in any spindle cell tumor in the lung

include a discohesive population of cells and lymphoglandular bodies, representing cytoplasmic fragments, in the background. On a touch preparation, the discohesion can be difficult to appreciate. Extensive pressure or manipulation on a smear, touch preparation, or core biopsy results in crush artifact mimicking that seen in small cell carcinomas, so care must be taken in handling these and other specimens alike.

Small cell lymphomas can be particularly difficult to distinguish from reactive lymphocytic infiltrates in the absence of flow cytometry or FISH studies to substantiate a clonal population, so a specimen demonstrating discohesive cells should raise suspicion for a lymphoproliferative process and prompt the appropriate workup [81] (Fig. 9.25). Some of the primary MALT lymphomas of the lung are heterogeneous and demonstrate plasma cells and granulomas, which also raise suspicion for an infection; thus, ancillary studies to resolve the proliferation are necessary [81].

Large cell lymphomas are more obviously malignant. However, immunostains are crucial to exclude poorly differentiated carcinoma, sarcoma, and melanoma, which may be in the differential diagnosis of a discohesive tumor with large, pleomorphic cells.

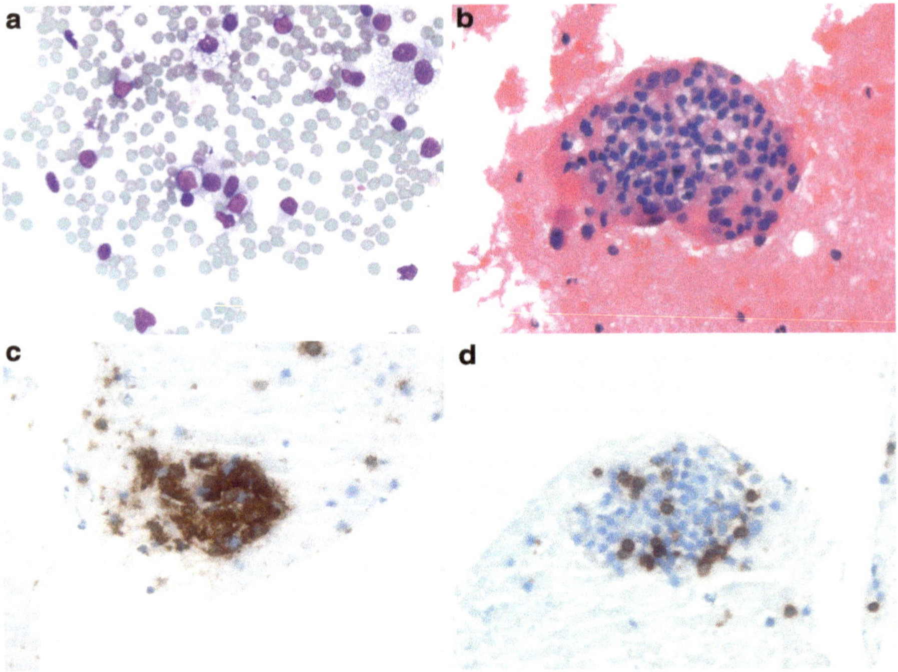

**Fig. 9.25** Extranodal marginal zone B-cell lymphoma [(**a**) DQ stain, high power; (**b**) H&E stain, medium power; (**c**) CD20 immunostain, medium power; (**d**) CD3 immunostain, medium power]. The aspirates from this lung lesion reveal a discohesive population of cells with lymphoglandular bodies and histiocytes (**a**, **b**). Occasional cells have a plasmacytoid appearance. Immunostains performed on the cell block reveal that the cells are positive for CD20 (**c**) and negative for CD3 (**d**). Flow cytometry confirmed a light-chain restricted B-cell population

In general lymphomas are typically positive for LCA/CD45, a lymphoid marker, and stain with CD20, given that most lymphomas involving the lung are of B-cell lineage. Additional immunostains and FISH studies can be performed based on the phenotype for further subtyping [81].

## Conclusions

The evaluation of patients with possible secondary and/or multiple lung tumors requires a multiparameter approach, incorporating a detailed clinical history, radiological findings, meticulous pathological review, and ancillary studies. The findings in various tumor types in the lung are summarized in Table 9.10. Given the emphasis on minimizing unnecessary loss of tissue in small biopsies and cytology specimens in today's era of personalized medicine, knowledge of the spectrum of entities to consider, in addition to the morphological clues, can be crucial in maximizing diagnostic accuracy and enhancing the yield from these minimally invasive specimens.

**Table 9.10** Differential diagnosis for tumors of unknown origin in cytopathology specimens and applicable ancillary studies

| Tumor type | Morphology | Immunostaining profile | Molecular studies and others |
|---|---|---|---|
| Adenocarcinoma | Cohesive, vacuolated cytoplasm, prominent nucleoli, glandular formation or other architectural types (signet ring, papillary, mucinous) | CK7 & CK20 profile, site-specific markers (e.g., TTF1, CDX2) | Molecular studies for theranostic information (e.g., lung (*EGFR*, *KRAS*, *ALK*), colon (*BRAF and KRAS*)) |
| Squamous cell carcinoma | Cohesive, dense cytoplasm, coarse chromatin, orangeophilia on Pap stain | p40/p63, CK5/6, site-specific markers (e.g., p16) | HPV CISH to exclude an HPV-related squamous cell carcinoma<br>FISH studies for FGFR amplification in primary lung squamous cell carcinomas |
| Lymphoma | Discohesive, lymphoglandular bodies | CD45, CD20, CD3, subtype-specific markers (e.g., CD30, ALK, EBV) | FC and FISH studies for clonality (e.g., IgH rearrangement or T-cell gene rearrangement) and subtyping (e.g., specific immunophenotype by FC or specific translocation by FISH) |
| Melanoma | Discohesive, binucleation, prominent nucleoli, intranuclear inclusions, melanin pigment | S100, MelanA, HMB45, tyrosinase, MiTF | Molecular studies for theranostic information (e.g., *BRAF and KRAS*) |
| Sarcoma | Discohesive, marked nuclear pleomorphism, scant-to-moderate amounts of cytoplasm | Vimentin, subtype-specific markers (e.g., desmin) | FISH studies for subtyping (e.g., *EWS* translocations) |
| Mesothelioma | Cohesive with spaces between cells, nucleoli, two-tone cytoplasm | WT-1, calretinin, D2-40, CK5/6, cytokeratin | FISH for diagnostic and prognostic information (e.g., *p16* deletion by FISH) |

*ICC* immunocytochemistry, *FISH* fluorescence in situ hybridization, *FC* flow cytometry, *CISH* chromogenic in situ hybridization

## References

1. Rivera MP, Mehta AC, Wahidi MM. Establishing the diagnosis of lung cancer: diagnosis and management of lung cancer, 3rd ed: American College of Chest Physicians evidence-based clinical practice guidelines. Chest. 2013;143:e142S–65S.
2. Hsiao SH, Chung CL, Lee CM, Chen WY, Chou YT, Wu ZH, Chen YC, Lin SE. Suitability of computed tomography-guided biopsy specimens for subtyping and genotyping of non-small-cell lung cancer. Clin Lung Cancer. 2013;14:719–25.

3. Travis WD, Brambilla E, Noguchi M, Nicholson AG, Geisinger K, Yatabe Y, Ishikawa Y, Wistuba I, Flieder DB, Franklin W, Gazdar A, Hasleton PS, Henderson DW, Kerr KM, Petersen I, Roggli V, Thunnissen E, Tsao M. Diagnosis of lung cancer in small biopsies and cytology: implications of the 2011 International Association for the Study of Lung Cancer/American Thoracic Society/ European Respiratory Society classification. Arch Pathol Lab Med. 2013;137:668–84.
4. Chang YL, Wu CT, Lee YC. Surgical treatment of synchronous multiple primary lung cancers: experience of 92 patients. J Thorac Cardiovasc Surg. 2007;134:630–7.
5. Martini N, Melamed MR. Multiple primary lung cancers. J Thorac Cardiovasc Surg. 1975;70:606–12.
6. Van Bodegom PC, Wagenaar SS, Corrin B, et al. Second primary lung cancer: importance of long term follow up. Thorax. 1989;44:778–93.
7. Wu CT, Lin MW, Hsieh MS, Kuo SW, Chang YL. New aspects of the clinicopathology and genetic profile of metachronous multiple lung cancers. Ann Surg. 2014;259(5):1018–24.
8. Monaco SE, Nikiforova MN, Cieply K, Teot LA, Khalbuss WE, Dacic S. A comparison of EGFR and KRAS status in primary lung carcinoma and matched metastases. Hum Pathol. 2010;41:94–102.
9. Son C, Lee SK, Choi PJ, Roh MS. Characteristics of additional primary malignancies in Korean patients with non-small cell lung cancer. J Thorac Dis. 2013;5:737–44.
10. Goldstraw P, Crowley J, Chansky K, Giroux DJ, Groome PA, Rami-Porta R, Postmus PE, Rusch V, Sobin L, International Association for the Study of Lung Cancer International Staging Committee; Participating Institutions. The IASLC Lung Cancer Staging Project: proposals for the revision of the TNM stage groupings in the forthcoming (seventh) edition of the TNM Classification of malignant tumours. J Thorac Oncol. 2007;2:706–14.
11. Dacic S. Dilemmas in lung cancer staging. Arch Pathol Lab Med. 2012;136:1194–7.
12. Clinical Lung Cancer Genome Project (CLCGP), Network Genomic Medicine (NGM). A genomics-based classification of human lung tumors. Sci Transl Med. 2013; 5: 209ra153.
13. Hida T, Ariyoshi Y, Sugiura T, Suyama M, Takahashi T, Ueda R. Synchronous lung cancer presenting with small cell carcinoma and adenocarcinoma. Chest. 1993;104:1602–4.
14. Gerlinger M, Rowan AJ, Horswell S, Larkin J, Endesfelder D, Gronroos E, Martinez P, Matthews N, Stewart A, Tarpey P, Varela I, Phillimore B, Begum S, McDonald NQ, Butler A, Jones D, Raine K, Latimer C, Santos CR, Nohadani M, Eklund AC, Spencer-Dene B, Clark G, Pickering L, Stamp G, Gore M, Szallasi Z, Downward J, Futreal PA, Swanton C. Intratumor heterogeneity and branched evolution revealed by multiregion sequencing. N Engl J Med. 2012;366:883–92.
15. de Biase D, Visani M, Malapelle U, Simonato F, Cesari V, Bellevicine C, Pession A, Troncone G, Fassina A, Tallini G. Next-generation sequencing of lung cancer EGFR Exons 18-21 allows effective molecular diagnosis of small routine samples (Cytology and Biopsy). PLoS One. 2013;8:e83607.
16. Ellison G, Zhu G, Moulis A, Dearden S, Speake G, McCormack R. EGFR mutation testing in lung cancer: a review of available methods and their use for analysis of tumour tissue and cytology samples. J Clin Pathol. 2013;66:79–89.
17. Vanderlaan PA, Yamaguchi N, Folch E, Boucher DH, Kent MS, Gangadharan SP, Majid A, Goldstein MA, Huberman MS, Kocher ON, Costa DB. Success and failure rates of tumor genotyping techniques in routine pathological samples with non-small-cell lung cancer. Lung Cancer. 2014;84(1):39–44.
18. Ocque R, Tochigi N, Ohori NP, Dacic S. Usefulness of immunohistochemical and histochemical studies in the classification of lung adenocarcinoma and squamous cell carcinoma in cytologic specimens. Am J Clin Pathol. 2011;136:81–7.
19. Sigel CS, Moreira AL, Travis WD, Zakowski MF, Thornton RH, Riely GJ, Rekhtman N. Subtyping of non-small cell lung carcinoma: a comparison of small biopsy and cytology specimens. J Thorac Oncol. 2011;6:1849–56.
20. Rodriguez EF, Monaco SE, Dacic S. Cytologic subtyping of lung adenocarcinoma by using the proposed International Association for the Study of Lung Cancer/American Thoracic Society/ European Respiratory Society (IASLC/ATS/ERS) adenocarcinoma classification. Cancer Cytopathol. 2013;121:629–37.

21. Varadhachary GR, Spector Y, Abbruzzese JL, Rosenwald S, Wang H, Aharonov R, Carlson HR, Cohen D, Karanth S, Macinskas J, Lenzi R, Chajut A, Edmonston TB, Raber MN. Prospective gene signature study using microRNA to identify the tissue of origin in patients with carcinoma of unknown primary. Clin Cancer Res. 2011;17:4063–70.
22. Billah S, Stewart J, Staerkel G, Chen S, Gong Y, Guo M. EGFR and KRAS mutations in lung carcinoma: molecular testing by using cytology specimens. Cancer Cytopathol. 2011;119: 111–7.
23. Jurado J, Saqi A, Maxfield R, Newmark A, et al. The Efficacy of EBUS-guided transbronchial needle aspiration for molecular testing in lung adenocarcinoma. Ann Thorac Surg. 2013;96(4):1196–202.
24. Coley SM, Crapanzano JP, Saqi A. Optimizing lung carcinoma diagnosis: FNA, core, or both. Mod Pathol. 2012;25(2):475A.
25. Kanagal-Shamanna R, Portier BP, Singh RR, Routbort MJ, Aldape KD, Handal BA, Rahimi H, Reddy NG, Barkoh BA, Mishra BM, Paladugu AV, Manekia JH, Kalhor N, Chowdhuri SR, Staerkel GA, Medeiros LJ, Luthra R, Patel KP. Next-generation sequencing-based multi-gene mutation profiling of solid tumors using fine needle aspiration samples: promises and challenges for routine clinical diagnostics. Mod Pathol. 2014;27:314–27.
26. Dacic S, Nikiforova MN. Present and future molecular testing of lung carcinoma. Adv Anat Pathol. 2014;21:94–9.
27. Khayyata S, Yun S, Pasha T, Jian B, McGrath C, Yu G, Gupta P, Baloch Z. Value of P63 and CK5/6 in distinguishing squamous cell carcinoma from adenocarcinoma in lung fine-needle aspiration specimens. Diagn Cytopathol. 2009;37:178–83.
28. Nicholson AG, Gonzalez D, Shah P, Pynegar MJ, Deshmukh M, Rice A, Popat S. Refining the diagnosis and EGFR status of non-small cell lung carcinoma in biopsy and cytologic material, using a panel of mucin staining, TTF-1, cytokeratin 5/6, and P63, and EGFR mutation analysis. J Thorac Oncol. 2010;5:436–41.
29. Rekhtman N, Ang DC, Sima CS, Travis WD, Moreira AL. Immunohistochemical algorithm for differentiation of lung adenocarcinoma and squamous cell carcinoma based on large series of whole-tissue sections with validation in small specimens. Mod Pathol. 2011;24: 1348–59.
30. Heyman BM, Chung MM, Lark AL, Shofer S. Endobronchial metastasis from primary anorectal melanoma. Am J Case Rep. 2013;14:253–7.
31. Kim JH, Min D, Song SH, Lee JH, Jeong HC, Kim EK. Endobronchial metastases from extrathoracic malignancies: recent 10 years' experience in a single university hospital. Tuberc Respir Dis (Seoul). 2013;74:169–76.
32. Mazziotta R, Borczuk AC, Powell CA, Mansukhani M. CDX2 immunnostaining as a gastrointestinal marker: expression in lung carcinomas is a potential pitfall. Appl Immunohistochem Mol Morphol. 2005;13(1):55–60.
33. Chen X, Mansukhani M, Borczuk AC, Singh B, He H, Hamele-Bena D. Diagnostic value of KRAS mutation in evaluation of synchronous or metachronous pancreatic and lung adenocarcinomas. J Am Soc Cytopathol. 2013;2(1 Suppl):S23.
34. Goldstein NS, Thomas M. Mucinous and nonmucinous bronchioloalveolar adenocarcinomas have distinct staining patterns with thyroid transcription factor and cytokeratin 20 antibodies. Am J Clin Pathol. 2001;116:319–25.
35. Montezuma D, Azevedo R, Lopes P, Vieira R, Cunha AL, Henrique R. A panel of four immunohistochemical markers (CK7, CK20, TTF-1, and p63) allows accurate diagnosis of primary and metastatic lung carcinoma on biopsy specimens. Virchows Arch. 2013;463:749–54.
36. Ye J, Hameed O, Findeis-Hosey JJ, Fan L, Li F, McMahon LA, Yang Q, Wang HL, Xu H. Diagnostic utility of PAX8, TTF-1 and napsin A for discriminating metastatic carcinoma from primary adenocarcinoma of the lung. Biotech Histochem. 2012;87:30–4.
37. Ordóñez NG. Value of PAX8, PAX2, napsin A, carbonic anhydrase IX, and claudin-4 immunostaining in distinguishing pleural epithelioid mesothelioma from metastatic renal cell carcinoma. Mod Pathol. 2013;26:1132–43.
38. Wang NP, Zee S, Zarbo RJ, Bacchi CE, Gown AM. Coordinate expression of cytokeratins 7 and 20 defines unique subsets of carcinomas. Appl Immunohistochem. 1995;3(2):99–107.

39. Kawaguchi KR, Lu FI, Kaplan R, Liu YF, Chadwick P, Chen Z, Brogi E, Shin SJ. In search of the ideal immunopanel to distinguish metastatic mammary carcinoma from primary lung carcinoma: a tissue microarray study of 207 cases. Appl Immunohistochem Mol Morphol. 2014;22(4):266–74.
40. Sica G, Wagner PL, Altorki N, Port J, Lee PC, Vazquez MF, Saqi A. Immunohistochemical expression of estrogen and progesterone receptors in primary pulmonary neuroendocrine tumors. Arch Pathol Lab Med. 2008;132(12):1889–95.
41. Siami K, McCluggage WG, Ordonez NG, et al. Thyroid transcription factor-1 expression in endometrial and endocervical adenocarcinomas. AJSP. 2007;31(11):1759–63.
42. Fujiwara S, Nawa A, Nakanishi T, et al. Thyroid transcription factor 1 expression in ovarian carcinomas is an independent prognostic factor. Human Pathol. 2010;41(4):560–5.
43. Lindeman NI, Cagle PT, Beasley MB, Chitale DA, Dacic S, et al. Molecular testing guideline for selection of lung cancer patients for EGFR and ALK tyrosine kinase inhibitors: guideline from the College of American Pathologists, International Association for the Study of Lung Cancer, and Association for Molecular Pathology. J Thorac Oncol. 2013;8(7):823–59.
44. Kawahara A, Akiba J, Abe H, Yamaguchi T, Taira T, Azuma K, Kage M. EML4-ALK-positive lung adenocarcinoma with signet-ring cells. Diagn Cytopathol. 2014;42(5):460–3.
45. Nishino M, Klepeis VE, Yeap BY, Bergethon K, Morales-Oyarvide V, Dias-Santagata D, Yagi Y, Mark EJ, Iafrate AJ, Mino-Kenudson M. Histologic and cytomorphologic features of ALK-rearranged lung adenocarcinomas. Mod Pathol. 2012;25:1462–72.
46. Rüschoff J, Hanna W, Bilous M, Hofmann M, Osamura RY, Penault-Llorca F, van de Vijver M. Viale G.HER2 testing in gastric cancer: a practical approach. Mod Pathol. 2012;25: 637–50.
47. Vazquez MF, Koizumi JH, Henschke CI, Yankelevitz DF. Reliability of cytologic diagnosis of early lung cancer. Cancer. 2007;111(4):252–8.
48. Silverman JF, Geisinger KR. Lung. Fine needle aspiration cytology of the thorax and abdomen. New York, NY: Churchill Livingstone Inc; 1996. p. 21–7.
49. Crapanzano JP, Loukeris K, Borczuk AC, Saqi A. Cytological, histological, and immunohistochemical findings of pulmonary carcinomas with basaloid features. Diagn Cytopathol. 2011;39(2):92–100.
50. Bishop JA, Teruya-Feldstein J, Westra WH, Pelosi G, Travis WD, Rekhtman N. p40 (ΔNp63) is superior to p63 for the diagnosis of pulmonary squamous cell carcinoma. Mod Pathol. 2012;25:405–15.
51. Collins BT, Wang JF, Bernadt CT. Utilization of p40 (ΔNp63) with p63 and cytokeratin 5/6 immunohistochemistry in non-small cell lung carcinoma fine-needle aspiration biopsy. Acta Cytol. 2013;57:619–24.
52. Faquin WC. Human papillomavirus (HPV) assays for testing fine-needle aspiration specimens in patients with head and neck squamous cell carcinoma. Cancer Cytopathol. 2014;122:92–5.
53. Yanagawa N, Wang A, Kohler D, da Cunha SG, Sykes J, Xu J, Pintilie M, Tsao MS. Human papilloma virus genome is rare in North American non-small cell lung carcinoma patients. Lung Cancer. 2013;79:215–20.
54. Flieder DB, Koss MN, Nicholson A, Sesterhenn IA, Petras RE, Travis WD. Solitary pulmonary papillomas in adults: a clinicopathologic and in situ hybridization study of 14 cases combined with 27 cases in the literature. Am J Surg Pathol. 1998;22:1328–42.
55. Singhi AD, Westra WH. Comparison of human papillomavirus in situ hybridization and p16 immunohistochemistry in the detection of human papillomavirus-associated head and neck cancer based on a prospective clinical experience. Cancer. 2010;116:2166–73.
56. Zengel P, Assmann G, Mollenhauer M, Jung A, Sotlar K, Kirchner T, Ihrler S. Cancer of unknown primary originating from oropharyngeal carcinomas are strongly correlated to HPV positivity. Virchows Arch. 2012;461(3):283–90.
57. Brambilla E, Travis WD. Adenosquamous carcinoma. In: Pathology and genetics tumours of the lung, pleura, thymus, and heart. Lyon, France: IARC Press, 2004.
58. Chaft JE, Rekhtman N, Ladanyi M, Riely GJ. ALK-rearranged lung cancer: adenosquamous lung cancer masquerading as pure squamous carcinoma. J Thorac Oncol. 2012;7(4):768–9.

59. Liao RG, Jung J, Tchaicha J, Wilkerson MD, Sivachenko A, Beauchamp EM, Liu Q, Pugh TJ, Pedamallu CS, Hayes DN, Gray NS, Getz G, Wong KK, Haddad RI, Meyerson M, Hammerman PS. Inhibitor-sensitive FGFR2 and FGFR3 mutations in lung squamous cell carcinoma. Cancer Res. 2013;73:5195–205.
60. Brandler TC, Aziz MS, Rosen LM, Bhuiya TA, Yaskiv O. Usefulness of GATA3 and p40 immunostains in the diagnosis of metastatic urothelial carcinoma in cytology specimens. Cancer Cytopathol. 2014;122(6):468–73.
61. Chang A, Amin A, Gabrielson E, Illei P, Roden RB, Sharma R, Epstein JI. Utility of GATA3 immunohistochemistry in differentiating urothelial carcinoma from prostate adenocarcinoma and squamous cell carcinomas of the uterine cervix, anus, and lung. Am J Surg Pathol. 2012;36:1472–6.
62. Molina JR, Aubry MC, Lewis JE, Wampfler JA, Williams BA, Midthun DE, Yang P, Cassivi SD. Primary salivary gland-type lung cancer: spectrum of clinical presentation, histopathologic and prognostic factors. Cancer. 2007;110:2253–9.
63. Monaco SE, Khalbuss WE, Ustinova E, Liang A, Cai G. The cytomorphologic spectrum of salivary gland type tumors in the lung and mediastinum: a report of 16 patients. Diagn Cytopathol. 2012;40:1062–70.
64. Seethala RR, Dacic S, Cieply K, Kelly LM, Nikiforova MN. A reappraisal of the MECT1/MAML2 translocation in salivary mucoepidermoid carcinomas. Am J Surg Pathol. 2010;34:1106–21.
65. Mitani Y, Rao PH, Futreal PA, Roberts DB, Stephens PJ, Zhao YJ, Zhang L, Mitani M, Weber RS, Lippman SM, Caulin C, El-Naggar AK. Novel chromosomal rearrangements and break points at the t(6;9) in salivary adenoid cystic carcinoma: association with MYB-NFIB chimeric fusion, MYB expression, and clinical outcome. Clin Cancer Res. 2011;17:7003–14.
66. Antonescu CR, Katabi N, Zhang L, Sung YS, Seethala RR, Jordan RC, Perez-Ordoñez B, Have C, Asa SL, Leong IT, Bradley G, Klieb H, Weinreb I. EWSR1-ATF1 fusion is a novel and consistent finding in hyalinizing clear-cell carcinoma of salivary gland. Genes Chromosomes Cancer. 2011;50:559–70.
67. Connor A, Perez-Ordoñez B, Shago M, Skálová A, Weinreb I. Mammary analog secretory carcinoma of salivary gland origin with the ETV6 gene rearrangement by FISH: expanded morphologic and immunohistochemical spectrum of a recently described entity. Am J Surg Pathol. 2012;36:27–34.
68. Cornolti G, Ungari M, Morassi ML, Facchetti F, Rossi E, Lombardi D, Nicolai P. Amplification and overexpression of HER2/neu gene and HER2/neu protein in salivary duct carcinoma of the parotid gland. Arch Otolaryngol Head Neck Surg. 2007;133:1031–6.
69. Solar AA, Schmidt BL, Jordan RC. Hyalinizing clear cell carcinoma: case series and comprehensive review of the literature. Cancer. 2009;115:75–83.
70. Saqi A, McGrath CM, Skovronsky D, Yu G. Cytomorphologic features of fine-needle aspiration of metastatic and recurrent melanoma. Diagn Cytopathol. 2002;27(5):286–90.
71. Riddle ND, Bui MM. When melanoma is negative for S100: diagnostic pitfalls. Arch Pathol Lab Med. 2012;136:237–9.
72. Chapman PB, Hauschild A, Robert C, Haanen JB, Ascierto P, Larkin J, Dummer R, Garbe C, Testori A, Maio M, Hogg D, Lorigan P, Lebbe C, Jouary T, Schadendorf D, Ribas A, O'Day SJ, Sosman JA, Kirkwood JM, Eggermont AM, Dreno B, Nolop K, Li J, Nelson B, Hou J, Lee RJ, Flaherty KT, McArthur GA. BRIM-3 Study Group. Improved survival with vemurafenib in melanoma with BRAF V600E mutation. N Engl J Med. 2011;364:2507–16.
73. Rahman AU, Salajegheh A, Smith RA, Lam AK. BRAF inhibitor therapy for melanoma, thyroid and colorectal cancers: development of resistance and future prospects. Curr Cancer Drug Targets. 2014;14:128–143.
74. Travis WD. Sarcomatoid neoplasms of the lung and pleura. Arch Pathol Lab Med. 2010;134:1645–58.
75. Rossi G, Cavazza A, Sturm N, Migaldi M, Facciolong N, et al. Pulmonary carcinomas with pleomorphic, sarcomatoid, or sarcomatous elements. Am J Surg Pathol. 2003;27(3):311–24.

76. Simone SB, Aubry MC, Yi ES, Boland JM. Immunohistochemical study of 36 pulmonary sarcomatoid carcinomas—sensitivity of TTF-1 is superior to napsin. Human Pathol. 2014;45(2):294–302.
77. Nuovo GJ, Schmittgen TD. Benign metastasizing leiomyoma of the lung: clinicopathologic, immunohistochemical, and micro-rna analyses. Diagn Mol Pathol. 2008;17(3):145–50.
78. Choi IH, Song DH, Han KM, Choi YS, Han J. Incidence of pulmonary non-epithelial tumors: 18 years' experience at a single institute. Pathol Res Pract. 2014;210:210–6.
79. Bégueret H, Galateau-Salle F, Guillou L, Chetaille B, Brambilla E, Vignaud JM, Terrier P, Groussard O, Coindre JM. Primary intrathoracic synovial sarcoma: a clinicopathologic study of 40t(X;18)-positive cases from the French Sarcoma Group and the Mesopath Group. Am J Surg Pathol. 2005;29:339–46.
80. Walia R, Jain D, Mathur SR, Iyer V. Spindle cell melanoma: a comparison of the cytomorphological features with the epithelioid variant. Acta Cytol. 2013;57(6):557–61.
81. Ko HM, Geddie WR, Boerner SL, Rogalla P, da Cunha SG. Cytomorphological and clinicopathological spectrum of pulmonary marginal zone lymphoma: the utility of immunophenotyping. PCR and FISH studies. Cytopathology. 2014;25(4):250–8.

# Chapter 10
# Mimickers of Lung Carcinoma in Cytology and Small Biopsy Specimens

**Elena Lucas and Sunati Sahoo**

A false-positive diagnosis of malignancy of 1 % has been reported in respiratory cytology even when the specimens were interpreted by highly experienced cytopathologists [1]. Discussed below are some of the common nonneoplastic and benign and low grade neoplastic lesions of the lung that mimic lung carcinoma in cytologic preparations and in small tissue biopsy.

## Nonneoplastic Lesions

### *Mimickers of Adenocarcinoma*

*Reactive type II pneumocytes* (*RPII*) are an important diagnostic pitfall of adenocarcinoma. In the normal lung, type II pneumocytes are small and account for only 5 % of alveolar lining cells. These cells undergo hyperplasia and reactive changes in response to injury resulting from conditions such as adult respiratory distress syndrome (ARDS), pulmonary infarction, embolism, infections, abscesses, organizing pneumonia, oxygen therapy, pulmonary drug toxicity, interstitial lung diseases with pulmonary fibrosis, alveolar hemorrhage, pulmonary Langerhans cell histiocytosis, radiation therapy, and chemotherapy, among others [2–9].

In *exfoliative cytology* specimens, RPII may be distributed singly or in clusters and show worrisome features that include large nuclei, macronucleoli, nuclear membrane irregularity, hyperchromasia, and coarse chromatin (Fig. 10.1). Although the nucleus

E. Lucas, M.D.
Department of Pathology, University of Texas Southwestern Medical Center, Dallas, TX, USA

S. Sahoo, M.D. (✉)
Department of Pathology, University of Texas Southwestern Medical Center, 5323 Harry Hines Blvd., Dallas, TX 75390, USA
e-mail: sunati.sahoo@utsouthwestern.edu



A.L. Moreira, A. Saqi (eds.), *Diagnosing Non-small Cell Carcinoma in Small Biopsy and Cytology*, DOI 10.1007/978-1-4939-1607-8_10

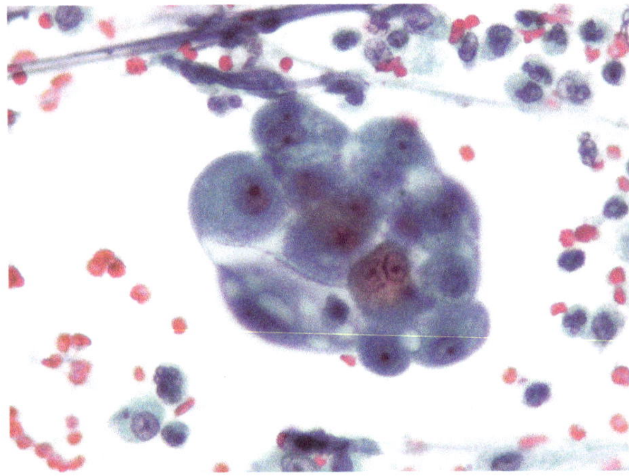

**Fig. 10.1** Reactive type II pneumocytes in a bronchoalveolar lavage specimen. Markedly enlarged nuclei, prominent nucleoli, and abundant vacuolated cytoplasm (cytospin, Papanicolaou stain)

to cytoplasm (N/C) ratio is usually low, it can be increased in some cases. The cytoplasm quality varies and can be delicately granular to dense squamoid or hypervacuolated. In some instances, if taken in isolation and out of the clinical context, the striking cytologic atypia can mimic adenocarcinoma to perfection [2–6, 8–13].

Morphologic features that favor RPII over malignant cells include lower cellularity, fewer single cells, smaller clusters without a great depth of focus, less uniformity among cell groups, tendency for a lower N/C ratio, scalloped borders, and intercellular windows in at least some cell clusters [3, 4, 6, 14] (Fig. 10.2a–f). In reactive conditions, careful examination usually reveals a spectrum of changes, whereas two distinct populations of normal and clearly malignant cells, are typically identified in adenocarcinomas. Unfortunately, no special immunohistochemical or cytochemical marker exists to reliably distinguish between these two conditions [15].

In *small tissue biopsy*, RPII usually do not pose the same diagnostic difficulty due to preservation of the architecture. However, prominent proliferation of type II pneumocytes can occasionally resemble in situ or invasive adenocarcinoma. Reactive hyperplasia in an area of atelectasis leading to a misdiagnosis of solid variant of adenocarcinoma has been reported [16]. Hyperplastic pneumocytes are cuboidal to columnar with large nuclei, vesicular chromatin, and prominent nucleoli, often protruding into the alveolar spaces in a hobnail fashion. Mitotic figures may be observed. The background parenchyma showing inflammation, diffuse alveolar damage, necrosis, organizing pneumonia, granulomas, fibrosis, or fibromyxoid changes often provides a clue to an underlying injurious process, but it can also be mistaken for a desmoplastic reaction (Fig. 10.3a–d).

The most important step in avoiding a misdiagnosis is to correlate the morphologic findings with clinical information and imaging studies. For example, in a setting of acute lung injury, a rapid clinical course and an absence of a mass lesion are strong indicators that the cytologic atypia may be of reactive nature. In such instances, it is appropriate to recommend a follow-up biopsy upon recovery to resolve the diagnostic dilemma.

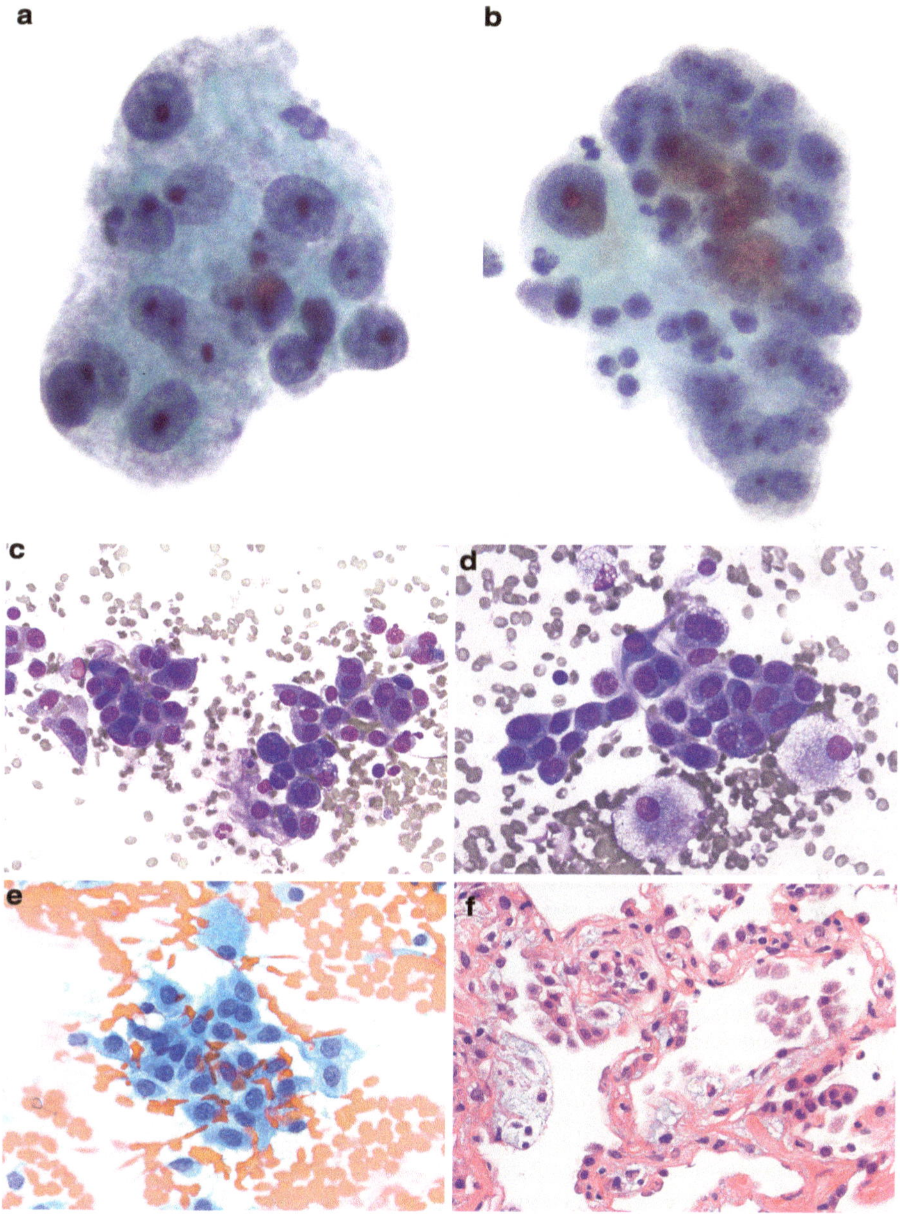

**Fig. 10.2** (**a, b**) Reactive type II pneumocytes in a liquid-based preparation. Clusters of cells with enlarged nuclei and macronucleoli arranged in three-dimensional clusters in a patient with acute respiratory failure (**a**, **b**) (ThinPrep, Papanicolaou stain). (**c**, **d**, **e**, and **f**) Reactive type II pneumocytes on FNA (**c**, **d**, and **e**) with corresponding biopsy (**f**). The pneumocytes on the FNA show flat sheets of loosely cohesive cells, vacuolated cytoplasm, and occasional intercellular windows. The core biopsy shows similar cells clinging to the alveolar walls (**f**) (Diff-Quik stain, Papanicolaou stain, H&E stain) (Photographs **c–f** courtesy of Dr. Anjali Saqi)

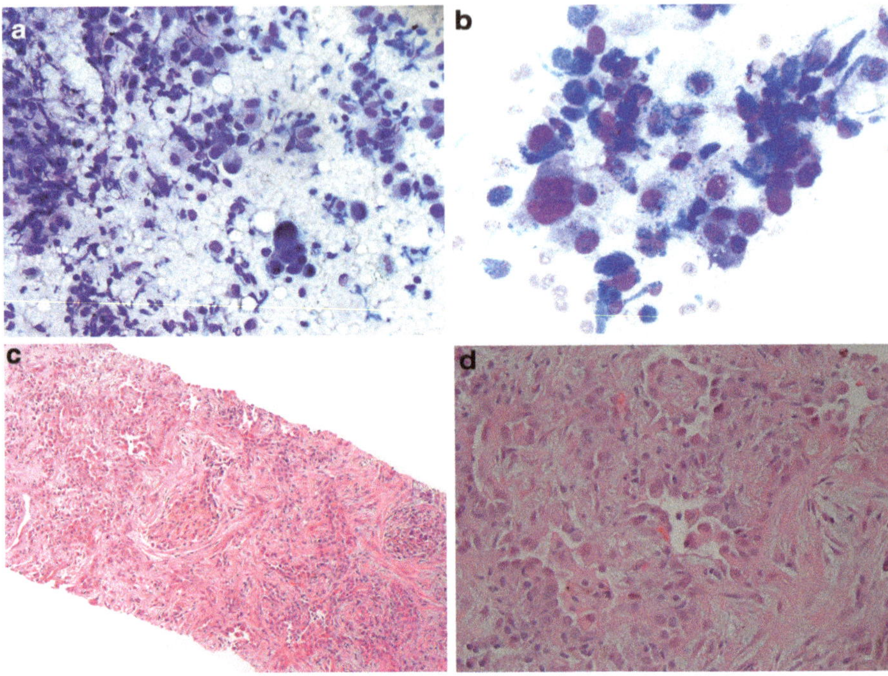


**Fig. 10.3** Organizing pneumonia. (**a**, **b**) Touch imprints of a CT-guided core biopsy showing enlarged, markedly atypical type II pneumocytes in an inflammatory background, originally interpreted as adenocarcinoma (Diff-Quik stain). (**c**, **d**) Core biopsy with reactive type II pneumocytes surrounded by fibromyxoid stroma (H&E stain)

*Reactive bronchial cells* are relatively common and occur as a response to a host of inflammatory and environmental stimuli, including infections, diffuse alveolar damage, pulmonary infarct, asthma, chronic obstructive airway disease, bronchiectasis, smoking, environmental toxins, chemotherapy, radiation treatment, and instrumentation [8]. Reactive atypia of bronchial cells can cause diagnostic difficulty. Their nuclei are enlarged, can be up to 6 times the size of a normal bronchial cell nucleus (Fig. 10.4a) and may contain prominent, sometimes irregular nucleoli [5, 17, 20]. Mitotic activity may be noted. The nuclear polarity is preserved, the nuclear contours are usually smooth, and the chromatin is fine. Often in this setting, there is a spectrum of changes ranging from small unremarkable to markedly reactive cells, without distinctive benign and malignant cell populations. Although mild nuclear contour irregularity and moderately course chromatin can be seen on occasion (Fig. 10.4b), very coarse and irregularly distributed chromatin with condensation underneath the nuclear membrane is distinctly uncommon and should raise a strong suspicion of malignancy.

Multinucleation is relatively common but the individual nuclei are identical to those of background single cells. The cells can be arranged in clusters and flat sheets or in a streaming pattern (Fig. 10.5a). Unlike carcinomas, dyscohesion and single

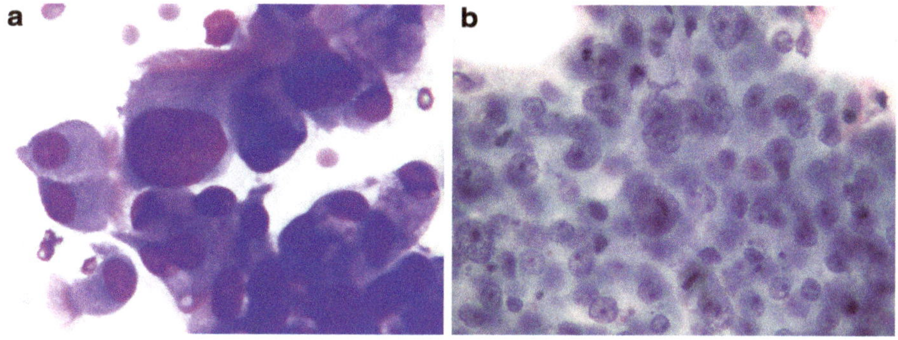


**Fig. 10.4** Reactive bronchial epithelial cells in a bronchial brushing specimen. (**a**) Nuclear enlargement can be up to six times the size of normal nucleus (smear, Diff-Quik stain). (**b**) Morphologic continuum of reactive changes including marked variation in size, macronucleoli, mild nuclear contour irregularity, and moderately course chromatin (smear, Papanicolaou stain)

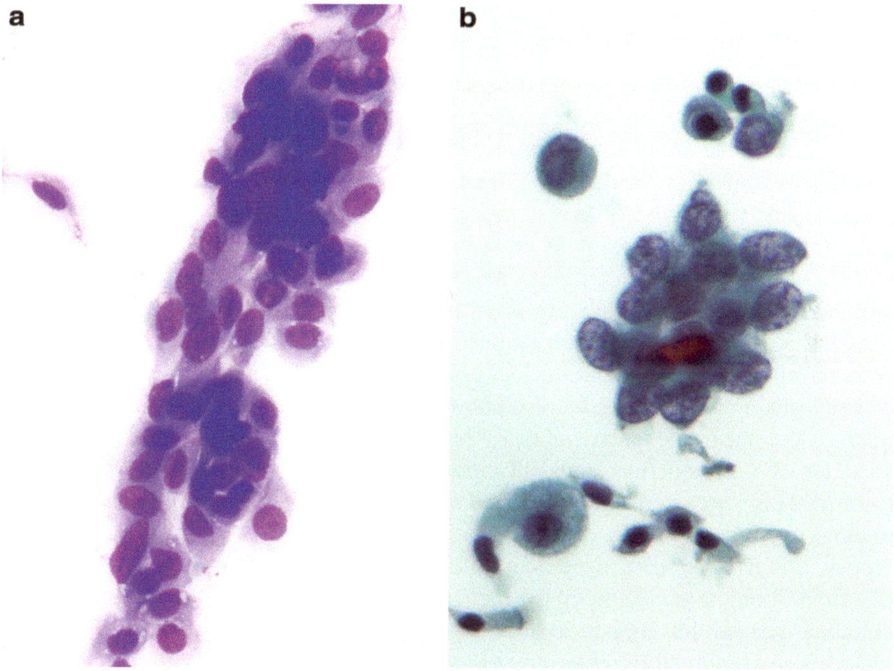


**Fig. 10.5** Reactive bronchial epithelial cells in a bronchial brushing and FNA. (**a**) The cells can be arranged in a streaming pattern (smear, Diff-Quik stain). (**b**) Nuclear enlargement, increased N/C ratio, and course chromatin. Focal retention of cilia or terminal bars helps with a benign diagnosis (ThinPrep, Papanicolaou stain)

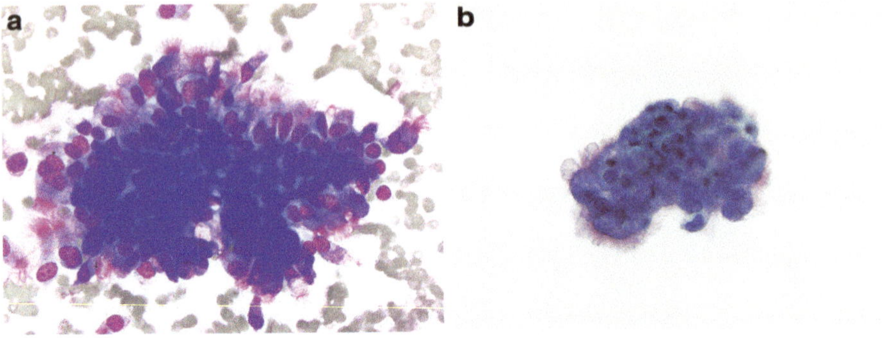

**Fig. 10.6** Creola body on FNA and in a liquid-based preparation. Three-dimensional cluster of bronchial epithelial cells. Smooth nuclear contours, light chromatin, cilia, and terminal bars (**a, b**) (Diff-Quik, ThinPrep, Papanicolaou stain) (Photographs courtesy of Dr. Anjali Saqi)

cells are uncommon. Reactive cells often retain cilia and terminal bars that aid with a benign diagnosis. In the absence of visible cilia or partial loss of cytoplasm, a benign diagnosis can be established by comparing the nuclear shape and chromatin quality of cells in question with other clusters containing benign ciliated cells (Fig. 10.5b) or identifying terminal bars (Fig. 10.5c).

*Bronchial cell hyperplasia* in exfoliative respiratory specimens can appear as tight papillary or spherical clusters called "Creola bodies." These clusters are encountered mostly in asthmatic patients; however, they have been described in other chronic respiratory diseases, viral infections, and instrumentation [20]. These cell clusters can be large, and the cells may show crowding and even nuclear molding. In inflammatory conditions, atypical nuclear features may be observed. Although the individual cells are often difficult to visualize due to multilayering, focusing at the periphery or sometimes in the center of the cluster usually reveals cilia, terminal bars, and bland nuclear features (Fig. 10.6).

*Peribronchiolar metaplasia*, also known as lambertosis, results from the replacement of the normal alveolar lining by bronchiolar epithelium that is connected to small airways through the canals of Lambert. This phenomenon occurs as a response to various unrecognized and recognized stimuli including smoking, chronic inflammation, obstructive airway disease, and interstitial lung disease. In surgical tissue biopsy, it is usually recognized as such due to the preservation of the architecture, retention of columnar shape by the metaplastic cells or a spectrum of cuboidal and columnar shapes. Rarely peribronchiolar metaplasia in a small biopsy may resemble atypical adenomatous hyperplasia or well-differentiated adenocarcinoma in situ. However, the retained architecture, the identification of cilia or terminal bars in some of the cells and the lack of nuclear atypia to the degree seen in adenocarcinoma help establish a benign diagnosis [21] (Fig. 10.7).

*Goblet cell hyperplasia* is another reactive change that can mimic primary or metastatic mucinous adenocarcinoma. In a quiescent bronchial lining, the ratio of goblet cells to ciliated cells is approximately 1:5 [22]. In chronic obstructive airway

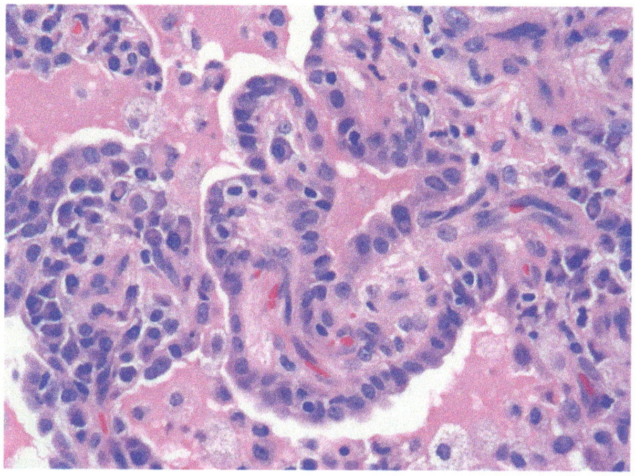

**Fig. 10.7** Peribronchiolar metaplasia (lambertosis) (H&E stain)

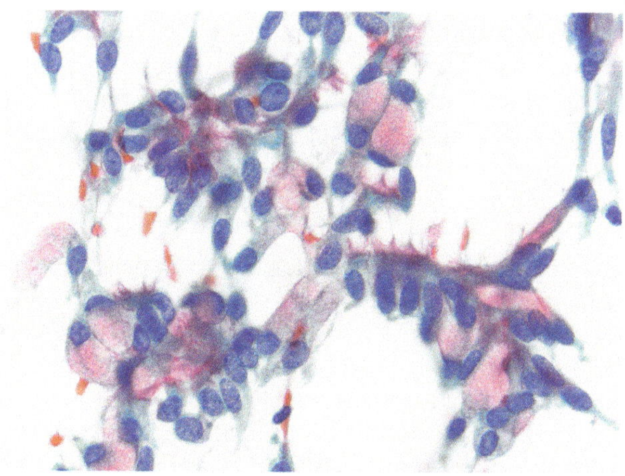

**Fig. 10.8** Goblet cell hyperplasia in a bronchial brushing. Small nuclei, smooth nuclear contours, featureless chromatin, and preserved nucleocytoplasmic polarity distinguish goblet cells from mucinous adenocarcinoma. Close association with ciliated columnar cells facilitates the diagnosis of benignity (smear, Papanicolaou stain) (Photograph courtesy of Dr. Anjali Saqi)

disease and asthma, goblet cells undergo proliferation as a compensatory response to airway obstruction. In exfoliative cytology specimens, goblet cells are increased in number and distributed singly, in sheets or small clusters. The features that distinguish benign goblet cell hyperplasia from a malignant process are: a clean background, cell uniformity, small basally located nuclei, smooth nuclear contours, and featureless chromatin (Fig. 10.8). Occasionally ciliated cells can be found amidst goblet cells, and their presence greatly facilitates the diagnosis of benignity. In a difficult case, clinical information may provide a clue. However, goblet cell hyperplasia in a patient with chronic airway disease presenting with a mass lesion may pose a diagnostic challenge requiring a tissue biopsy.

## *Mimickers of Squamous Cell Carcinoma*

*Reactive squamous changes and atypical squamous metaplasia* of respiratory epithelium occur in response to a wide variety of irritants. Some of the common inciting factors include cigarette smoking, chronic inflammation, inhalants, pulmonary infarction, diffuse alveolar damage, cavitary infections, radiation therapy, chemotherapy, instrumentation, and tracheostomy [5, 22–25].

Exaggerated reparative or degenerative changes in metaplastic squamous cells may raise a suspicion for squamous dysplasia or invasive carcinoma (Fig. 10.9a–e). Additionally, high-grade squamous dysplasia arising in metaplastic squamous mucosa may be indistinguishable from invasive carcinoma in superficial biopsy or cytologic preparations. Atypical metaplastic squamous cells can show enlarged hyperchromatic nuclei and nuclear pleomorphism. The cytoplasm can be brightly eosinophilic or orangeophilic. Usually these cells are scant in number and show poor nuclear detail due to smudgy or degenerative chromatin (Fig. 10.9a,b). In some cases, a distinction between squamous metaplasia, dysplasia, and invasive squamous carcinoma may not be possible. In the absence of unequivocally malignant cells, great care should be taken not to label these as squamous cell carcinoma.

*Prolonged tracheostomy or intubation* leading to atypical squamous metaplasia may extend to the mucosa distant from the stoma site and be seen years or even decades following laryngectomy or tracheostomy. Presence of atypical and degenerated squamous cells with dense, highly keratinized cytoplasm with nuclear karyorrhexis and karyolysis can potentially mimic squamous cell carcinoma. Clinical history and the absence of well-preserved cells with unequivocal features of malignancy are helpful in reaching an accurate interpretation [2, 19, 26].

*Cavitary infections* due to fungi or mycobacteria can be associated with markedly atypical squamous cells. In cytologic preparations, these cells can be single or arranged in clusters demonstrating worrisome features described above [2, 19]. In contrast to squamous cell carcinoma, the chromatin tends to be smudgy, the cytoplasm is more eosinophilic than orangeophilic, and atypical cells are few in number [11] (Fig. 10.9d). Correlation with the clinical findings, presence of inflammatory background, or identification of microorganisms (e.g., fungal hyphae) is helpful in establishing a benign diagnosis. On the contrary, truly dysplastic or malignant cells should not be overlooked or dismissed since squamous cell carcinoma often undergoes cavitation and can be associated with necrosis and inflammation. Furthermore, squamous cell carcinoma can sometimes arise in infectious cavities, or, alternatively, a cavitary tumor can be secondarily colonized by fungus [27–29].

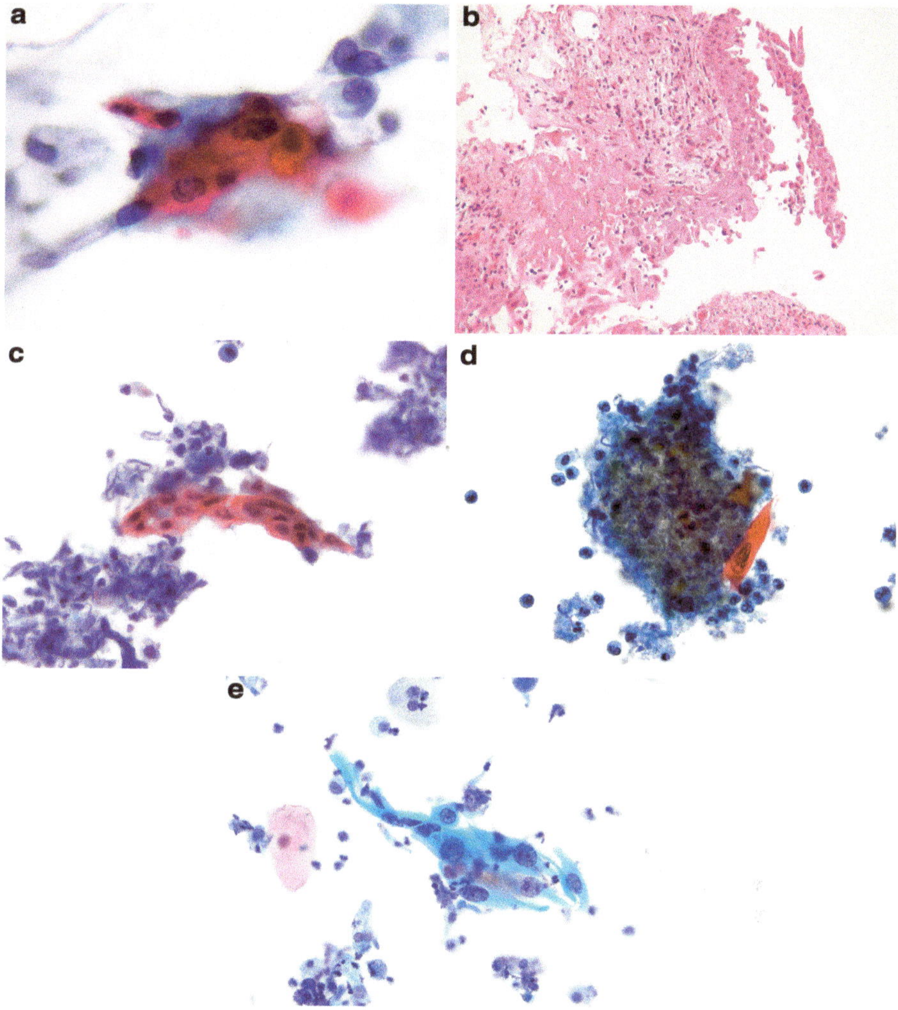


**Fig. 10.9** Atypical squamous metaplasia. (**a**) Squamous metaplastic cells associated with an airway injury show enlarged hyperchromatic nuclei, nuclear pleomorphism, and orangeophilic cytoplasm. Usually these cells are scant (smear, Papanicolaou stain). (**b**) Reactive atypical squamous metaplasia of bronchial mucosa adjacent to an ulcer may be difficult to differentiate from dysplasia (H&E stain). (**c**) Atypical squamous cells associated with inflammation. (**d**) Atypical squamous cells in a case of Aspergillus (organisms not shown). (**e**) Atypical squamous cells in a streaming pattern; Candida infection (not shown) present [Photographs courtesy of Dr. John Crapanzano (**c**) and Dr. Anjali Saqi (**d**, **e**)]

*Diffuse alveolar damage* (*DAD*), a histologic manifestation of ARDS, can rarely induce extensive squamous metaplasia of the alveolar lining cells. These metaplastic cells may display significant cytologic atypia, leading to a misdiagnosis of carcinoma in cytologic or small biopsy specimens even by experienced pathologists [25].

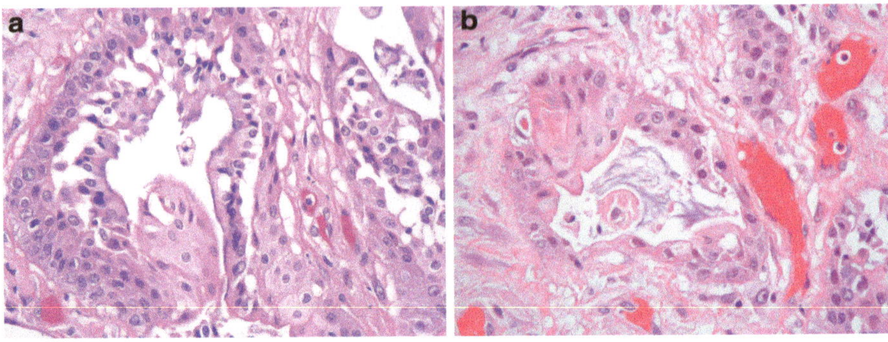

**Fig. 10.10** Atypical squamous metaplasia in diffuse alveolar damage. (**a**) In this case the normal alveolar lining underwent both bronchial and squamous metaplasia (H&E stain). (**b**) Higher magnification shows reactive changes in metaplastic squamous cells (H&E stain)

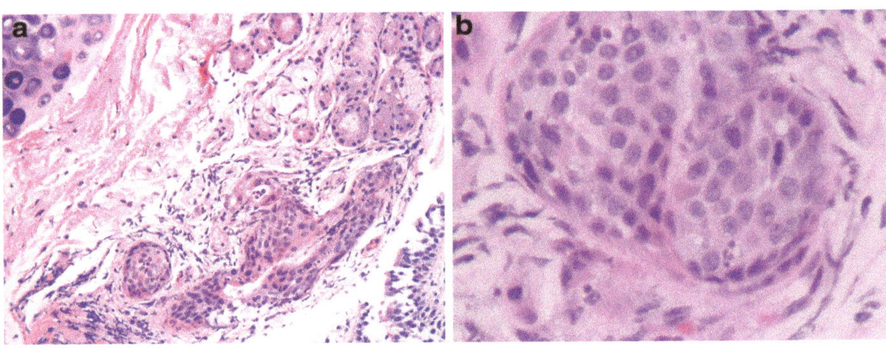

**Fig. 10.11** Necrotizing sialometaplasia. (**a**) Squamous nests usually retain lobular architecture (H&E stain). (**b**) Under higher magnification, metaplastic squamous cells have benign nuclear features without evidence of dysplasia (H&E stain)

Clinical history of acute lung injury and histologic features of DAD, if present, should prompt a pathologist to be extremely cautious in diagnosing malignancy [25] (Fig. 10.10a, b).

*Necrotizing sialometaplasia*, a reactive process that occurs as a response to bronchial injury, appears as nests of squamous epithelium replacing bronchial submucosal salivary-type glands. These nests usually retain lobular architecture, occasionally taking irregular shapes with a pseudoinfiltrative appearance and resembling well-differentiated squamous cell carcinoma. However, under higher magnification, metaplastic squamous nests display benign morphologic features (Fig. 10.11a, b). In endobronchial biopsy material, necrotizing sialometaplasia can be confused with carcinoma only if taken out of clinical context since no mass lesion is usually present.

## *Miscellaneous Conditions Mimicking Adenocarcinoma or Squamous Cell Carcinoma*

Some benign lesions and contaminants can rarely be misdiagnosed as adenocarcinoma or squamous cell carcinoma.

*Therapy-related changes* secondary to radiation, chemotherapy, and, less commonly, other therapeutic agents are a potential source of diagnostic pitfalls. Pronounced reactive changes can be seen in different types of respiratory epithelium, stromal cells, and pulmonary macrophages after chemotherapy or radiation therapy. These changes can rarely be mistaken for either adenocarcinoma or squamous cell carcinoma [1, 5, 17–19, 31]. The appearance or disappearance of reactive changes in relation to the timing of therapy varies. Changes associated with chemotherapy may be noted as early as a few weeks after the initiation of therapy and be resolved by a month after the discontinuation of treatment [17, 31]. Some radiation-induced changes may persist throughout life [20] and may be seen outside of radiation field [32]. Occasionally radiation changes may result in pulmonary consolidation, a potential confounding factor in the diagnosis.

The common cytomorphologic changes of chemotherapy and acute radiation injury (i.e., within 6 months of treatment) in bronchial cells include large nuclei, macronucleoli, and irregular distribution of chromatin. These atypical cells are seen singly or within a group of more normal-appearing cells (Fig. 10.12a,b). On occasion cilia and terminal bars are lost after chemotherapy, further hindering the diagnosis [32]. Similar atypia are evident in pneumocytes and macrophages. In fine-needle aspiration (FNA) specimens, cohesive flat sheets of cells with a "streaming" appearance resembling reparative changes can be seen. The cells are large and often polygonal with dense cytoplasm and occasionally have perinuclear clearing or vacuoles. The nuclei are hyperchromatic with macronucleoli and wrinkled nuclear contours. Multinucleation is common. Despite the nuclear enlargement, the N/C ratio is usually low, although it may be increased [5, 17, 19, 20, 31].

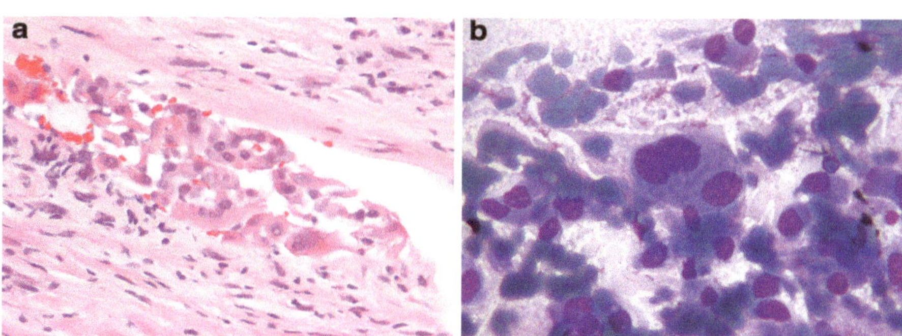


**Fig. 10.12** Glandular cells after radiation. (**a**) Bronchial epithelial cells with nuclear enlargement, cytomegaly, and occasional multinucleation (H&E stain). (**b**) Radiation atypia in bronchial brushing following radiation therapy for lung carcinoma (smear, Diff-Quik stain)

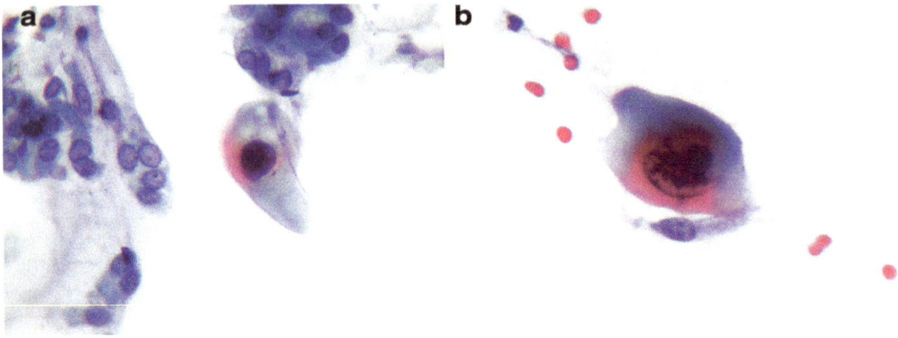


**Fig. 10.13** Metaplastic squamous cells post acute radiation. (**a**) Cells with nuclear enlargement, hyperchromasia, two-tone cytoplasm, and low N/C ratio. (**b**) Nuclear contour and chromatin irregularity can be seen in radiation changes (smear, Papanicolaou stain)

Changes in metaplastic squamous cells from chemotherapy or acute radiation injury result in nuclear enlargement, hyperchromasia, amphophilic or two-tone cytoplasm, nuclear contour irregularity, and, occasionally, perinuclear clearing or vacuolization (Fig. 10.13a, b). The N/C ratio can be low or high, but smudgy chromatin with poor nuclear detail is typical. Bizarre cells and mitoses, including atypical forms, can be seen. In chronic radiation changes, the findings are nonspecific: the cytoplasm may be brightly eosinophilic, cellular shapes distorted, and nuclei pyknotic. In summary, awareness of the above morphologic changes as well as clinical presentation and a history of treatment will help in avoiding a misdiagnosis of malignancy.

*Pulmonary infarct* deserves a special mention since it can closely mimic malignancy not only clinically but also on cytology. A radiologic finding of a wedge-shaped, pleural-based infiltrate and symptoms of hemoptysis, chest pain, cough, dyspnea, and fever are typical of pulmonary infarct. However, it can present without typical symptoms or with a radiologic impression of a neoplasm with occasional cavitation. In these situations, the presence of markedly atypical cells in an exfoliative or FNA cytology specimen is fraught with a danger of misdiagnosis, particularly in individuals with a history of smoking [8, 10, 13, 30]. Reactive cells derived from bronchial or alveolar epithelium can closely resemble adenocarcinoma [10, 20, 30].

Occasionally single keratinized metaplastic squamous cells with hyperchromatic degenerative and smudgy nuclei can be seen along with reactive bronchial cells simulating squamous cell carcinoma [5, 10]. If pulmonary infarct is suspected clinically but the cytology is suspicious for malignancy, careful review of the slides may reveal subtle features that favor benign diagnosis. In difficult cases, a repeat sample should be obtained in several weeks.

*Viral infections* (e.g., Herpes simplex, Cytomegalovirus) of the respiratory tract can cause nuclear enlargement and hyperchromasia. In exfoliative specimens, infected cells are usually distributed singly but sometimes can form clusters which under low magnification may mimic malignancy. Careful examination under higher

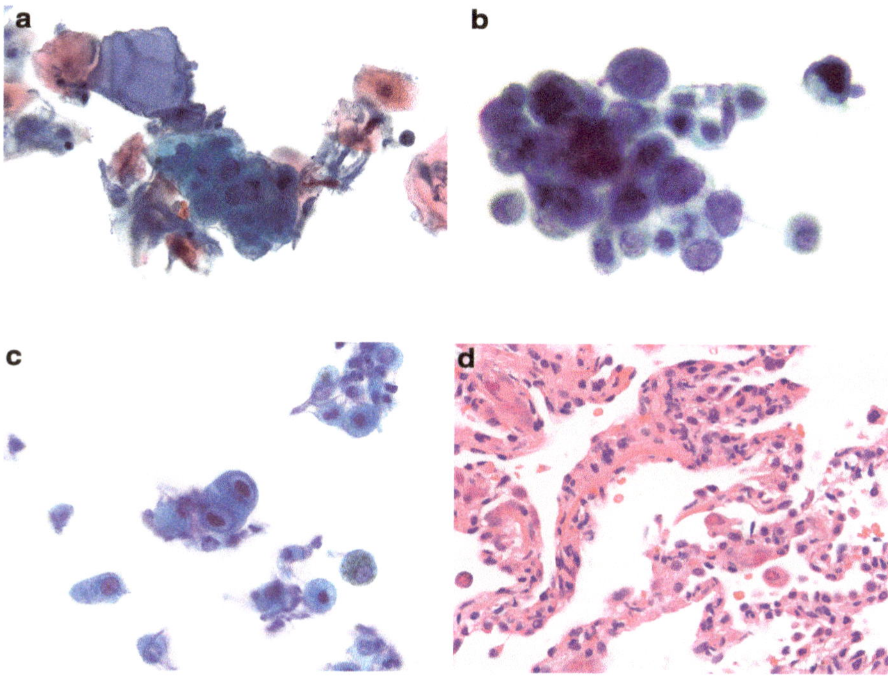

**Fig. 10.14** Bronchoalveolar lavage of a case with HSV infection (**a**, **b**). A cell cluster with large hyperchromatic nuclei on close examination reveals intranuclear viral inclusions with ground-glass appearance and margination of chromatin (ThinPrep and cytospin, Papanicolaou stain). CMV in bronchoalveolar lavage and core biopsy (**c**, **d**). Inclusions of the CMV-infected cells potentially mimic a malignancy (Papanicolaou stain, H&E stain) [Photographs (**c**, **d**) courtesy of Dr. Anjali Saqi]

magnification usually allows identification of viral inclusions and cytopathic effect in some of the cells (Fig. 10.14). Ancillary studies can be used to confirm the diagnosis in questionable cases.

*Mesothelial cells* from pleura are incidentally sampled during transthoracic or a deep transbronchial biopsy [33, 34]. Reactive mesothelial cells can have large nuclei and prominent nucleoli. When arranged in flat sheets, they can be confused with squamous cell carcinoma or a focus of lepidic pattern from a well-differentiated adenocarcinoma. Uniform honeycomb arrangements, intercellular windows, and the absence of keratinization favor a mesothelial origin (Fig. 10.15). Occasionally mesothelial cells can be vacuolated and distributed as single cells, small groups, or, in cases of mesothelial hyperplasia, papillary clusters closely resembling adenocarcinoma. In doubtful cases, immunohistochemical stains can confirm the mesothelial origin. Calretinin, WT-1, HBME-1, and D2-40 are positive in mesothelial cells and usually negative in adenocarcinoma, while MOC-31, Ber-EP4, B72.3 (BRST-3), and CEA are positive in adenocarcinoma and usually negative in mesothelial cells. Cytokeratin 5/6, although positive in mesothelial cells, is of little help

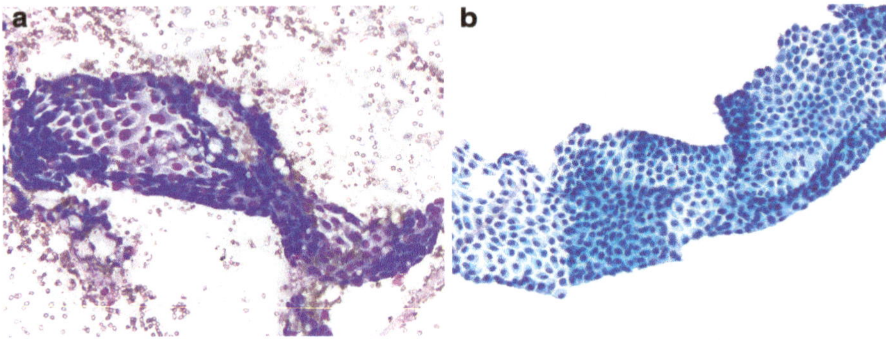


**Fig. 10.15** (**a**, **b**) Mesothelial cells with squamoid appearance from FNA. Uniform honeycomb arrangement and intercellular windows are seen (smears, Diff-Quik stain, Papanicolaou stain) (Photographs courtesy of Dr. Anjali Saqi)

in differentiating them from squamous cell carcinoma since squamous cells are also positive for this marker. None of the immunohistochemical markers are entirely sensitive or specific; therefore, it is prudent to use a combination of two markers from each group.

*Hepatocytes* can be sampled inadvertently during FNA and core biopsy targeting the right lower lobe of the lung. In such instances, benign hepatocytes potentially can be misinterpreted as cells of adenocarcinoma. A heightened awareness of this sampling helps to avoid such diagnostic error [30].

*Granulomas* can mimic epithelioid neoplasms, both adenocarcinoma and squamous cell carcinoma [35], as well as spindle cell neoplasms. In fact, granulomatous inflammation is one of the most common lesions that result in false-positive diagnosis. This error occurs largely due to the presence of cohesive three-dimensional clusters. The presence of epithelioid and spindle-shaped histiocytes and the lack of single neoplastic cells in the background are clues to the diagnosis (Fig. 10.16).

## *Mimickers of Neuroendocrine Carcinoma*

*Reserve cell hyperplasia* occurs in response to various noxious stimuli including inflammation and inhaled irritants. Hyperplastic reserve cells may appear in bronchial washing and brushing specimens as tight crowded clusters of small cells with a rim of dense basophilic cytoplasm, high N/C ratio, hyperchromatic nuclei, and occasional nuclear molding. The distinction is usually straightforward, since reserve cells have the nuclear size of small lymphocytes and are smaller than the cells of small cell carcinoma. Their chromatin is dark and featureless unlike granular, neuroendocrine-type chromatin of small cell carcinoma. Mitotic figures, apoptotic bodies, and necrosis are absent. The cell clusters are cohesive with tight appearance and, in contrast to small cell carcinoma, with no cell dissociation.

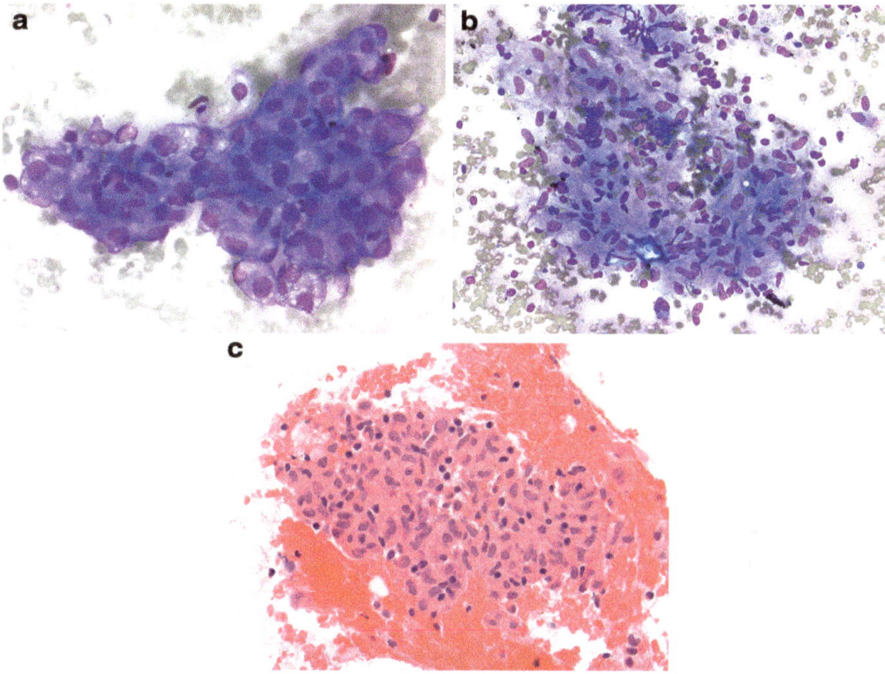


**Fig. 10.16** FNAs of granulomas with epithelioid and spindle-shaped cells (**a**, **b**, **c**). Granulomas form cohesive clusters with epithelioid cells (**a**) and/or spindle-shaped cells (**b**, **c**). The presence of boomerang- and spindle-shaped cells is a clue to the diagnosis (**a**, **b**, **c**) (Diff-Quik stain, H&E stain) (Photographs courtesy of Dr. Anjali Saqi)

Although there may be nuclear molding, the crush artifact or chromatin streaks characteristic of small cell carcinoma are not present (Fig. 10.17a, b).

In surgical biopsy material, the hyperplastic reserve cells are located underneath the normal bronchial cell lining without an invasive growth pattern and are easily recognized as benign, although at times due to tangential sectioning, they may pose diagnostic difficulty (Fig. 10.17c).

*Lymphocytes* in small tissue specimens, particularly when crushed, can be mistaken for small cell carcinoma. The distinction must be made on cells that are better preserved. Lymphocytes are smaller, with darker staining clumped chromatin. In contrast, cells of small cell carcinoma are larger than lymphocytes and have finely granular to smooth neuroendocrine-type chromatin. In doubtful cases, immunostains (CD45 for lymphocytes versus cytokeratin, synaptophysin, chromogranin, and CD56 for small cell carcinoma) will provide a diagnostic solution.

*Naked nuclei of degenerating bronchial cells* with stripped cytoplasm can be confused with small cell carcinoma or low-grade neuroendocrine carcinoma (carcinoid). These nuclei can be seen in the sputum of patients with asthma, chronic bronchitis, or other benign conditions [5]. The differentiating features are fine chromatin without "salt and pepper" granularity of neuroendocrine-type chromatin, the

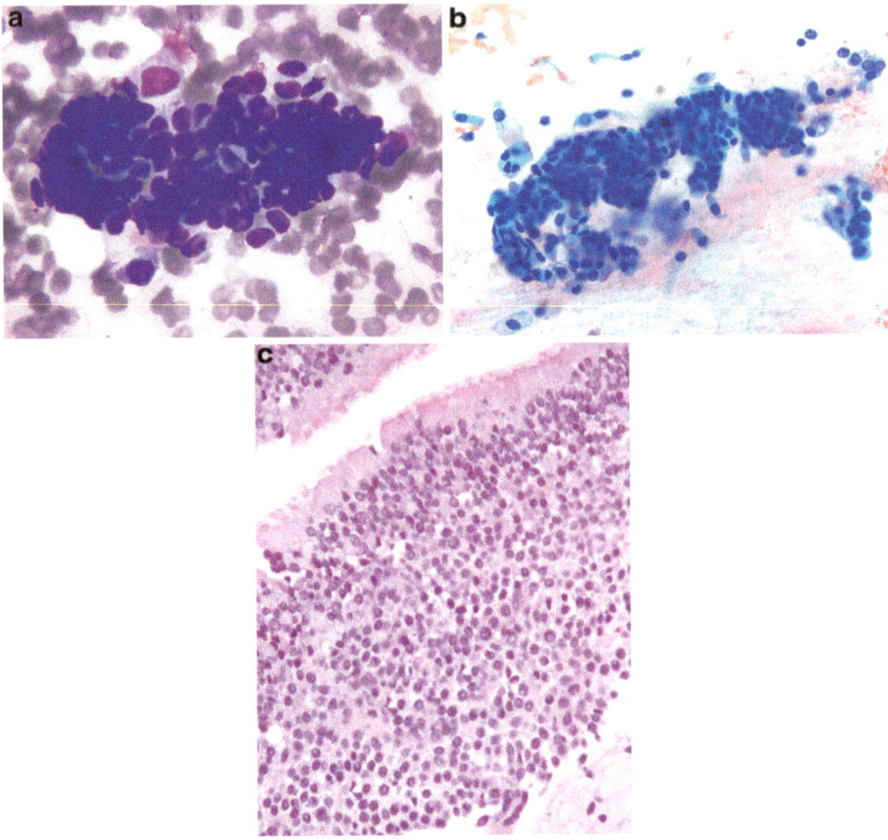


**Fig. 10.17** Reserve cell hyperplasia (**a**, **b**). Tight clusters of small uniform cells with hyperchromatic nuclei and a thin rim of basophilic cytoplasm. Some areas appear to have nuclear molding; however, no crush artifact or necrosis is seen (smears, Diff-Quik and Papanicolaou stain). (**c**) Reserve cell hyperplasia with overlying ciliated epithelial cells (H&E stain) [Photograph (**b**) courtesy of Dr. Anjali Saqi]

absence of molding or necrosis, and the similarity of the naked nuclei to those of better-preserved benign bronchial cells. A diagnosis of malignancy should not be made on degenerated cells or naked nuclei regardless of the level of atypia.

## Tumorlike Lesions and Low-Grade Neoplasms

### *Meningothelial-Like Nodules*

Meningothelial-like nodules usually are incidental findings in resection specimens. Rarely they can be found in a lung biopsy performed for nonneoplastic conditions (e.g., in a transbronchial biopsy of a transplant recipient). These lesions consist of

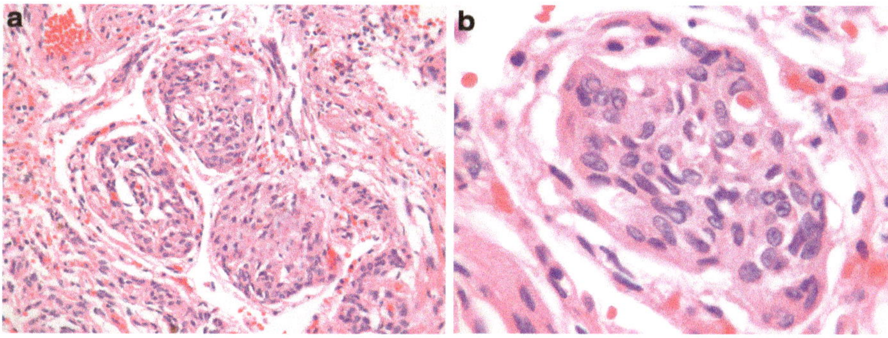


**Fig. 10.18** Meningothelial-like nodules. (**a**) Whorled nests of cells with bland nuclei and eosinophilic cytoplasm. (**b**) Some cells show nuclear grooves and intranuclear inclusions (H&E stain)

whorls or nests of elongated medium-sized cells with eosinophilic cytoplasm and oval nuclei with fine chromatin. Architecturally the whorls or nests may resemble squamous cells or neuroendocrine carcinoma. On close inspection, the absence of keratinization, poorly defined cytoplasmic borders, bland ovoid nuclei with inconspicuous nucleoli, occasional nuclear grooves, and intranuclear inclusions provide clues to a correct diagnosis. By immunohistochemistry, these cells are positive for vimentin, EMA, CD56, and progesterone receptor but negative for keratin, S100, or neuroendocrine markers [20, 36, 37] (Fig. 10.18a, b).

## *Pulmonary Hamartoma*

The question whether pulmonary hamartomas are malformations arising from embryonic rests or true neoplasms is unresolved. Despite the discovery of chromosomal aberrations in some of these lesions [38, 39], they are still considered to be tumorlike malformations by many.

Pulmonary hamartoma is characterized by an overgrowth of mesenchymal tissue including cartilage, smooth muscle, and fat, intermixed with epithelial cells arranged mostly in tubular structures. The epithelial cells, which are typically cuboidal or low columnar, are not an inherent component of this lesion, but rather represent entrapment of small airways by expanded mesenchymal tissue.

In surgical biopsy material, biphasic sarcomatoid carcinoma with heterologous elements or primary intrapulmonary chondrosarcoma may enter the differential diagnosis. In FNA specimens, occasionally emphasis on epithelial cells showing reactive features or intranuclear inclusions, while underrecognizing the subtleness of the mesenchymal component, can lead to a false-positive diagnosis of low-grade neuroendocrine carcinoma (carcinoid), adenocarcinoma, or even small cell carcinoma [40, 41] (Fig. 10.19).

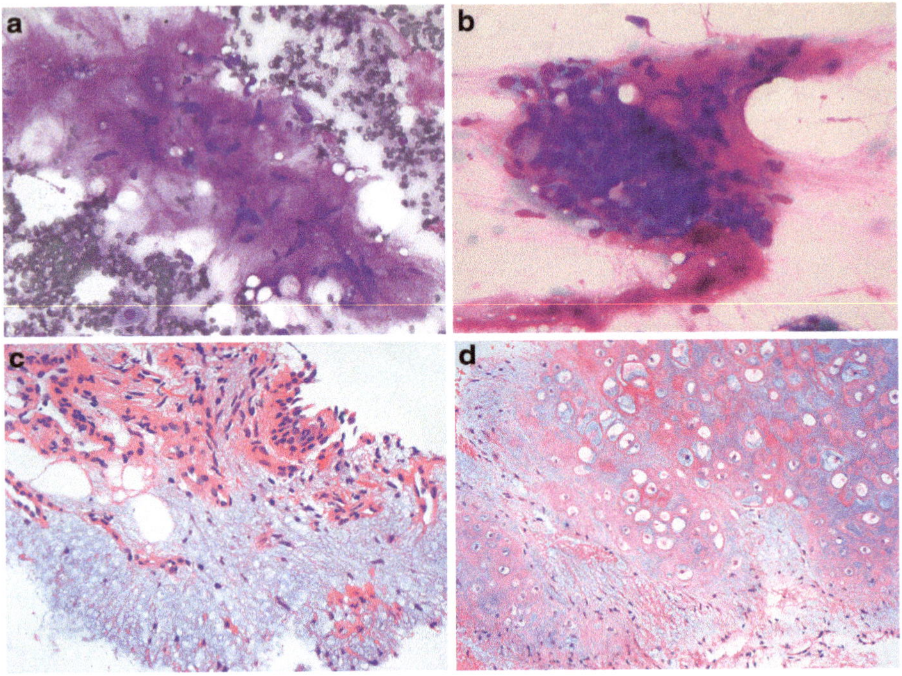


**Fig. 10.19** Pulmonary hamartoma. (**a**) FNA of hamartoma showing fibromyxoid stroma with spindle-shaped cells (Diff-Quik stain). (**b**) Touch imprint of the core biopsy showing fibromyxoid stroma with entrapped benign epithelial cells (Diff-Quik stain). (**c, d**) Cartilage and fibromyxoid stroma are intimately attached. No atypical or malignant cellular features are present (H&E stain) [Photographs (**a, c, d**) courtesy of Dr. Anjali Saqi]

## *Clear Cell (Sugar) Tumor of the Lung*

Clear cell tumor of the lung, also known as "sugar tumor," is a rare pulmonary neoplasm that belongs to the perivascular epithelioid cell tumor (PEComa) family and potentially can be confused with a clear cell variant of lung adenocarcinoma or metastatic carcinomas. The tumor cells demonstrate both smooth muscle and premelanocytic differentiation evidenced by immunohistochemical staining pattern and ultrastructural studies [42]. Large polygonal, elongated, or spindle cells with abundant clear to lightly eosinophilic cytoplasm grow around small sinusoidal-type blood vessels that can rarely be sclerotic [43]. The neoplastic cell nuclei are round to oval and have fine chromatin, small to inconspicuous nucleoli, and occasional single to multiple intranuclear inclusions. Typically they lack significant cytologic atypia, high mitotic activity or necrosis (Fig. 10.20a, b). In cytologic smears, the cells are distributed in cohesive clusters (Fig. 10.20c); however, the cytoplasm is

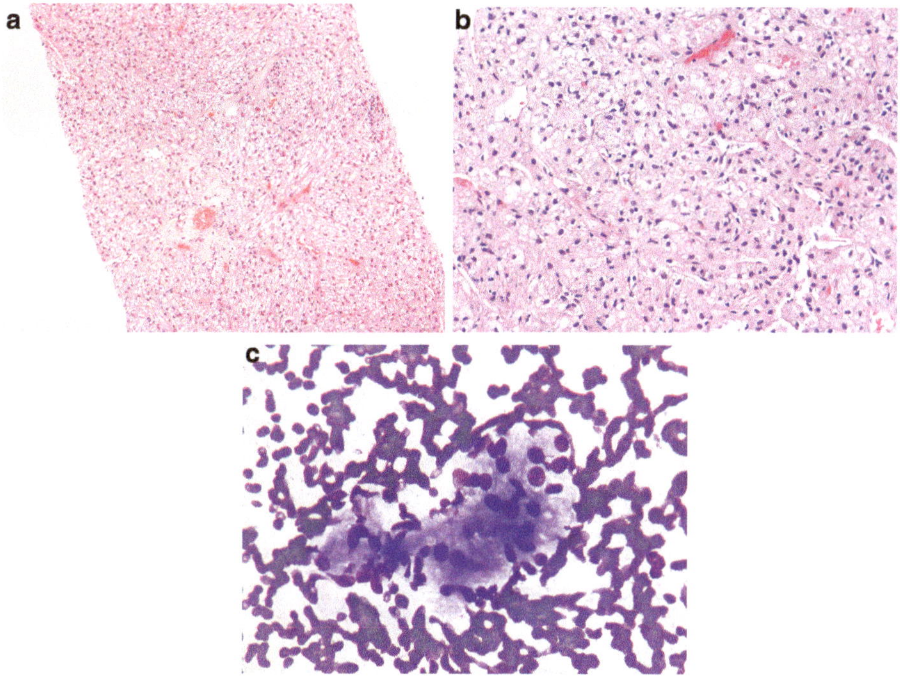


**Fig. 10.20** Clear cell (sugar) tumor of the lung. (**a**, **b**) Core biopsy shows large polygonal cells with abundant cytoplasm growing around small sinusoidal-type blood vessels (H&E stain). (**c**) Touch imprint of the core biopsy shows cohesive groups of cells with abundant foamy cytoplasm that is easily stripped (Diff-Quik stain)

easily stripped, leaving naked nuclei and a foamy or granular background [44, 45]. Like PEComas of other sites, these tumors are negative for keratin but are positive for vimentin and melanocytic markers such as HMB-45, MART1/Melan-A, and microphthalmia transcription factor-1 [42]. Reactivity for smooth muscle and muscle-specific actin is inconsistent. The tumor cytoplasm contains glycogen that is highlighted by PAS positivity that disappears following diastase digestion.

## *Granular Cell Tumor*

Primary granular cell tumors of the lung are rare. Usually these lesions are endobronchial but may arise peripherally [46]. The cells are large, with ill-defined borders, small- to medium-sized nuclei, and abundant eosinophilic to amphophilic cytoplasm filled with granules that are ultrastructurally proven to be lysosomes.

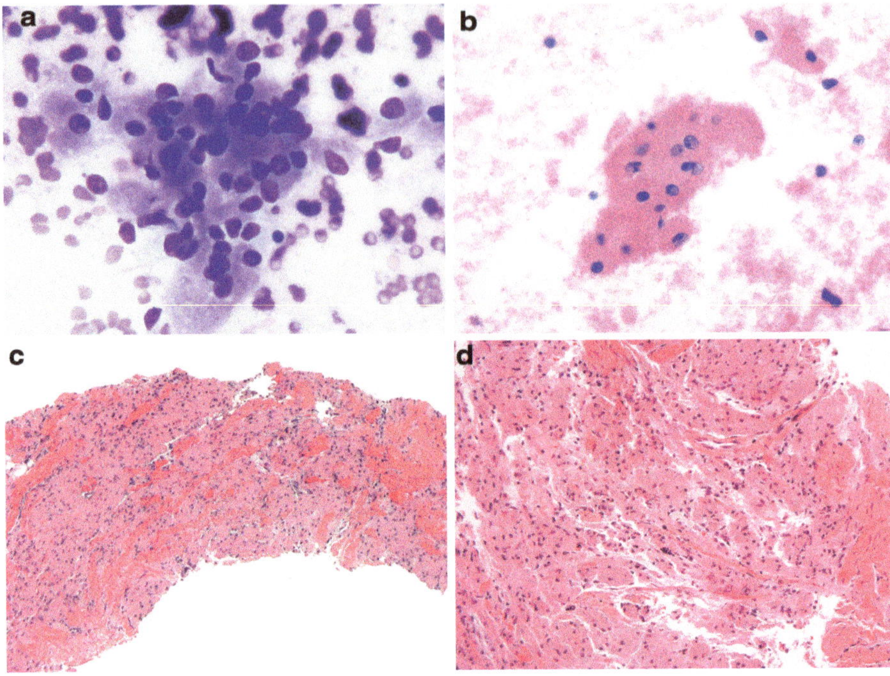


**Fig. 10.21** Granular cell tumor. (**a**) FNA shows loosely cohesive clusters and single cells with abundant granular cytoplasm that is easily stripped and degranulated, giving the background a granular appearance (smear, Diff-Quik stain). (**b**) Clusters of cells with abundant granular cytoplasm and low-grade nuclei (cell block, H&E stain). (**c, d**) Similar cells with low N/C are evident on the core biopsy (H&E stain) [Photographs (**c, d**) courtesy of Dr. Andre Moreira]

The nuclear features are bland, the chromatin is fine, and the nucleoli are small to inconspicuous. In biopsy specimens, these tumors grow as single cells and irregular nests. In cytologic smears, they appear as thick syncytial clusters or sheets [47]. The cells often lose their cytoplasm due to degranulation, giving the background a vacuolated or granular appearance [20]. Granular cell tumors are of Schwann cell origin and are positive for S-100 as well as CD68. They can be mistaken as oncocytic carcinoid, adenocarcinoma, or acinar cell carcinoma of the bronchial submucosal glands. Characteristic cytoplasmic granularity and bland nuclear features point toward a correct diagnosis that can be confirmed with immunostains [20, 47] (Fig. 10.21).

## *Pneumocytoma (Sclerosing Hemangioma)*

Pneumocytoma, also known as sclerosing hemangioma, is an unusual benign pulmonary neoplasm that arises from the primitive uncommitted respiratory

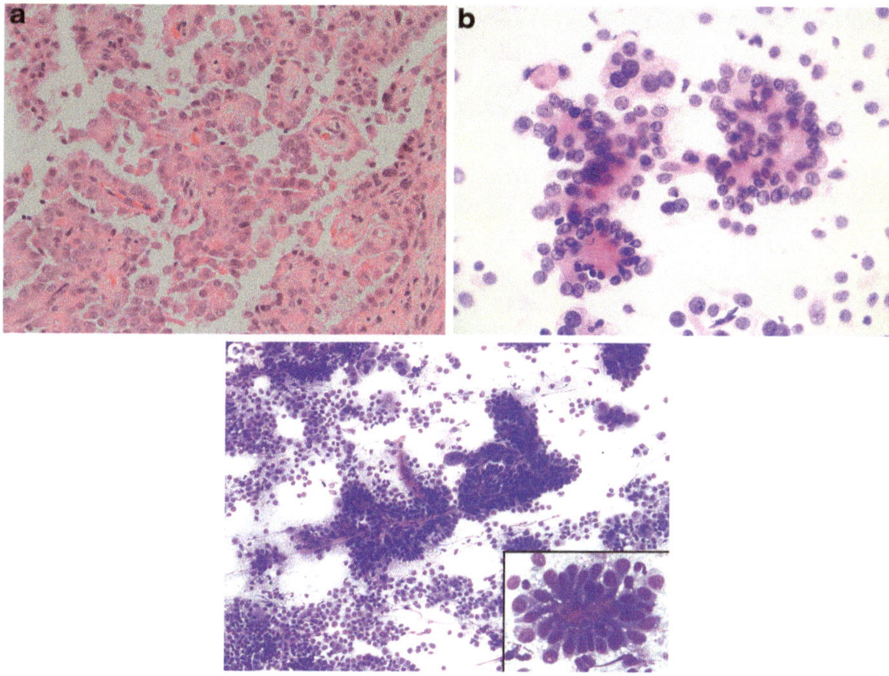


Fig. 10.22 Pneumocytoma (sclerosing hemangioma). (a) Plump cells resembling type II pneumocytes line fibrovascular cores, some of which contain round to polygonal cuboidal cells (H&E stain). (b) Papillary structures composed of cells with bland chromatin and occasional nuclear grooves (cell block, H&E stain). (c) FNA shows markedly cellular smear with papillary clusters. The papilla is composed of bland cells (inset) (smear, Diff-Quik stain) [Photographs courtesy of Dr. Anjali Saqi]

epithelial cells and can very closely resemble well-differentiated adenocarcinoma. These tumors are histologically heterogeneous with four characteristic architectural patterns (papillary, solid, sclerotic, and vascular), two to three of which are often present in a majority of tumors [48]. The cellular component is comprised of two cell types: surface and stromal cells. The surface cells are plump cuboidal, resemble reactive type II pneumocytes and have light eosinophilic or clear cytoplasm and oval nuclei with fine to coarse chromatin and variably prominent nucleoli. Intranuclear pseudoinclusions and multinucleation can be encountered. These cells are positive for cytokeratin, EMA, and TTF-1 by immunohistochemistry. The second cell type is round, polygonal, or spindle stromal cells that feature well-defined borders, oval or round nuclei, fine chromatin, and inconspicuous nucleoli. The nuclei may have smooth contours or show nuclear grooves. These cells are also positive for TTF-1 and EMA but negative or only focally positive for cytokeratin [49]. In the papillary pattern, the cuboidal cells typically line papillae that have cores filled with the second type of cells (Fig. 10.22a). Alternatively, two cell types can intermix in a solid pattern with cuboidal cells surrounding sheets of round/polygonal cells. Foamy or hemosiderin-laden macrophages may be observed in the background. Psammoma bodies and lamellar concretions have been described.

In cytologic smears and cell block preparations, this lesion recapitulates the classic histologic patterns. The cells are typically bland; however, cuboidal surface cells may be indistinguishable from well-differentiated adenocarcinoma [50] (Fig. 10.22b, c). Mild cytologic atypia, prominent nucleoli, and mitotic figures can be seen in both tumors. However, marked atypia, significant pleomorphism, or necrosis is not characteristic of pneumocytoma.

The diagnosis of pneumocytoma on FNA or small biopsy requires recognition of two distinctive cell types that can be confirmed by immunostains [51]. Rarely pneumocytoma can be confused with low-grade neuroendocrine carcinoma (carcinoid); however, pneumocytoma cells lack typical "salt and pepper" chromatin characteristic of neuroendocrine tumors.

## *Solitary Papillomas and Invasive Papillomatosis*

Papillomas are rare endobronchial lesions that in a small biopsy specimen can be confused with lung carcinoma. Solitary squamous papillomas usually occur in elderly smokers, while multiple papillomas tend to occur in children (juvenile papillomatosis) [52]. Depending on the predominant epithelial type, papillomas can be squamous, glandular, or mixed (Fig. 10.23). Squamous papillomas are associated with both low-risk (HPV 6/11) and high-risk (HPV 18) human papillomavirus. They can exhibit exophytic or endophytic growth pattern and the epithelium can be dysplastic. In endophytic or inverted growth pattern, nests of squamous epithelium invaginate and proliferate in the submucosa. When cytologic atypia or dysplasia is present within such a variant, it can closely simulate well-differentiated squamous cell carcinoma. Unlike squamous cell carcinoma, the nests of a papilloma are invested with a basement membrane and lack destructive invasive growth pattern and desmoplastic stromal reaction. Prominent nuclear atypia, pleomorphism, and dyskeratosis typical of squamous cell carcinomas are not seen in squamous papilloma [53].

In *invasive papillomatosis*, squamous papillary proliferations extend into the pulmonary parenchyma and spread between alveolar spaces through the pores of Kohn, leading to the formation of complex endophytic lesions that can simulate invasive squamous carcinoma [52].

Glandular papillomas can be mistaken for well-differentiated adenocarcinoma. The distinguishing features are the endobronchial location and arborizing fibrovascular cores lined by benign columnar or cuboidal glandular epithelium. The epithelium can be pseudostratified but does not show cellular atypia or proliferation unsupported by stromal cores. In contrast to adenocarcinomas, no intraparenchymal growth is present [53].

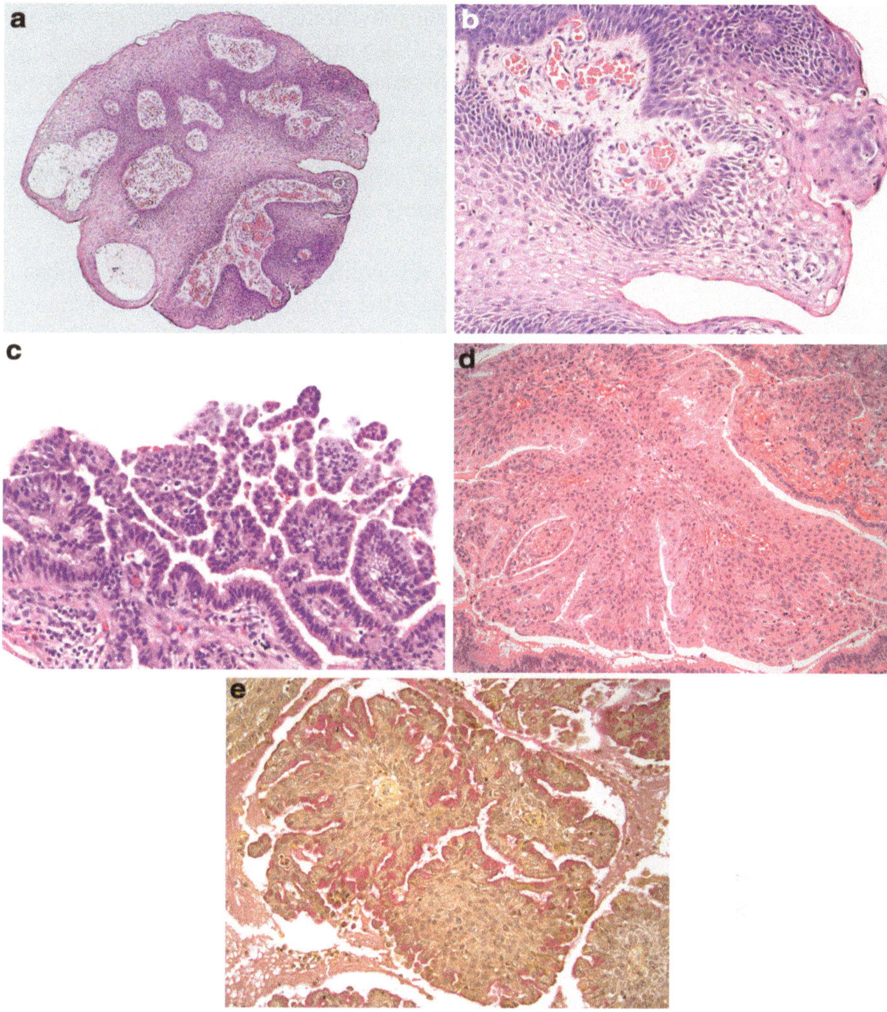


**Fig. 10.23** Papillomas. (**a, b**) Squamous papilloma consisting of a fibrovascular core lined by squamous epithelium. (**c**) Glandular papilloma surfaced by columnar to cuboidal cells. (**d**) Mixed squamous and glandular papilloma with mucicarmine stain (**e**) highlighting the mucin-containing cells (H&E stain) [Photographs courtesy of Dr. William Travis (**a, b**), Dr. Andre Moreira (**c**), and Dr. Anjali Saqi (**d, e**)]

## *Primary Pleuropulmonary Thymoma*

Primary pleuropulmonary thymomas are rare and can present as mass lesions in different parts of the lung and pleura [54]. Although the origin of these tumors is debatable, embryological displacement or development from pluripotent stem cells has been proposed [55]. The rarity, clinical presentation, and wide morphologic spectrum of these lesions pose significant diagnostic difficulty both on cytology and small biopsy. When faced with the diagnosis of a primary pleuropulmonary thymoma, a pathologist must exclude the presence of a mediastinal mass or history of prior thymomas/mediastinal mass. Metastatic thymomas to the pleura are more common than a primary tumor in this location. In addition, thymomas have indolent behavior with metastases appearing many years following the initial diagnosis.

Similar to their thymic counterparts, pleuropulmonary thymomas are biphasic and composed of a mixture of neoplastic epithelial cells and nonneoplastic lymphocytes. The proportion of these two components varies from lesion to lesion: lymphocyte-predominant lesions, lesions containing exclusively epithelial cells, or a mixture of both [56]. Architecturally, these tumors can exhibit different growth patterns including diffuse sheets sometimes separated by fibrous bands, organoid pattern, pseudorosettes, or even gland formation. The tumors demonstrate variable vascularity and may have prominent perivascular spaces with serum lakes. The different schemes used for the classification of these tumors are beyond the scope of this chapter.

The neoplastic epithelial cells can show a wide morphologic variation. They can range from spindle or oval with indistinct cytoplasmic borders, finely dispersed chromatin, and indistinct nucleoli to round or polygonal with well-defined cell borders and enlarged nuclei with smooth to irregular nuclear contours (Fig. 10.24). The nuclei can be hyperchromatic with conspicuous nucleoli. Mitotic activity is variable.

In cytologic preparations, a similar morphologic spectrum is evident including the dual population of cells as seen in biopsy material (i.e., spindle to oval to round epithelial cells with nuclei ranging from bland to atypical). The smears usually contain small cohesive clusters of cells (Fig. 10.24a), but occasionally it may contain large cohesive sheets as well as single cells [57, 58]. The epithelial cells can be mistaken for lung primary or metastatic squamous carcinoma, adenocarcinoma, or neuroendocrine carcinoma. The number of lymphoid cells is variable as is their morphology with small lymphocytes containing dark clumped chromatin to larger lymphoid cells with more immature or reactive-appearing nuclei that potentially can be confused with lymphoblastic lymphoma.

An accurate diagnosis can be reached with awareness of the entity, identification of two cell populations, and appropriate use of immunohistochemistry. While the epithelial cells stain with keratins including high-molecular-weight CK 5/6 and p63 (nuclear staining), the tumor lymphoid component expresses CD1a, CD99, and TdT (terminal deoxynucleotidyl transferase).

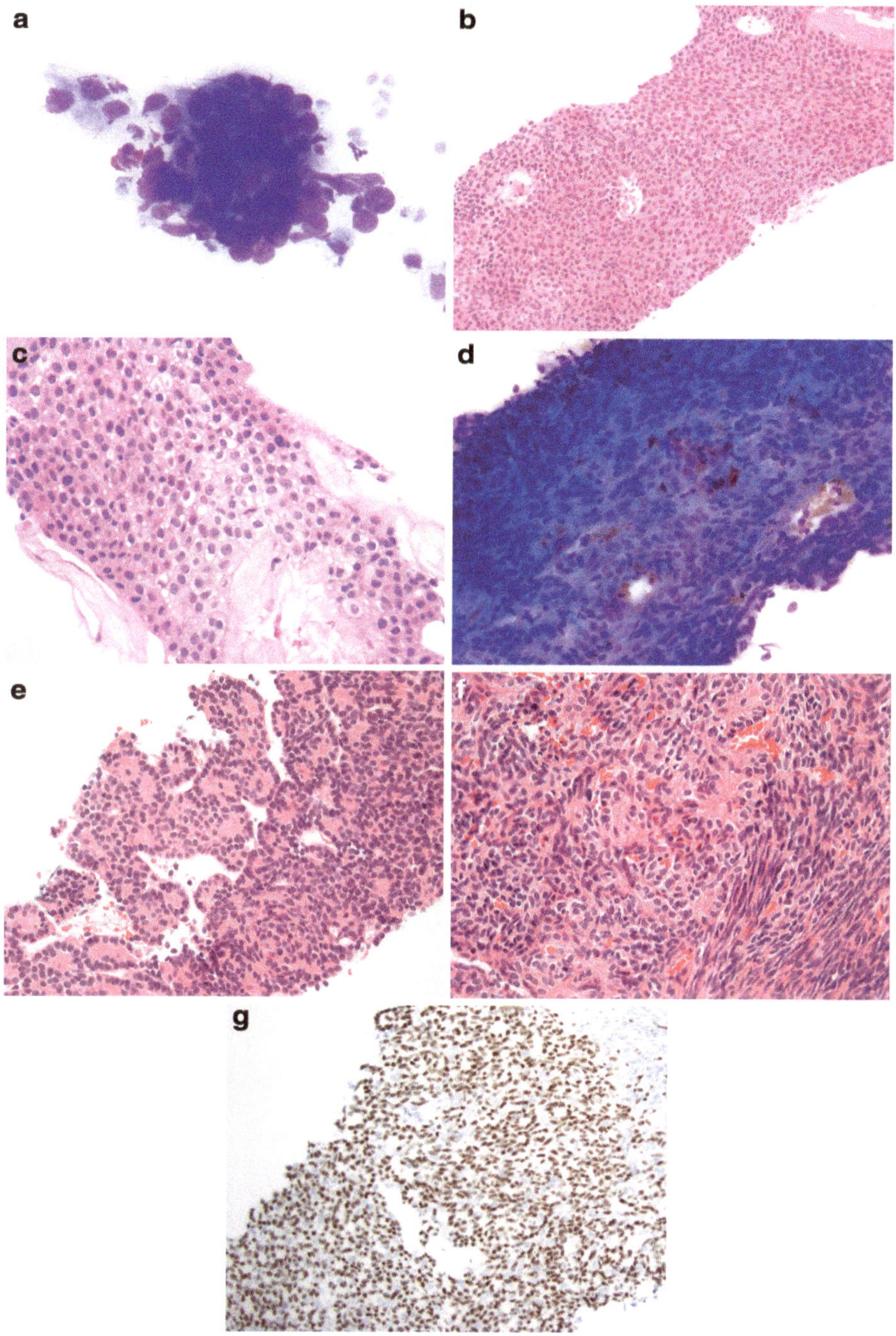

**Fig. 10.24** Type B3 thymoma (**a**–**c**). Touch imprint (**a**) of the core biopsy shows tight clusters of epithelial cells and a few loosely cohesive cells with variably conspicuous nucleoli. No definite lymphocytes are seen (Diff-Quik stain). The core biopsy (**b**, **c**) shows predominantly round epithelial cells with distinct cell borders, round nuclei, and conspicuous nucleoli. Lymphocytes are scant (H&E stain). Type A thymoma (**d**–**g**). Touch imprint (**d**) of a core biopsy showing mostly epithelioid cells and scattered ovoid cells (Diff-Quik). The corresponding core biopsy shows predominantly epithelioid cells in one focus and a combination of epithelioid and spindle-shaped cells in another (**e**, **f**). An immunostain for p63 highlights the epithelial cells [Photographs (**d**–**g**) courtesy of Dr. Anjali Saqi]

## References

1. Thivolet-Bejui F. Cytological pitfalls in bronchopulmonary tumors. Diagn Cytopathol. 1997;17(6):412–6.
2. Saad RS, Silverman JF. Respiratory cytology: differential diagnosis and pitfalls. Diagn Cytopathol. 2010;38(4):297–307.
3. Grotte D, et al. Reactive type II pneumocytes in bronchoalveolar lavage fluid from adult respiratory distress syndrome can be mistaken for cells of adenocarcinoma. Diagn Cytopathol. 1990;6(5):317–22.
4. Stanley MW, et al. Hyperplasia of type II pneumocytes in acute lung injury. Cytologic findings of sequential bronchoalveolar lavage. Am J Clin Pathol. 1992;97(5):669–77.
5. Naryshkin S, Young NA. Respiratory cytology: a review of non-neoplastic mimics of malignancy. Diagn Cytopathol. 1993;9(1):89–97.
6. Zaman SS, et al. Distinction between bronchioloalveolar carcinoma and hyperplastic pulmonary proliferations: a cytologic and morphometric analysis. Diagn Cytopathol. 1997;16(5): 396–401.
7. Selvaggi SM, Gerber M. Pulmonary cytology in patients with the acquired immunodeficiency syndrome (AIDS). Diagn Cytopathol. 1986;2(3):187–93.
8. Lawther RE, et al. Pulmonary infarct cytologically mimicking adenocarcinoma of the lung. Ann Thorac Surg. 2002;73(6):1964–5.
9. Beskow CO, et al. Diffuse alveolar damage. Morphologic features in bronchoalveolar lavage fluid. Acta Cytol. 2000;44(4):640–6.
10. Bewtra C, Dewan N, O'Donahue Jr WJ. Exfoliative sputum cytology in pulmonary embolism. Acta Cytol. 1983;27(5):489–96.
11. Crapanzano JP, Zakowski MF. Diagnostic dilemmas in pulmonary cytology. Cancer. 2001;93(6):364–75.
12. Kaminsky DA, Leiman G. False-positive sputum cytology in a case of pulmonary infarction. Respir Care. 2004;49(2):186–8.
13. Scoggins WG, et al. False-positive cytological diagnosis of lung carcinoma in patients with pulmonary infarcts. Ann Thorac Surg. 1977;24(5):474–80.
14. Saqi A, Coley SM, Crapanzano JP. Granulomatous inflammation and organizing pneumonia: role of computed tomography-guided lung fine needle aspirations, touch preparations and core biopsies in the evaluation of common non-neoplastic diagnoses. CytoJournal. 2014;11:2.
15. Linssen KC, et al. Reactive type II pneumocytes in bronchoalveolar lavage fluid. Acta Cytol. 2004;48(4):497–504.
16. Shilo K, et al. Exuberant type 2 pneumocyte hyperplasia associated with spontaneous pneumothorax: secondary reactive change mimicking adenocarcinoma. Mod Pathol. 2007;20(3):352–6.
17. Naryshkin S, Bedrossian CW. Selected mimics of malignancy in sputum and bronchoscopic cytology specimens. Diagn Cytopathol. 1995;13(5):443–7.
18. Saito Y, et al. Cytologic study of tissue repair in human bronchial epithelium. Acta Cytol. 1988;32(5):622–8.
19. Policarpio-Nicolas ML, Wick MR. False-positive interpretations in respiratory cytopathology: exemplary cases and literature review. Diagn Cytopathol. 2008;36(1):13–9.
20. Idowu MO, Powers CN. Lung cancer cytology: potential pitfalls and mimics – a review. Int J Clin Exp Pathol. 2010;3(4):367–85.
21. Fukuoka J, et al. Peribronchiolar metaplasia: a common histologic lesion in diffuse lung disease and a rare cause of interstitial lung disease: clinicopathologic features of 15 cases. Am J Surg Pathol. 2005;29(7):948–54.
22. Demay RM. The art and science of cytopathology, vol. 1. 2nd ed. Chicago, IL: American Society for Clinical Pathology; 2011. p. 201–28.
23. Peters EJ, et al. Squamous metaplasia of the bronchial mucosa and its relationship to smoking. Chest. 1993;103(5):1429–32.

24. Ritter JH, et al. False-positive interpretations of carcinoma in exfoliative respiratory cytology. Report of two cases and a review of underlying disorders. Am J Clin Pathol. 1995;104(2): 133–40.
25. Ogino S, et al. Extensive squamous metaplasia with cytologic atypia in diffuse alveolar damage mimicking squamous cell carcinoma: a report of 2 cases. Hum Pathol. 2002;33(10):1052–4.
26. Berman JJ, Murray RJ, Lopez-Plaza IM. Widespread posttracheostomy atypia simulating squamous cell carcinoma. A case report. Acta Cytol. 1991;35(6):713–6.
27. Kita Y, et al. Resected early lung cancer with pulmonary aspergilloma. Jpn J Thorac Cardiovasc Surg. 2000;48(8):540–1.
28. Tomioka H, et al. Undiagnosed lung cancer complicated by intracavitary aspergillosis. Nihon Kokyuki Gakkai Zasshi. 1999;37(1):78–82.
29. Nakajima K, et al. A case of combined squamous cell carcinoma and aspergilloma arising in a cyst wall. Nihon Kokyuki Gakkai Zasshi. 2001;39(12):961–5.
30. Silverman JF, et al. Fine needle aspiration cytology of pulmonary infarct. Acta Cytol. 1985;29(2):162–6.
31. Ness M, Hansen S, Armitage JO, Rennard SI, Vaughan WP, Stahl MG, Linder J. Acute effects of chemotherapy on cellular composition and cytomorphology of bronchial lavage specimens [abstract]. Acta Cytol. 1987;31:647–8.
32. Ali SZ, Yang GCH. Lung and mediastinum cytohistology, Cytohistology of small tissue samples. 1st ed. Cambridge, UK: Cambridge University Press; 2012. p. 65.
33. Bejarano PA, Garcia MT, Ganjei-Azar P. Mesothelial cells in transbronchial biopsies: a rare complication with a potential for a diagnostic pitfall. Am J Surg Pathol. 2007;31(6):914–8.
34. Cagle PT, Allen TC. Transbronchial and endobronchial biopsies. 1st ed. Philadelphia, PA: Lippincott Williams & Wilkins; 2008. p. 3.
35. Auger M, Moriarty AT, Laucirica R, Souers R, Chmara BA, Fatheree LA, Wilbur DC. Granulomatous inflammation-an underestimated cause of false-positive diagnoses in lung fine-needle aspirates: observations from the college of american pathologists nongynecologic cytopathology interlaboratory comparison program. Arch Pathol Lab Med. 2010;134(12): 1793–6.
36. Mizutani E, et al. Minute pulmonary meningothelial-like nodules: clinicopathologic analysis of 121 patients. Hum Pathol. 2009;40(5):678–82.
37. Niho S, et al. Immunohistochemical and clonal analysis of minute pulmonary meningothelial-like nodules. Hum Pathol. 1999;30(4):425–9.
38. Johansson M, et al. Recombinations of chromosomal bands 6p21 and 14q24 characterise pulmonary hamartomas. Br J Cancer. 1993;67(6):1236–41.
39. Tallini G, et al. HMGI-C and HMGI(Y) immunoreactivity correlates with cytogenetic abnormalities in lipomas, pulmonary chondroid hamartomas, endometrial polyps, and uterine leiomyomas and is compatible with rearrangement of the HMGI-C and HMGI(Y) genes. Lab Invest. 2000;80(3):359–69.
40. Hughes JH, et al. Fine-needle aspiration of pulmonary hamartoma: a common source of false-positive diagnoses in the College of American Pathologists Interlaboratory Comparison Program in Nongynecologic Cytology. Arch Pathol Lab Med. 2005;129(1):19–22.
41. Saqi A, Shaham D, Scognamiglio T, Murray MP, Henschke CI, Yankelevitz D, Vazquez MF. Incidence and cytological features of pulmonary hamartomas indeterminate on CT scan. Cytopathology. 2008;19(3):185–9.
42. Gaffey MJ, et al. Clear cell tumor of the lung. Immunohistochemical and ultrastructural evidence of melanogenesis. Am J Surg Pathol. 1991;15(7):644–53.
43. Hornick JL, Fletcher CD. PEComa: what do we know so far? Histopathology. 2006;48(1): 75–82.
44. Nguyen GK. Aspiration biopsy cytology of benign clear cell ("sugar") tumor of the lung. Acta Cytol. 1989;33(4):511–5.
45. Policarpio-Nicolas ML, et al. Fine needle aspiration cytology of clear cell "sugar" tumor (PEComa) of the lung: report of a case. Diagn Cytopathol. 2008;36(2):89–93.

46. Deavers M, et al. Granular cell tumors of the lung. Clinicopathologic study of 20 cases. Am J Surg Pathol. 1995;19(6):627–35.
47. Husain M, Nguyen GK. Cytopathology of granular-cell tumor of the lung. Diagn Cytopathol. 2000;23(4):294–5.
48. Katzenstein AL, Gmelich JT, Carrington CB. Sclerosing hemangioma of the lung: a clinicopathologic study of 51 cases. Am J Surg Pathol. 1980;4(4):343–56.
49. Devouassoux-Shisheboran M, et al. A clinicopathologic study of 100 cases of pulmonary sclerosing hemangioma with immunohistochemical studies: TTF-1 is expressed in both round and surface cells, suggesting an origin from primitive respiratory epithelium. Am J Surg Pathol. 2000;24(7):906–16.
50. Ng WK, et al. Sclerosing hemangioma of lung: a close cytologic mimicker of pulmonary adenocarcinoma. Diagn Cytopathol. 2001;25(5):316–20.
51. Blanco LZ, et al. Cytologic features of sclerosing hemangioma of the lung on crush preparations. Diagn Cytopathol. 2013;41(3):242–6.
52. Churg A, Myers J, Tazelaar H, Wright J. Thurlbeck's Pathology of the Lung. 3rd ed. New York: Thieme; 2005. p. 481–2.
53. Zander D, Farver C. Pulmonary pathology: a volume in foundations in diagnostic pathology series. 1st ed. Philadelphia, PA: Churchill Livingstone; 2008. p. 679–82.
54. Leslie KO, Wick MR. Practical pulmonary pathology. A diagnostic approach. Philadelphia, PA: Saunders; 2011.
55. Marchevsky AM. Lung tumors derived from ectopic tissues. Semin Diagn Pathol. 1995;12(2):172–84.
56. Moran CA, et al. Primary intrapulmonary thymoma. A clinicopathologic and immunohistochemical study of eight cases. Am J Surg Pathol. 1995;19(3):304–12.
57. Shabb NS, et al. Fine-needle aspiration of the mediastinum: a clinical, radiologic, cytologic, and histologic study of 42 cases. Diagn Cytopathol. 1998;19(6):428–36.
58. Chhieng DC, et al. Cytology of thymomas: emphasis on morphology and correlation with histologic subtypes. Cancer. 2000;90(1):24–32.

# Index





A.L. Moreira, A. Saqi (eds.), *Diagnosing Non-small Cell Carcinoma in Small Biopsy and Cytology*, DOI 10.1007/978-1-4939-1607-8

**T**

FSC
www.fsc.org
MIX
Papier | Fördert
gute Waldnutzung
FSC® C083411

Kolibri 360 GmbH
Ferdinand-Jühlke-Straße 7
99095 Erfurt, Deutschland
produktsicherheit@kolibri360.de